TYLER ENGLISH

Men'sHealth

NATURAL BODYBUILDING BIBLE

A COMPLETE 24-WEEK PROGRAM FOR SCULPTING MUSCLES THAT SHOW

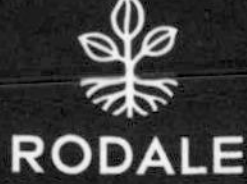

RODALE

The information in this book is meant to supplement, not replace, proper exercise training. All forms of exercise pose some inherent risks. The editors and publisher advise readers to take full responsibility for their safety and know their limits. Before practicing the exercises in this book, be sure that your equipment is well-maintained, and do not take risks beyond your level of experience, aptitude, training, and fitness. The exercise and dietary programs in this book are not intended as a substitute for any exercise routine or dietary regimen that may have been prescribed by your doctor. As with all exercise and dietary programs, you should get your doctor's approval before beginning.

Direct and trade editions are being published simultaneously with the same title.
The direct edition contains exclusive content.

Rodale books may be purchased for business or promotional use or for special sales.
For information, please write to:
Special Markets Department, Rodale, Inc., 733 Third Avenue, New York, NY 10017

Printed in the United States of America
Rodale Inc. makes every effort to use acid-free ♾, recycled paper ♲.

Historical photo credits: Brand X Pictures/Getty Images *(page 20)*; Popperfoto/Getty Images *(page 21)*; Popperfoto/Getty Images *(page 23)*; Gene Lester/Getty Images *(page 24)*; Hulton Archive/Getty Images *(page 25)*; Robert Cianflon/Getty Images *(page 26)*; and Illustration by Alix Nicholaeff *(page 39)*

Book design by Mark Michaelson

Library of Congress Cataloging-in-Publication Data is on file with the publisher.
978–1–60961–877–3 trade paperback
978–1–60961–969–5 direct hardcover

Distributed to the trade by Macmillan

4 6 8 10 9 7 5 trade paperback
2 4 6 8 10 9 7 5 3 1 direct hardcover

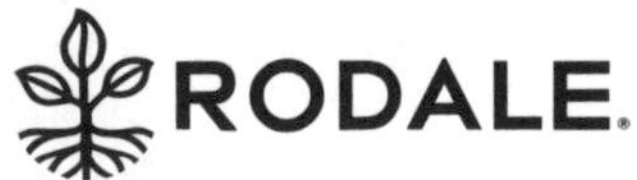

Contents

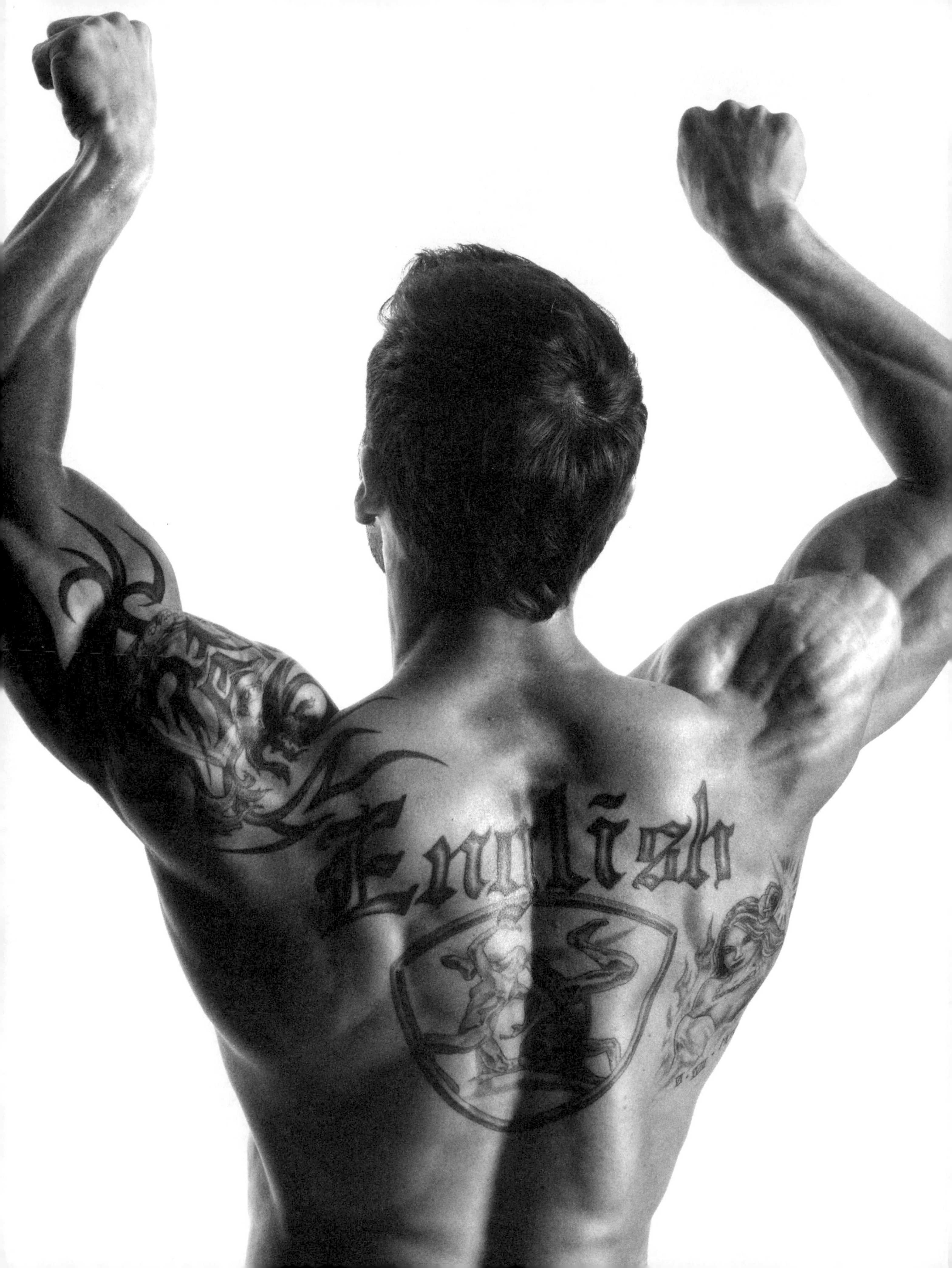
English

Introduction
What Bodybuilding Can Do for You

REMEMBER THE FIRST time you stood in front of the bathroom mirror and made a muscle? You were probably 9 or 10, wondering if you would ever get as big as your older brother or cousin. Your biceps looked pretty puny at the time. But you knew they had potential—you had potential—to get bigger and stronger.

So you started doing pushups and curling your brother's dumbbells. Maybe you hung a poster of Arnold Schwarzenegger or Lou Ferrigno in your garage for motivation. You probably turned a lined notebook into a workout log and started recording repetitions and sets and, go ahead admit it, the size of your arms and chest measured with a tape. (We all did that.) And through all this effort you learned a grand lesson: that hard work and dedication to a goal paid off in spades. And the payoff didn't just come in the form of bigger biceps.

Some people believe bodybuilding is for the insecure or narcissistic, but that's a narrow view. Anyone who has tried to build muscle and strength knows this. The sport of bodybuilding brings with it a rewarding experience that can provide the bodybuilder with a vast array of benefits beyond the sense of accomplishment that comes from winning the recognition of peers through competition. Natural bodybuilding delivers incredible health benefits regardless of whether you decide to compete against others or just challenge yourself.

I encourage you to try competition. Competing in a bodybuilding event takes a serious commitment. When done correctly, it can have a profound life-altering effect. It has in my life, as you'll learn in the first chapter. I've had the pleasure of meeting some amazing people, many of whom I now call dear friends, who define the true essence of the sport of natural bodybuilding and make it such an awesome and inspiring lifestyle.

From my experience and from the experience of many others, here are some of the ways bodybuilding can benefit you that go far beyond impressing that 9-year-old kid looking back at you in the mirror:

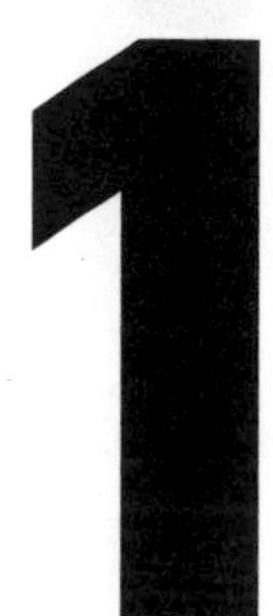

Mental clarity and focus

You've heard the expression "Give it 110 percent." When a person makes the decision to compete in a bodybuilding competition, he or she is doing just that. There are no shortcuts, no quick fixes. When you make the decision to compete in bodybuilding, you are flipping on a switch inside your body that signals it's time to get serious. It fosters a mental clarity and focus of purpose that will flood into all other aspects of your life.

One of the first things I tell a prospective physique competitor—man or woman, figure competitor or bodybuilder—is that he or she needs to be 100 percent ready to make the mental connection and to do what it takes to compete. It's a decision that will help shape every aspect of your life and determine the body and health benefits you receive.

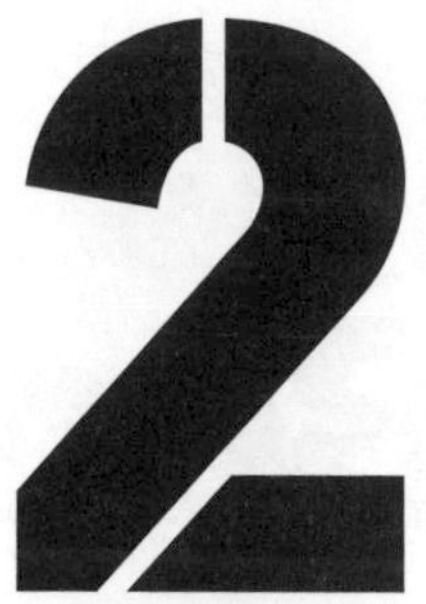

Physical strength and spirit

The human body was meant to be active every day. It was designed for work. Building lean muscle, burning body fat, and pushing your body to the limit—in the gym and outside of it—are what make the physical aspect of bodybuilding so unique.

We are not only training to train, or training to lose body fat, or training to look better. No, we are training to bring our bodies to a point at which they rival the ancient Greece sculptures—the images of the Greek gods, the embodiments of perfection.

We may want the ultimate lean, conditioned, and muscular body—but it's the physical effort that will get us there.

Bodybuilding is about the physical body, the physical mind, and the physical spirit—the improvement of each can have its own benefit for the bodybuilder.

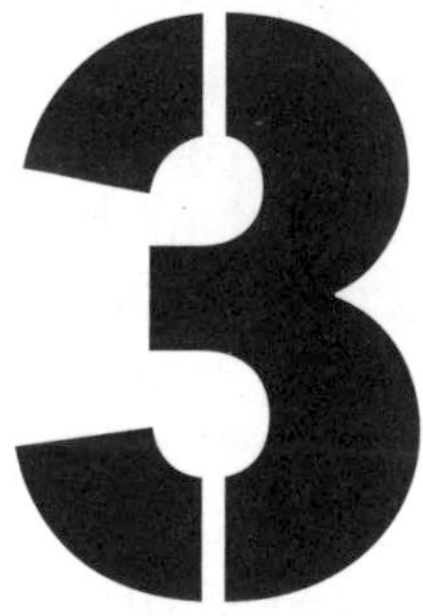

Discipline and commitment

Why do diets fail?

It's not the diet or the food that fails. Nine times out of 10 it's the person who gives up. The person simply lacks the discipline and commitment to see it through to the end. It's not that it is always the individual's fault—he or she might have been set up for failure from the beginning by the wrong plan or family life situation, time restraints, and the list goes on. This is not a criticism of the weakness of people who fall off their fitness and diet plans; it's just a fact of human nature. The only way to overcome it is through this X factor: discipline and commitment.

The bodybuilder must make a commitment to discipline. There is no other way. The ability to make an amazing commitment may be the reason that many bodybuilders are stereotyped as type A personalities. A successful bodybuilder will always have discipline and will always understand the true meaning of commitment.

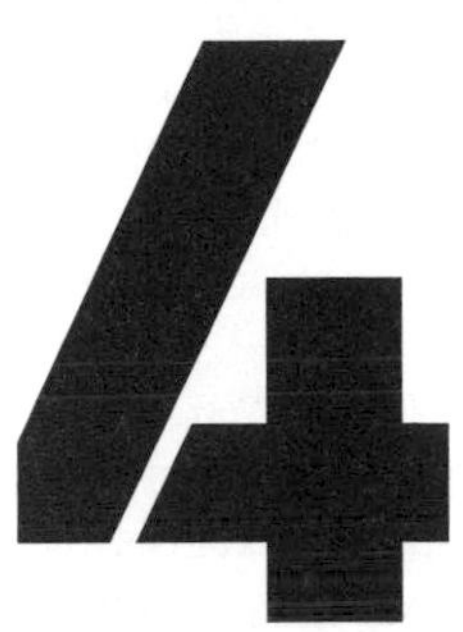

The ideal physique

Much of the world is facing a frightening epidemic of obesity and the diseases triggered by sedentary lifestyles. For most of these people the goal is simply to improve their health. For a bodybuilder, the goal is optimization.

The human body is a work of art that when given the correct guidance can become an amazing real-life sculpture. Bodybuilding provides the physical element like no other sport out there. You are judged on your ability to present a physique that you have sculpted for others to see and ultimately reward.

Nothing else offers the same blank canvas on which to create that your body can provide. Your muscles are there, ready to be shaped and fine-tuned into the exact form you wish to achieve. Just think of the sense of accomplishment that you'll feel when you present a physique that you have brought to its ultimate potential.

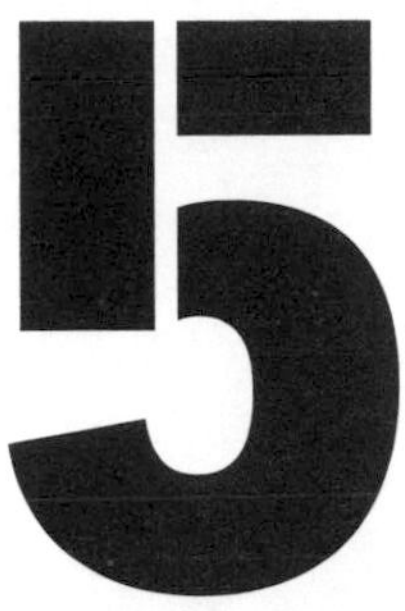

The aesthetic of symmetry

Aesthetics are what make up a well-balanced bodybuilder. Bodybuilders such as Frank Zane—of the sport's golden era—brought to the stage a very aesthetically pleasing physique at only 170 pounds. A bodybuilder's ability to present a symmetrical, conditioned, muscular physique will make him aesthetically pleasing to the human eye—especially when shirtless. This is something people drawn to bodybuilding training want to achieve even if they have no intention of ever competing. They appreciate the confidence that developing a strong and fit body of symmetrical muscle gives them when wearing a bathing suit at the beach or a business suit in the boardroom.

Optimum nutrition

They say that 80 percent of weight-loss success comes from nutrition. In bodybuilding, nutrition is closer to 90 percent of the game of sculpting the best body possible. Most weight-loss attempts fail. In bodybuilding you cannot fail your diet and expect to achieve your goal. The food you consume impacts how your body responds to training. The proper nutritional plan is what will separate you from those who move through the process with no structure. Imagine what your physique would look like if you were to commit to a strict diet for a minimum of 12 weeks or even a maximum of 24 weeks. Your physique would reach a level you've never seen before. Guaranteed. That's what this book will help you to do.

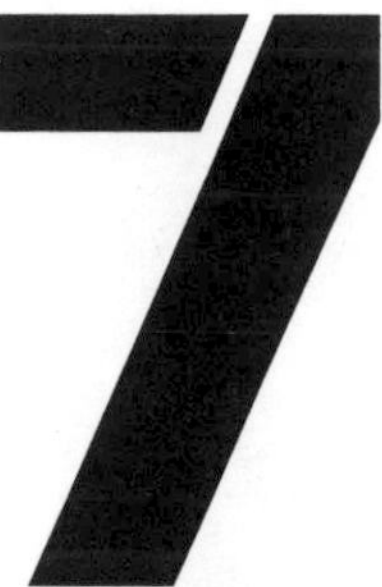

The thrill of competition

We humans thrive on competition. Developing a physique to showcase is a competition in its own right—even before you step onstage wearing posing trunks. Bodybuilding brings out a new level of competitive spirit. For some, it's about finding a way to reenergize their lives with the kind of competition they first experienced as high school athletes. For others, it's about creating a competition within themselves to test self-discipline and measure self-improvement. No matter the level of competition, bodybuilding brings out the best of the competitor in each of us. And that sense of drive and purpose often carries over to other aspects of life—business, relationships, and charitable causes.

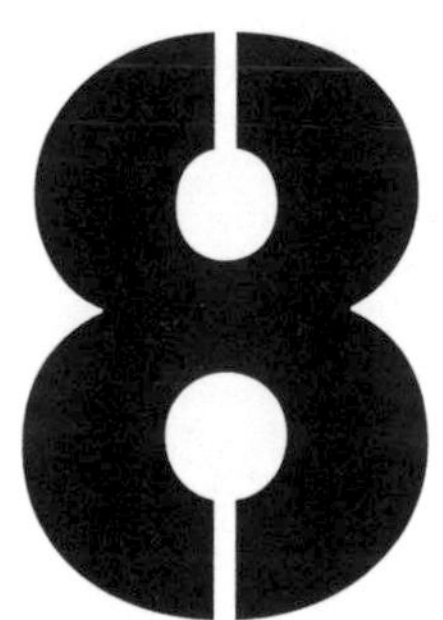

Top-notch health

A natural bodybuilder is the ideal specimen of peak conditioning and health. Building lean muscle mass, maintaining low body fat levels and sculpted muscles, boosting the cardiovascular system, and eating a whole-food based diet will help you avoid the diseases of aging— cancer, diabetes, and heart disease—as well as fighting obesity, high blood pressure, stress, depression, and fatigue. Through rigorous fitness and nutrition efforts you will dramatically stall the aging process and protect yourself from the physical decline that comes from sarcopenia (muscle atrophy) and a decreasing metabolic rate.

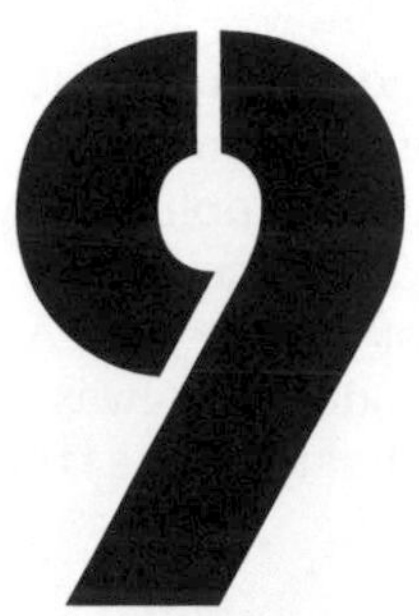

The power of the journey

Throughout our lives we will embark upon numerous journeys. Committing to compete as a bodybuilder can prove to be the greatest journey of all. Giving your all to transform your physique—for some this means remaking their entire lives—can truly clarify how important the body is and how we must take care of it. When the journey is complete, the greatest sense of accomplishment will come from the connection between mind and body. For many, bodybuilding is much more than a competition, it's a life-altering experience, not unlike a spiritual awakening.

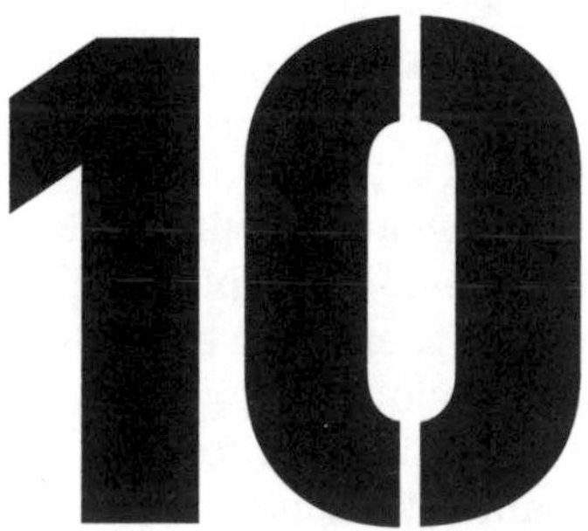

The ultimate lesson

Win or learn, never lose—I firmly believe that an understanding of these words sets apart those who commit to bodybuilding as a lifestyle from those who choose to compete solely for the sake of winning. The lessons natural bodybuilding will teach you about your body, mind, heart, soul, and spirit will be components of an even greater part of your life if you approach bodybuilding as a lifestyle in which the journey itself is the ultimate victory.

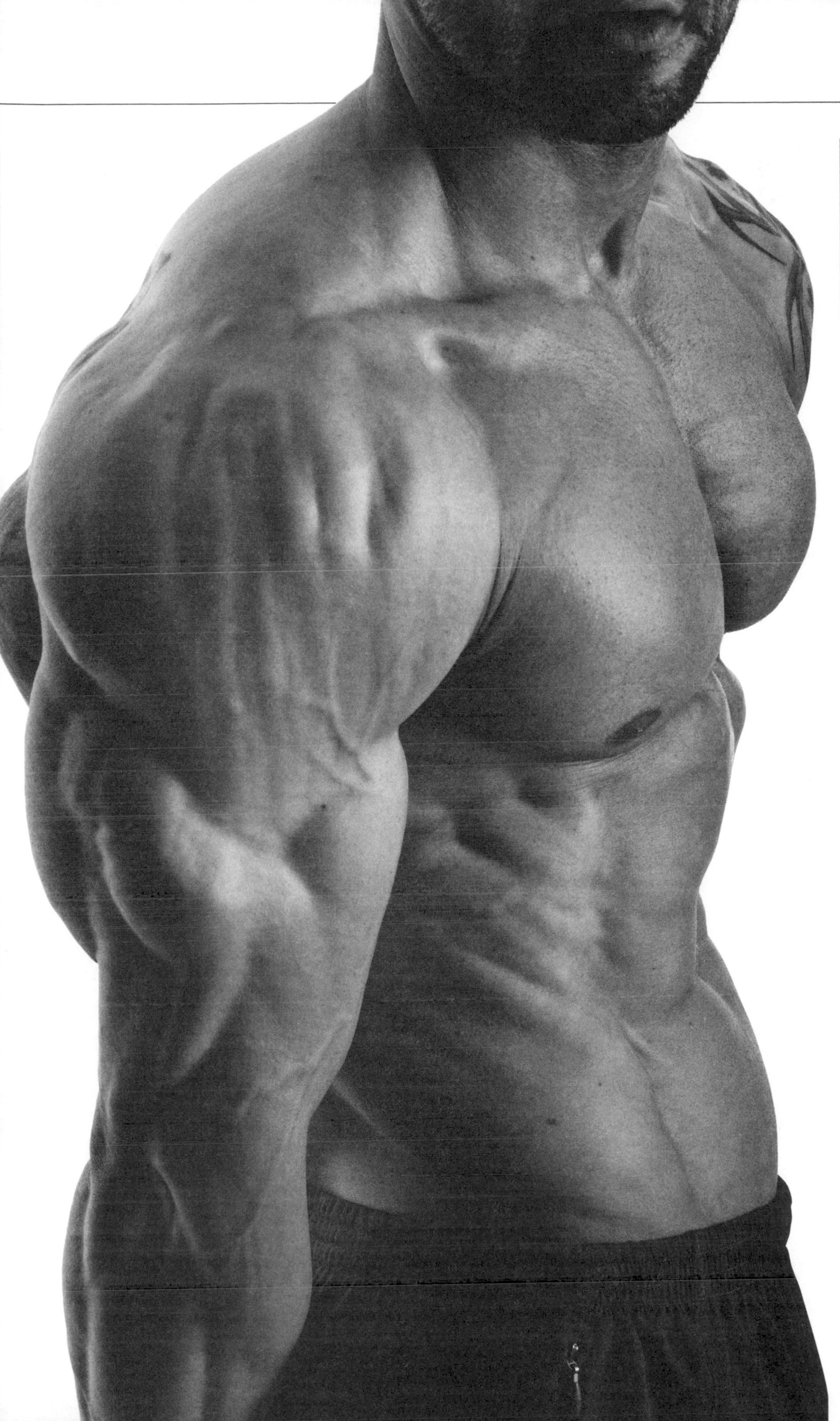

Mind-Body Connection. Bodybuilding can be a spiritual awakening.

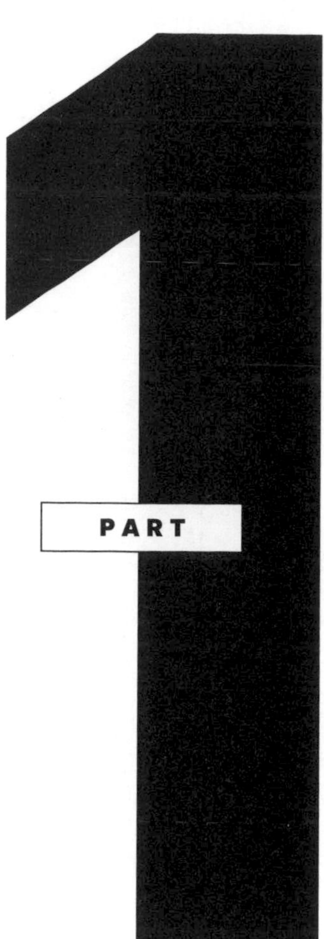

PART

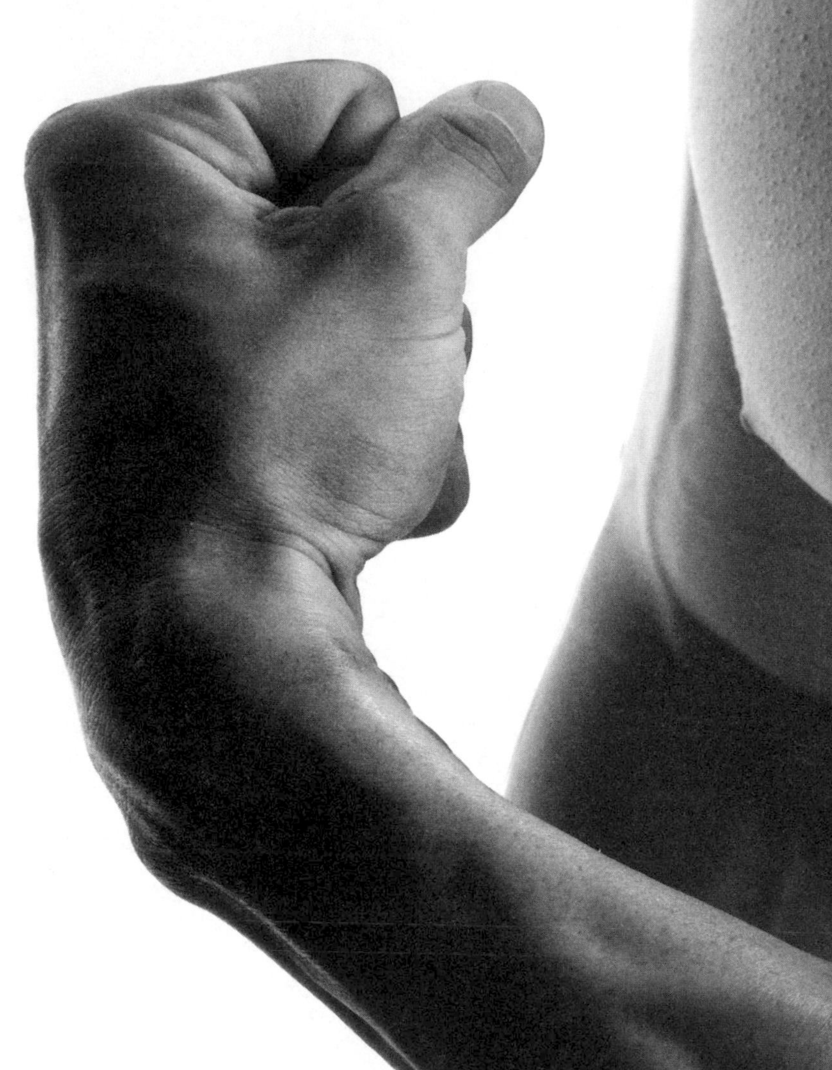

Understanding Bodybuilding

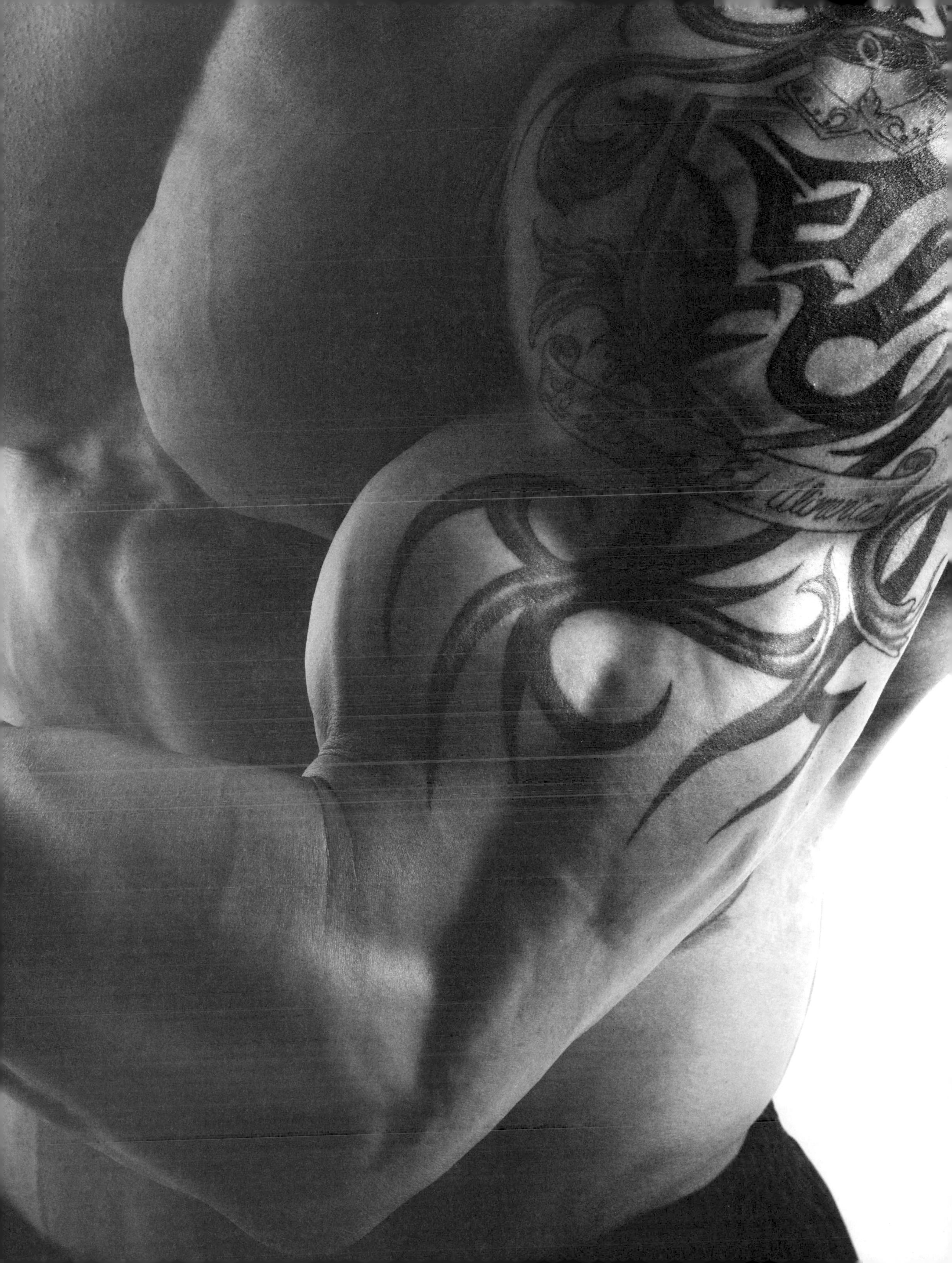

PART 1

CHAPTER 1

How to Become a Competitive Bodybuilder

One man's story; yours will be different but just as rewarding

I'VE BEEN AN ATHLETE ALL MY LIFE. From the time I could walk, I was playing some sort of sport. And now, at 30, I'm still playing, still using my body, my muscles, and my lungs to have fun in my career. I own two fitness facilities near Hartford, Connecticut. My coaches and I help people lose weight, build muscle, reduce stress, and improve their lives through fitness. We have more than 700 clients, everyone from stay-at-home moms to working professionals, teenage athletes to 6-year-olds. That's my job: fitness training and running a growing business. My hobby and love is bodybuilding.

I feel extremely fortunate that my vocation and my avocation are so closely entwined. But that doesn't mean you have to work in the fitness industry to be a bodybuilder. You don't even have to be a lifelong athlete, growing up playing lots of different sports and doing physical things 24–7 as I did to become a bodybuilder. I know hundreds of bodybuilders. Some weren't athletic at all as teens. Some were video-game playing kids who rarely saw the sun. Some were intellectually

Scrawny to Brawny. As a kid, I could curl my nephew Austin, but couldn't put on muscle weight no matter how hard I tried.

driven youngsters who never tossed a ball or ran around on the grass. Some were fit, active kids who turned into overweight workaholics who ate fast food every night. Others became obese couch potatoes who eventually found the path to weight loss and fitness and discovered a love of training their bodies later in life.

My point is that there are no prerequisite lifestyles for becoming a bodybuilder. There's only hard work and dedication. The story of how I became one is just one story. I share it here to provide some background about me and how bodybuilding changed my life. Your story will likely be much different. One of the remarkable things about the sport of bodybuilding is that almost anyone can do it on one level or another. Sure, genetics plays a role in success. Some people are blessed with a physiology that makes sculpting lean muscle easier for them. But with grit and determination—and the right individual plan—anyone can make his or her body stronger, healthier, and better looking. That's the essence of bodybuilding and my hope for you in this book.

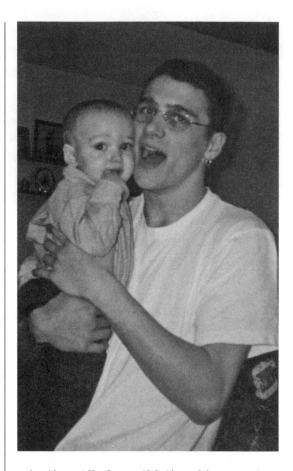

The Skinny Kid

When I look at my transition into the world of bodybuilding, I can't help but think about the rich history that is bodybuilding and how bodybuilding has helped shape the fitness industry. My first experiences with weight training are what eventually brought me to the sport, and my growth as a fitness professional is what has continued to expand my love for bodybuilding.

Growing up I loved sports, and I was always involved in organized athletics, everything from swimming and gymnastics to soccer, wrestling, and baseball. I don't think a day went by when my mother, Maura, wasn't driving my sister, Tara, my brother, Robert, or me, to a practice or a game. It was what we English children did, and we did it well. As a kid, I was very athletic, super competitive, and naturally strong and fast. What I lacked in overall size, I made up for in hard work and determination. All of my athletic achievements came not from inborn talent or strength, but from my sheer desire to be the best at whatever I did.

I was never a big kid, instead I was the skinny athlete who could eat whatever he wanted and not gain weight. That's not saying I ate unhealthily—I could just get away with more. At the start of sophomore year of high school, I weighed 114 pounds sopping wet. I couldn't gain weight even though I ate all the crap that teenagers eat. It was only through natural growth spurts and a little bit of weight lifting that I was able to bulk up to around 125 pounds by my junior year.

In the basement of my house my father, Bobby, kept an assortment of plastic weights that were filled with concrete. He was a recreational boxer who stayed in good shape with weight lifting and fighting. Though I didn't realize it until later in my life, my fascination with his weights would be my gateway into strength training and ultimately bodybuilding. At first, all this skinny kid wanted to do was to pack on muscle. I saw the potential in those concrete-filled weights, but there was a problem—I had no idea what I was doing. So I just started benching, curling, and pressing to "get big." My experimentation with strength training or "lifting," as I called it back then, was inconsistent at best. There were periods when I'd go hard, committing to three or four lifting sessions per week in that basement, and other weeks (or months) when I'd never go down there because I was too busy being a kid.

In high school, the weight room seemed to be a way of life. I took part in "team workouts," which seemed more like social hour. We talked a lot about girls. We admired our biceps. But we didn't get much lifting done. Like a lot of teen guys I got sidetracked by the high school social scene. I became consumed with being part of the in-crowd, going to parties, and trying to maintain my social status. I lost my focus for playing sports. Peer pressure affected my attitude, my athletic ability, and ultimately my schoolwork. During my sophomore year, I had to walk away from wrestling, due to poor grades.

Then, the summer before my junior year, I started working in a warehouse, moving furniture. It was hard, heavy-lifting work, but it felt good to use my muscles (and to make some money). About the same time, a good friend who was a standout on our football team encouraged me to start lifting. And we visited the weight room on a regular basis, this time to actually lift. In a few months, I began weight training 5 or 6 days a week.

Lifting became my obsession.

By my senior year of high school I had grown to 155 pounds of solid lean muscle. When I showed up for preseason soccer practice, my coach couldn't believe his eyes. I had packed on close to 30 pounds of muscle in less than a year. He was amazed, yet I wasn't satisfied.

As my nutritional needs grew, so did my hunger for reading everything I could get my hands on about weight lifting and nutrition. I read every major muscle magazine there was, and I saw ads for all the different types of supplements. The targeted messages regularly called out to me: Take this to build muscle mass. *Take this to increase your lean muscle by 300 percent!*

These supplements cost anywhere between $40 and $100. That was a lot of dough for a high school teenager to dish out, but I had a solid part-time job working in the furniture warehouse so I had the cash. I went on a spending spree, buying supplements and more supplements! I believed that one of these powders or pills was going to be the way to the physique I desperately desired. The local GNC became a second home for me. Gold Card Tuesdays were my opportunity to buy the latest and greatest while saving some money. At my peak, I was spending $200 to $400 per month on supplements. I was swallowing and experimenting with everything from mass-building powders to so-called natural testosterone boosters (even though at 17 I had plenty of naturally occurring testosterone) to the latest and greatest pre- and post-workout drinks. As I continued reading hundreds of online articles about supplements, I still wanted more muscle and strength.

Natural for Life—The Steroids That Never Happened

Then the same friend who reintroduced me to the weight room told me he could get us "a cycle" of testosterone. A simple cycle, I thought, how hard could that be to do? My thoughts were, *I'll be bigger, stronger, and I'll be able to do it so much faster!*

My friend set up the entire process and actually drove us to meet "the seller," who just so happened to be someone we both already knew. The entire situation just didn't feel right. I mean, does secretly meeting a person in a shopping plaza parking lot to illegally purchase steroids sound right to you?

We bought two cycles, one for him and one for me. I remember not being able to afford the steroid cycle, because I was already spending so much money on supplements and food, so my friend fronted me the money. But in my heart, I knew the steroids were never mine or meant to be mine.

Well, he immediately started his cycle and began to see strength and size gains. He updated me almost daily about the changes he was seeing. As for me, I hid my vial in a secret compartment in the dresser in my room. An entire 3 weeks passed and I never attempted to administer the steroids. There were days I would come home from school and take out the vial, stare at it, but nothing came of it. When I look back at it all today, I think, *Did this happen for a reason? Did somewhere, deep down inside, I know that my life would lead me to a healthy lifestyle and natural bodybuilding?*

The whole steroid thing seemed wrong from the start, and the thought of sticking myself with a needle freaked me out! NO WAY! As a kid I was deathly afraid of getting a flu shot. Maybe that's why I never sought out the tool I would need to administer the steroids. I would sit in my room staring at the vial, wondering if I would ever get a syringe. After my friend had completed his cycle, he knew I hadn't taken the step. So, I gave him my vial.

Did the thought of attempting this again ever cross my mind? I'd be lying if I told you no. Even in college I still bought supplements, only then I became obsessed with finding the "Holy Grail" of the supplement world. Despite my early frustrations and experiments, the industry continued to tempt me with promises of "bigger, faster results." Total BS.

As I continued spending money on supplements, I stepped over the line into a dangerous area. In college I began to hear about these things called prohormones. These are precursors to anabolic steroids like testosterone. The prohormone 4-androstenedione is a common one. It is designed to boost the body's available hormone supply. These prohormones are available in most supplement stores and online, which of course I thought made them okay to take.

Still, in the back of my mind I kept thinking these were too good to be true. They were being marketed as having steroid-like results without the nasty side effects. Even better, they were in pill form. No nasty needles. Since I initially worked in journalism in college, I used the skills I'd learned and began researching everything there was to know about prohormones. I found ways to stack and cycle. I experimented for about 3 months with prohormones and thought I'd found the key to success. I began to see my weight increase, my strength increase, and, ultimately, my muscle mass increase. I weighed 206 pounds; I was benching 225 pounds for 23 repetitions and squatting close to 400 pounds. And I was only 20 years old. In college, the weight room became my temple. It was my place of peace, my place of reckoning; it became my sanctuary from the madness that a young man endures. There was no pressure of a test, no one to tell me what to do, no deadlines like those associated with working on the student newspaper, and I could push my physical self to new places. I'd train in the early morning, before the start of class, for the sheer feeling of dedication and commitment I gained from training while everyone else was still sleeping.

But there was a downside. My obsession took control of me. I remember seeing an ESPN special on these prohormones and steroidal precursors. Major League Baseball stars were taking them. NFL standouts were taking them. How bad could they be? Then I began to see a change in my attitude. My mood. My energy levels. This was only from 3 months of use! I learned a lot about myself during those 3 months of use, and I realized I needed to change my ways. I stopped taking the prohormones cold turkey.

Upon graduating from college in 2004, I followed my passion for weight lifting into the fitness industry. I started working as a personal trainer in two gyms. I became a research-aholic. I would read and research everything about the human anatomy, physiology, nutrition, fat loss, and muscle growth. One aspect I became quite fond of was the effect of proper nutrition and diet.

I began to change the way I approached exercise, nutrition, and supplementation. What I had failed to realize early on was that there is a way to properly use the right supplements to help you maximize your body's potential without falling prey to all the hype and spending lots of money on powders and pills. I learned that there is a healthy, safe, and effective way to achieve the physique you desire.

I began to discover the need for essential nutrients. Even though many of the essential nutrients are found in our food, a large portion of the population falls short of the proper intake. I truly believe that introducing essential nutrient supplements into people's daily lives can help to develop a healthier population, becoming a long-lasting strategy for healthier lifestyles.

Becoming a Natural Bodybuilder

As I began to grow as a personal trainer, my obsession with transforming my physique continued. Conversations with colleagues and a local amateur bodybuilder convinced me to try competing in my first natural bodybuilding competition, the Fitness Atlantic, in April of 2005. It was a show promoted by Musclemania, an organization that has since accepted athletes who have failed drug tests in other natural competitions.

I didn't know what I was getting into. I had just 11 weeks to prepare. I trained 6 days a week doing cardio four or five times per week all the way up to the contest day. My diet, training, and entire preparation were self-designed. I'll never forget the support I received that day from friends, family, and coworkers who came out to watch me.

The prejudging portion of the competition was harder than I'd ever imagined. I had to hold poses to what felt like no end, over and over again. It didn't feel like how I had practiced. Looking back on it now, I'd truly underestimated how important it was to practice posing. Despite what I thought was a long battle in the beaming lights on stage, the judges noticed my physique. That day I took home two second-place trophies, one in the junior men division and the other in novice heavyweight (the novice classes were split at 165 to create two classes). I felt a great sense of accomplishment, especially when the crowd began to boo in disapproval of my placings; they believed I should have been awarded the first place trophy.

Later, I was approached by Nancy Andrews outside the auditorium. She told me about her upcoming International Natural Bodybuilding Federation (INBF) Northeast Classic competition a few weeks down the road in Marlborough, Massachusetts. She congratulated me on my first show and handed me a registration form. She told me I had a great look and physique and could go far in the world of natural bodybuilding if I stuck with it. Her words still stay with me today.

A few weeks afterward I traveled to Marlborough for the INBF competition and won the junior class and finished third in the open middleweight class, out of 16 competitors. I was hooked. That night, I dedicated myself to natural bodybuilding. I still wonder whether I'd have found my direction in natural bodybuilding if Nancy Andrews hadn't been in attendance at my first competition. I've told Nancy this personally: that she had a major impact on my bodybuilding career.

Later in 2005, I competed again in Nancy's INBF Monster Mash, taking fifth place in open middleweight, and the following week in the INBF Amateur World Championships, held in conjunction with the WNBF (World Natural Bodybuilding Federation) Professional World Championships in New York City, taking another fifth-place finish. This time in a field that included many international competitors in my middleweight class.

At this time, I took a job as a personal trainer in a new health club. I remember showing up for my initial interview wearing my first coat of tan for my next bodybuilding competition. It didn't go over very well with my future boss; he said he didn't like to hire bodybuilders, but I got the job and stayed for 4 years. Fast forward to 2008, and I had become their top personal trainer, after taking off from competition for an entire season. I guess some bodybuilders make great coaches after all.

During 2007 I grew tremendously as a personal trainer, but I found myself torn between the world of functional training, which was attacking the world of

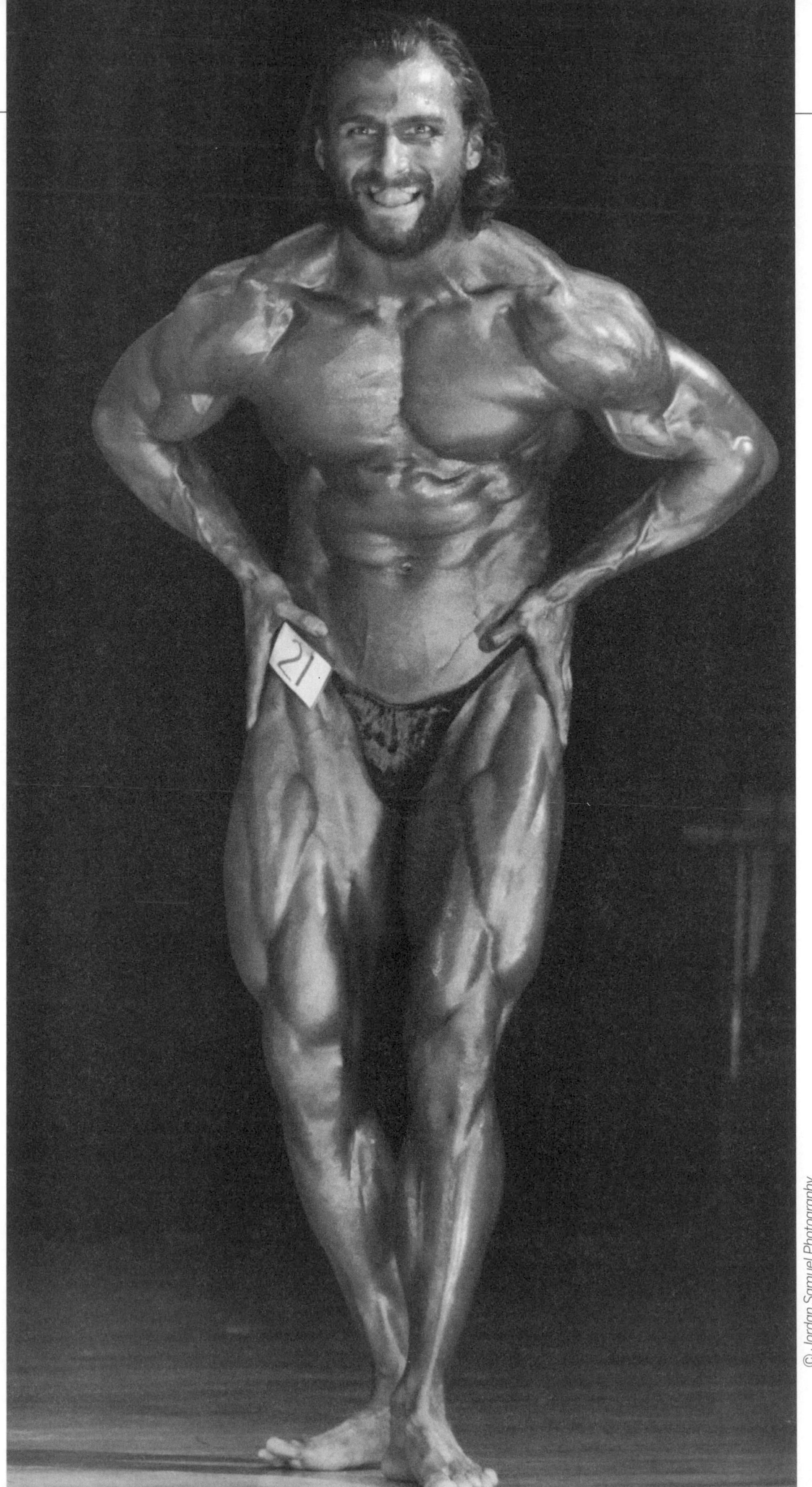
© Jordan Samuel Photography

All Natural Except for the Tan. Striking a hands-on-hips "most muscular" pose at the 2010 WNBF World Championships.

bodybuilding, and my desire to become a professional natural bodybuilder. The best thing that happened to me that year was finding the balance between the two.

Competing as a Professional Natural Bodybuilder

In 2009, I entered the World Natural Bodybuilding Federation (WNBF) as professional bodybuilder. This was a whole new level of competition. My goal wasn't to come in first, it was simply to survive and build up enough confidence to get me to the next competition and the next.

During this same time I was in the middle of growing my own personal training business, which was quickly expanding. The easy choice would have been to place competition on the backburner until things slowed down. But that isn't my style.

The 2009 contest season was a learning experience in my personal, professional, and bodybuilding life. Only 3 months after winning my pro card, I was a business owner doing it all: coaching, answering calls, responding to e-mails, building my Web site, networking, bookkeeping, and marketing my services. I was the business, and therefore I had to spend a great amount of time on all aspects of it.

During this early growth period of my new venture, I made the decision to compete again. I began my preparation in February for the WNBF Pro American Championships in Massachusetts that June. From the start the determination was there and the desire to compete as a professional was there, but looking back at it I'm positive that I never did give 100 percent of what I was capable of. As a result, I took fourth out of eight WNBF pros in the heavyweight division. My true weight class is middleweight, so I was pretty happy with my performance.

After taking some much-needed time off from contest preparation from June through September, I decided to compete

In 2008 I returned to the competitive stage—pushing the fine line between winning and overdoing it. I'd compete in seven competitions in 6 months. Here's what I accomplished in 2008:

APRIL 26
MUSCLEMANIA FITNESS ATLANTIC
Second-place open welterweight

MAY 3
INBF NORTHEAST CLASSIC
Third-place open middleweight

MAY 10
OCB NY STATE NATURAL
Second-place in open middle-weight "B" class

JUNE 14
INBF CONNECTICUT CHAMPIONSHIPS
Second-place in open middle-weight

JUNE 28
INBF HERCULES CHAMPIONSHIP
Second-place middleweight (I lost by a single point. This event was a Super Pro Qualifier, meaning if I had won, I would have earned professional status. It was during the preparation for this contest that I recognized the benefits of dieting longer.)

SEPTEMBER 13
OCB NORTHERN ATLANTIC STATES
First-place tall division and overall winner

SEPTEMBER 20
INBF NATURALMANIA (SUPER PRO QUALIFIER)
First-place middleweight class and third overall (I won my WNBF professional status!)

for the first time at the WNBF World Championships that November. As my business began to grow—with my assistant Kristy Bilodeau and my brother, Robert, on board as a coach—focusing on my contest preparation just wasn't a priority. On a daily basis, training was always the third, fourth, or even fifth priority, and finding the time to prepare food and get my cardio work done just wasn't commonplace. I did my best to accomplish what I could in a 3-month span, and I stepped on stage knowing I could have done more. The outcome spoke for itself: I finished eighth out of 16 middleweight competitors, a mere point from reaching the finals. I sat in the crowd that night watching my competition perform their evening posing routines and pondered what my future in this sport would bring.

After the World Championships, I didn't feel defeated; I was now much more aware of the level I'd need to reach in order to compete in the professional ranks. So I took close to a month off, and I completely focused on the business, trained sparingly, ate whatever I wanted, and waited for a new beginning.

Then on January 3, 2010, I started to experience ridiculous pains in my lower abdominal region. My initial thought was that I was upset from watching New England Patriot Wes Welker tear his MCL and ACL during the Patriots final regular-season game against the Houston Texans. I am a passionate fan of Boston sports, especially Pats football. I even named my dog Bruschi after the great Patriots linebacker Tedy Bruschi. As the day continued, the pain didn't subside and it only increased into the night. It was a new year, and a new 4-week phase of our fitness boot camp was to begin that Monday at my gym, Tyler English Fitness. I was in such pain, I only slept about 90 minutes that night, and then I taught back-to-back training sessions at 6:00 and 7:00 a.m. I called my brother to help me teach the 9:30 session because I felt so bad. A couple of hours later I was doubled over in pain. I went to an urgent care center to get checked out, and they sent me straight to the emergency room. Six hours later, I was in surgery to have my appendix removed.

Following surgery I felt like hell, but I refused to take pain medication. My body weight dropped to 172 pounds from 185 pounds in a little over a week. I compete around 170 to 175 pounds, and gaining weight wasn't going to be easy with a limited appetite. To make matters worse, I wouldn't be able to lift anything over 5 pounds for a minimum of 6 weeks. No weight-bearing movements whatsoever, the surgeon said. I couldn't even do bodyweight exercises for fear of abdominal stress and the possibility of a hernia.

I feared that I wouldn't be able to coach, train, or compete in bodybuilding anytime soon. The next month and a half was by far the worst period of my life. I ate horribly, had a hard time sleeping, and—now that I think back on it—was definitely suffering from some level of depression.

As I struggled with not being able to coach and not eating right, I lost my focus on some parts of my business and on my own well-being. Even after returning to teaching boot camps, my mind-set wasn't the same. Not being able to lift heavy iron, drip sweat from intense workouts, and feel the euphoric aftermath of a brutal strength training session was draining me.

Two weeks after surgery, I returned to my doctor, and he told me exactly what I didn't want to hear. I had to wait 4 more weeks. I waited out the remainder of my recovery. Upon returning to training, it took only 6 weeks of moderate workouts for me to realize that I needed to change everything. I needed to go back to the drawing board. I made a promise to reinvent myself, my training, my diet, my recovery, and my work habits. My first step was to get help. In April of 2010 I engaged the services of Joe Klemczewski, PhD, "The Diet Doc," who is a renowned bodybuilding contest prep coach. Dr. Joe has made all the difference in the world to my training. Sure, I design my own workouts, I design my own meal plans, but I could now turn to Joe for tweaks in my macronutrients and especially for guidance during my peak week leading up to my competition. Joe has become more than my coach. He's become a mentor in my approach to bodybuilding nutrition.

With Joe in my corner I was focused once again and would make one hell of a run in 2010, including finishing fifth in a tough heavyweight class at the 2010 WNBF Pro America on only 9 weeks of prep, winning the 2010 WNBF Mid-America Pro Am lightweight class 9 weeks later, and finishing second via a tiebreaker at the US Cup in the lightweight class. I entered the 2010 WNBF World Championships as a legitimate contender and finished two points out of second place, taking home the third-place middleweight honors in the world.

Earning the title Natural Bodybuilding Champion doesn't happen overnight. It takes time. Bodybuilding has brought me to personal heights I never imagined when I began competing in this sport. The sport of bodybuilding has also brought me back from some of the lowest times in my life.

It took me close to 5 years to truly understand the importance of bodybuilding. I can associate my desire to compete against the best natural bodybuilders in the world with my desire to be recognized as a leader in the fitness industry. Since first stepping onstage as a professional natural bodybuilder, I've worked hard to grow my personal-training business from a small fitness boot camp with six clients inside a karate studio, into two personal-training facilities: Tyler English Fitness, a 9,100-square-foot gym that is home to more than 500 clients, and its sister location, the 2,700-square-foot Fitness Revolution, which services more than 200 clients.

While I train a number of competitive bodybuilders, the majority of our clients are moms, dads, business owners, and everyday working professionals who are looking for the ultimate fitness solution for transforming their health, body, mind, and lifestyle. Combining hybrid functional strength training, metabolic training, and nutritional support in small and large group formats, we provide our clients with the tools they need to succeed.

As I've grown as a bodybuilder and fitness professional, I've worked hard to make both fit into my life so that I can share my training and nutrition philosophies to help thousands of people transform their own lives.

I wouldn't be where I am today, either personally or professionally, without the life lessons I've been taught by natural bodybuilding. The sport first introduced me to the fitness industry, and the fitness industry has allowed me to pursue my love for bodybuilding. For this reason, the two will always have a profound effect on each other in my life.

PART 1

CHAPTER 2

From Strongmen to Bodybuilders

A brief history of the making of muscle culture and sport

BODYBUILDING IS DEEPLY layered in a rich history and tradition that begins in antiquity. Chinese texts dating back to 2600 BC and Greek texts from 2500 to 200 BC reference the importance of strength training for military preparedness. In ancient Egyptian and Greek societies the sport of weight lifting had developed from stone lifting, where men would heft stones of various sizes and weights. It began as a form of entertainment for the masses and grew from displaying feats of great strength to showcasing aesthetically carved physiques. It became a celebration of the perfection of the human body.

In the 13th century, muscle building became wildly popular in India, with gyms sprouting up throughout the country where men would exercise with weights to enhance health and stamina. In Italy, in 1569, the physician Hieronymus Mercurialis published an illustrated medical book called *De Arte Gymnastica,* showing muscular men lifting dumbbells.

In the American colonies, in the 18th century, even Ben Franklin attributed his longevity to "daily exercise of the dumbbell." The modern evolution of muscle building began in earnest toward the end of the 19th century in Europe and the United States when professional strongmen emerged as a form of entertainment. This new style of weight lifting for entertainment was all about strength. The physique didn't matter. What did matter was how much iron a man could press above his head. Many of these competitors had thick, protruding stomachs and fatty limbs. Their physiques didn't need to appeal to their audiences because

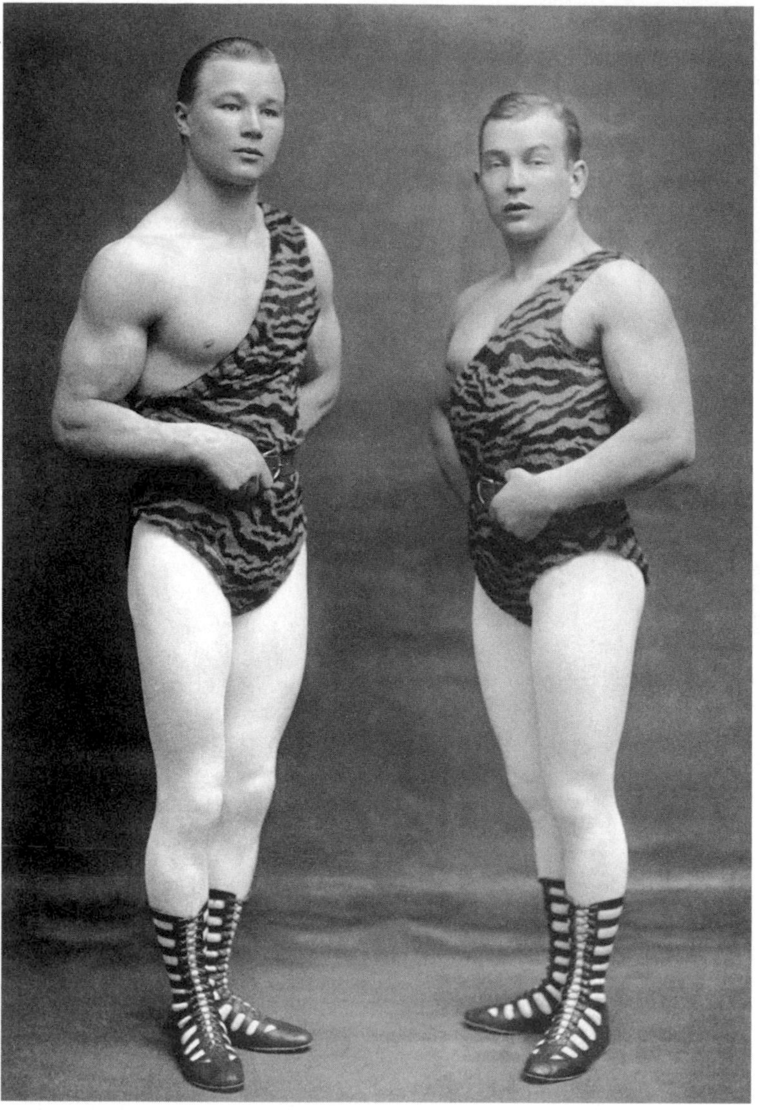

Men in tights. The modern-day bodybuilder evolved from strongmen entertainers who emphasized pure brawn over body shape.

pure power was what the crowds came to see. The strongmen entertainers would pull heavy carts loaded with boulders, lift cows and other animals on their backs, and heft a variety of odd but heavy objects aloft with their arms and sometimes only one arm.

From the 1890 through the 1920s strongman competitions thrived in the United States and sparked an intense interest in weight training. Then, in 1894, a German man named Louis Durlacher opened Professor Attila's Studio of Physical Culture in New York City. Professor Attila was a pioneer of strength training and bodybuilding. He preached the gospel of repetitive lifting of light weights to build muscle. He even invented fitness equipment, such as the globe barbell and the Roman chair.

Two of Attila's students were Warren Lincoln Travis, the "Coney Island Strongman" who once lifted 667 pounds with one finger and did a verified backlift of 4,140 pounds, and Eugen Sandow, the father of modern bodybuilding.

A Different-Looking Strongman

To the turn-of-the-century bodybuilder the terms *symmetry* and *aesthetics* were foreign. Enter Sandow, who bridged the gap between the unsightly strongman and the bodybuilder of today. Sandow had made a reputation in Europe as a vaudeville strongman who would outdo other strongmen at their own stunts. But because his chiseled physique was so well proportioned, he was able to begin transforming a raw and rogue sport into a healthy lifestyle that celebrated the aesthetic of the human form. Sandow was a beauty among beasts; he was as much an exhibitionist as he was a strongman. He enjoyed having people marvel (and the women ooh and aah) at his muscular development. Sandow's muscular symmetry set him apart from all other strongman and made him an instant hit. He would ultimately position himself as the first real bodybuilder and become a promoter of bodybuilding. Sandow's influence led to increased sales of barbells and dumbbells. His magazine and books were wildly popular, and he even developed some of the first weight-lifting machines.

From 1891 to 1901, Sandow toured the United States and Europe performing his muscle poses and promoting strength and bodybuilding shows, including in 1901, the first major bodybuilding contest called "The Great Show." To compete in the contest, all competitors would need to place in smaller regional shows that were held throughout England. The culminating event took place on Saturday, September 14, 1901, at Royal Albert Hall. Spectators were entertained by displays of wrestling, gymnastics, and fencing and, finally, the bodybuilding competition. Sixty men wearing black tights, some in jockey

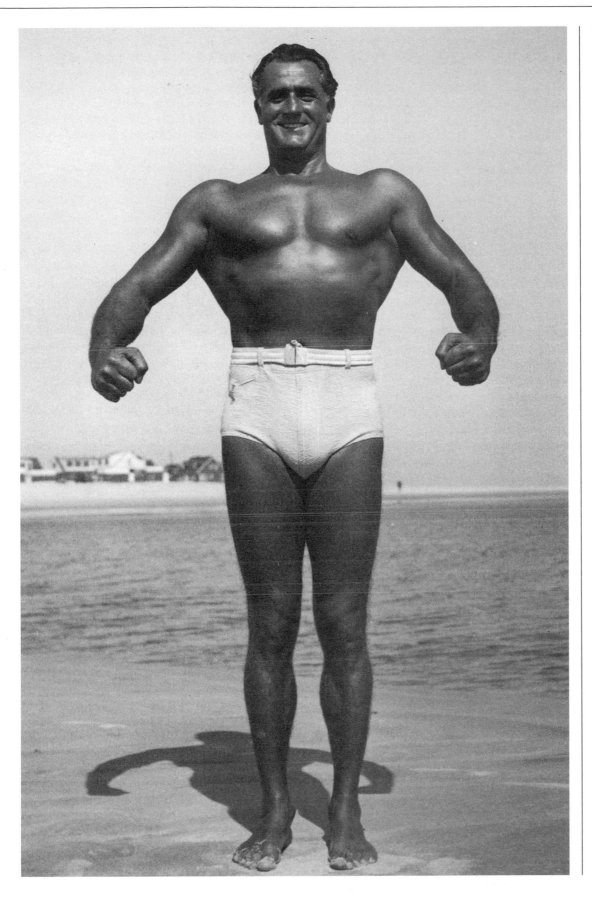

Marketing Muscle. In 1929—using advertisements declaring, "Hey Skinny!...Yer Ribs Are Showing!" and "I Can Make You a New Man!"—Charles Atlas successfully marketed a mail-order fitness course aimed toward the "97-pound weakling." It was called Dynamic Tension.

belts and others in leopard skins were judged on muscle size, balance of muscular development, muscle tone, general health, and condition of the skin. The total prize money that day equaled 1,000 guineas, or more than $5,000. The first-place finisher, William L. Murray of Nottingham, Great Britain, received $2,500 and a gold statue designed to resemble Sandow's physique.

Sandow promoted weight lifting and bodybuilding up until his death from a fatal brain hemorrhage in 1925 when, it is said, he tried to show off by pulling his car from a ditch. Today, Sandow's legacy lives on—his likeness has been immortalized in the Mr. Olympia award statue.

The "Father of Physical Culture"

Also at the turn of the century, businessman Bernarr Macfadden published the first bodybuilding magazine: *Physical Culture.* Macfadden was a great promoter, and, beginning in 1903, he presented a series of contests at Madison Square Garden in New York City to find the "Most Perfectly Developed Man in the World."

Macfadden's influence on bodybuilding lasted for decades, as did his contests and magazine. Even though Macfadden might not have approved of the emphasis on visual development over athletic skill, his contests helped promote a growing interest in muscle appearance versus strength.

In 1921, Angelo Siciliano won a Macfadden contest and strived to capitalize on his new fame by changing his name to Charles Atlas and acquiring the rights to a mail-order course entitled the Dynamic-Tension system, a workout program of muscle-against-muscle exercises developed by Macfadden 20 years before. According to the story Siciliano liked to tell, when he was younger and only weighed 97 pounds, a bully kicked sand in his face at the beach in front of a girl. Humiliated, he joined a YMCA,

Did the Fitness Industry Kill Bodybuilding?

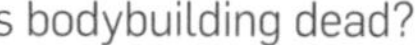

Is bodybuilding dead?

Some people in the health and wellness community feel that bodybuilding is an archaic practice and no longer has a place in the modern fitness industry.

To many, bodybuilding is merely a muscle-flexing competition, not a valid exercise program. I argue that it was the exercise programs developed by bodybuilders that created the foundation for many of today's classic strength-training programs.

As the owner of fitness-training centers, I know for a fact that 9 out of 10 of my clients exercise because they want to look better in a bathing suit. Often the traditional fitness industry gets hung up on treating clients like rehab patients when the ultimate goal for most people who exercise is to look younger, leaner, and healthier.

From that time back in grade school when I first lifted weights in my basement to that day during my junior year of high school when I made a commitment to strength training that ultimately led me to my life's mission, bodybuilding has always been a major part of my journey into the fitness industry. Bodybuilding has forever helped to shape me as a man, friend, competitor, business owner, strength coach, and fitness professional.

I encourage you to look past the tired stereotypes of bodybuilding to discover what it really is—a way to achieve a healthy body and a physique that you can feel good about.

As human beings we each carry with us the need for self-pride and self-satisfaction. This need can be achieved by simply changing the way you feel about your body by making it lean and fit. Deep down, every one of us truly cares about the way he or she looks. It's the reason you picked up this book.

Men, do you want a six-pack? Bigger arms? A bigger back and a thicker chest?

Women, do you want a tighter butt? A toned upper back? Leaner arms and sleek shoulders? I hate to break it to the naysayers, but all of these goals are about bodybuilding.

People want to look better, they want to feel better, and they want to build an aesthetically pleasing physique.

The fitness industry can provide the tools to help them reach those goals. For that reason alone, bodybuilding will always have a place in the fitness industry.

determined to build his body and strength. Atlas used this story to market his exercise in advertisements that arguably still influence the self-help industry today. In one magazine ad, a hulking Atlas in leopard-print swim trunks challenges readers: "Skinny! Give Me 15 Minutes a Day and I'll Give You a New Body." The advertisements for this exercise program inspired a generation of boys and men to try bodybuilding with dynamic tension.

By the end of the 1920s and the start of the 1930s the general public's interest had grown to acknowledge the importance of becoming healthy, fit, and strong.

Training knowledge was very limited during this time, but bodybuilders began to learn a great deal about the importance of weight training from the competitors of the strongman era. Even Atlas used lifting weights over his dynamic tension moves to achieve his physique.

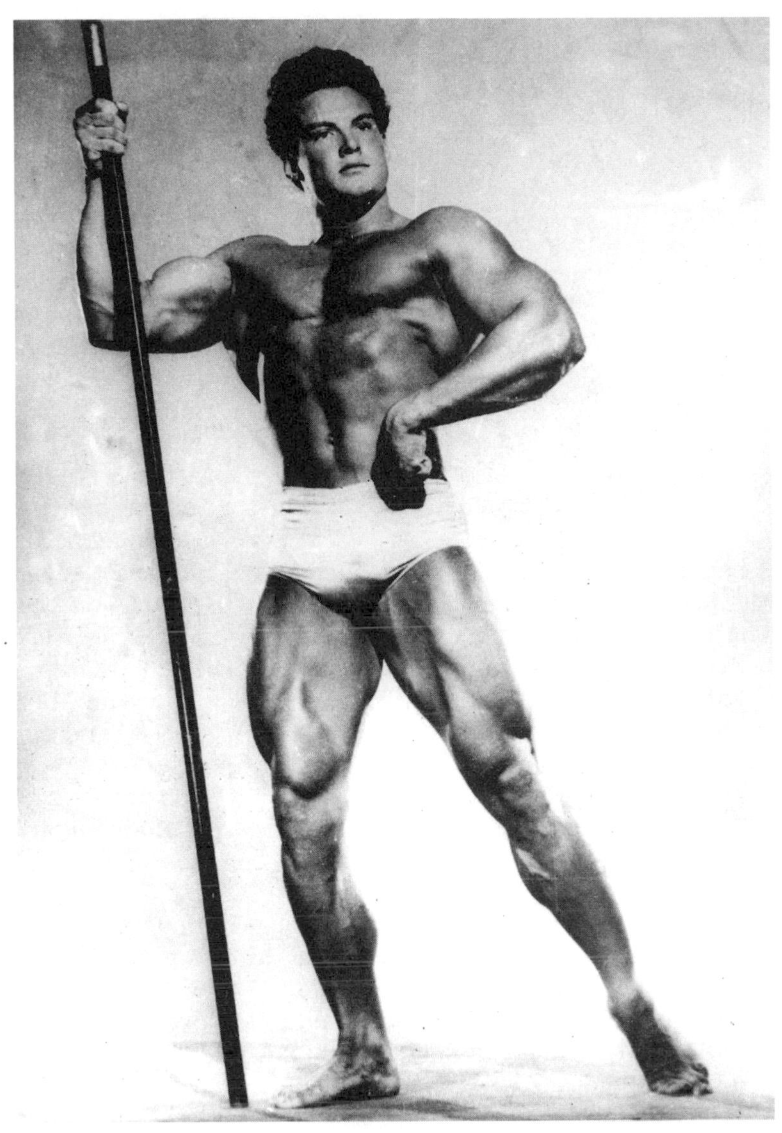

Leading man. Five major bodybuilding titles propelled Steve Reeves on to Hollywood's big screen where the muscleman appeared in sword-and-sandal movies like the 1959 film *Hercules*.

Bodybuilding continued to grow in the 1930s and began to even further separate itself from strongman training. Now men wanted to develop balanced muscular physiques with lower body fat. Training techniques and further advancements in exercise equipment made this transition more apparent. This was the beginning of the "golden age" of bodybuilding, when gyms promoted the idea of group training and posing in front of mirrors.

Thanks to men like Sandow, Macfadden, and Atlas, people began to turn their attention to training to produce an aesthetically muscular physique. Bodybuilder Sigmund Klein was influential through his writing about training and the nutrition aspects of bodybuilding. Klein used nutrition and special training methods to develop a physique based on muscular shape and symmetry (having muscles on one side of the body appear symmetrical to those on the other side), and increased definition due to low body fat.

In 1936, Jack LaLanne opened his first fitness studio in Oakland, California. The following year, a Canadian-born weightlifting champion named Joe Weider started publishing his first magazine, the influential *Your Physique*. By 1939, bodybuilding developed into a structured sport. The

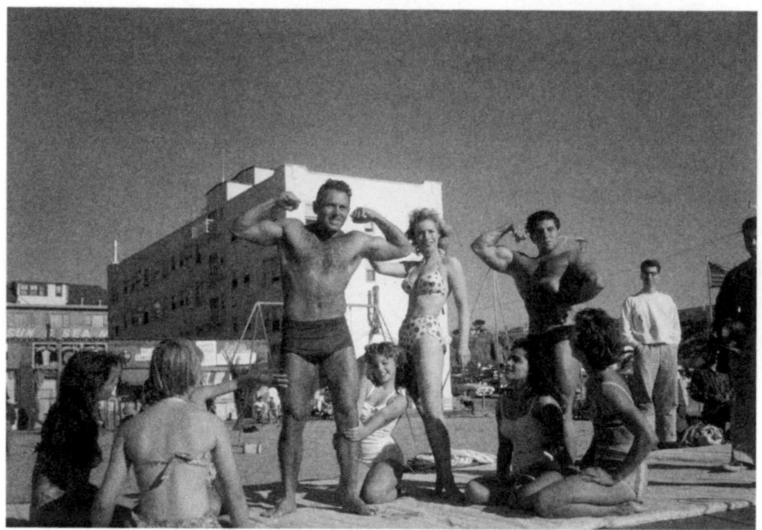

Muscle Beach. In the 1950s, Santa Monica's sandy shore became a mecca for strength training and showing off.

Amateur Athletic Union (AAU) created a Mr. America contest on July 4 in Chicago. The competitors were not true-to-form bodybuilders, instead coming from all different athletic backgrounds. Some competed in boxer shorts, others in jockstraps. The winner was a man named Roland Essmaker.

In 1940 and 1941, John Grimek was crowned Mr. America. Grimek trained solely by lifting weights in the gym, and those who were to compete against him realized they too must do the same. Grimek was also the man who would put to rest the belief that this new generation of bodybuilders were muscle-bound and nonathletic—he would often perform lifts and poses simultaneously, showcasing both his muscular strength and athleticism.

The Birth of Modern Bodybuilders

In 1945 the winner of the Mr. America title was a man by the name of Clarence "Clancy" Ross. Ross's physique rivaled that of today's bodybuilders. Ross possessed round shoulders, wide lats, a tiny waist, sharp abs, and balanced calves—all derived from lifting weights to build shapely and symmetrical muscles. Though Ross never gained much notoriety with the general public, he was a pioneer in his use of weight training to develop the unique physique of the bodybuilder we know today.

Along the California coast in the late 1940s and early 1950s weight training on the beach became ultra popular among both amateur and professional bodybuilders. The most famous beach-based gym was centered in Santa Monica and affectionately called Muscle Beach. Bodybuilding was still a rather obscure sport, but then Steve Reeves came along and won the Mr. America and Mr. Universe titles. Reeves, with his amazingly balanced physique and handsome looks, became the first bodybuilder to be embraced by the general public. Crowds would flock to Muscle Beach to admire his exceptional physique. With the exception of Charles Atlas, Steve Reeves was the only truly famous bodybuilder during the 1950s. He would become an international star in movies such as *Hercules, Morgan the Pirate,* and *The Thief of Baghdad*.

Taking over where Reeves left off was Reg Park, who won the Mr. Universe titles in 1958 and 1965. Park was built with density and mass that made his physique overpowering when paired against other bodybuilders of this era.

Bodybuilding began to expand exponentially with the continued success of the IFBB (International Federation of Bodybuilders) and the NABBA (National Amateur Bodybuilders Association), which was founded in 1950 in England. These organizations held the first large-scale bodybuilding competitions, first with the Mr. Universe in 1950 by the NABBA and later the Mr. Olympia in 1965 by the IFBB.

The mid '60s also saw the emergence of arguably the most influential bodybuilder of all time, Arnold Schwarzenegger, who won the Jr. Mr. Europe title that year, the first of 19 bodybuilding and powerlifting titles he'd claim.

In 1967, Schwarzenegger won the Mr. America title. He went on to win Mr. Universe on five occasions and Mr. Olympia seven times. In 1975, he was filmed training and competing in the Mr. Olympia contest for the famed docudrama *Pumping Iron,* which helped to popularize bodybuilding and made Schwarzenegger a household name. Lou Ferrigno, Arnold's costar in the film, did likewise, appearing in film and TV as *Hercules* and *The Incredible Hulk.*

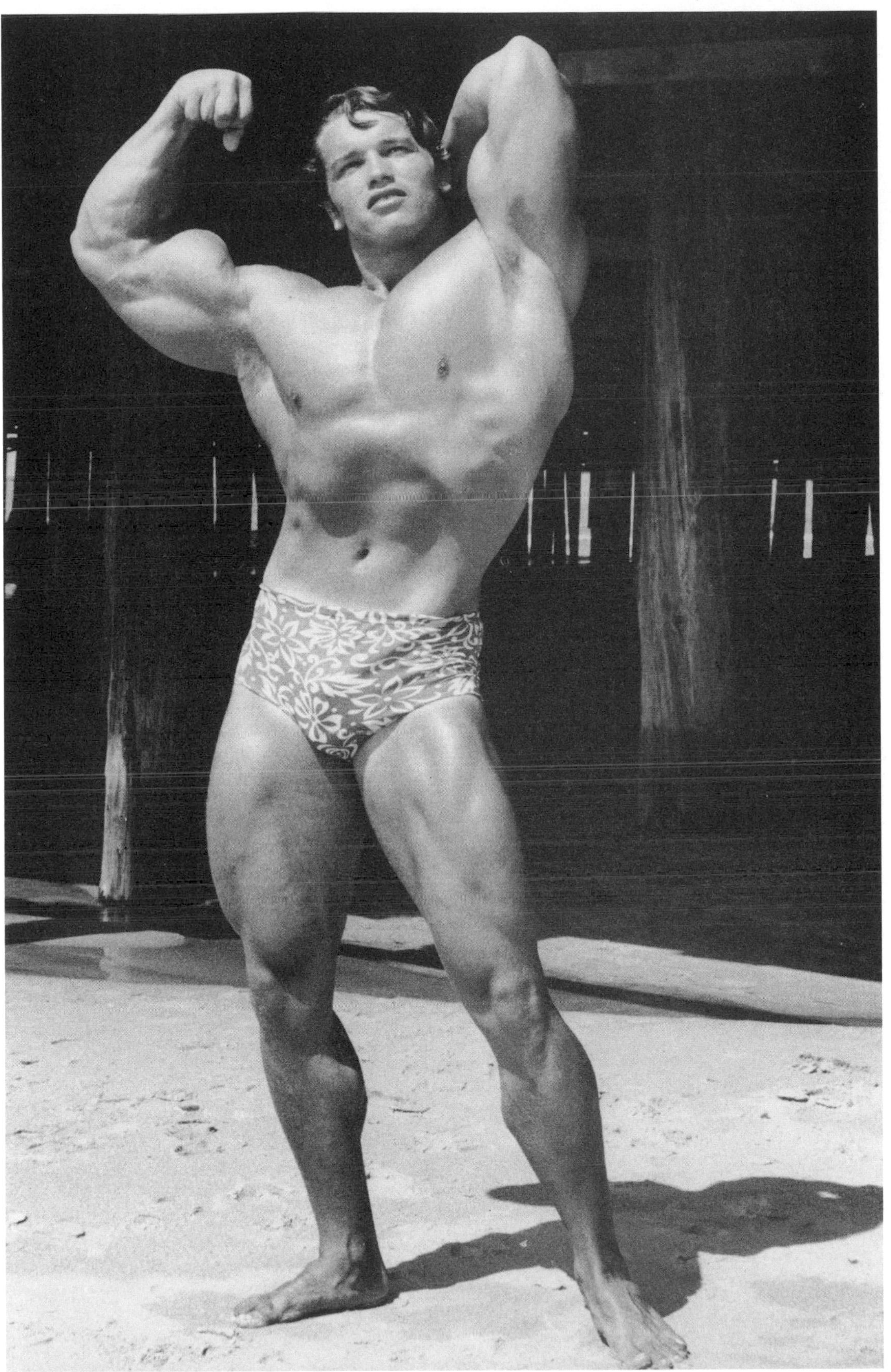

Young Terminator (circa 1975): *Pumping Iron* (and 19 bodybuilding and powerlifting titles) gave Arnold Schwarzenegger blockbuster status.

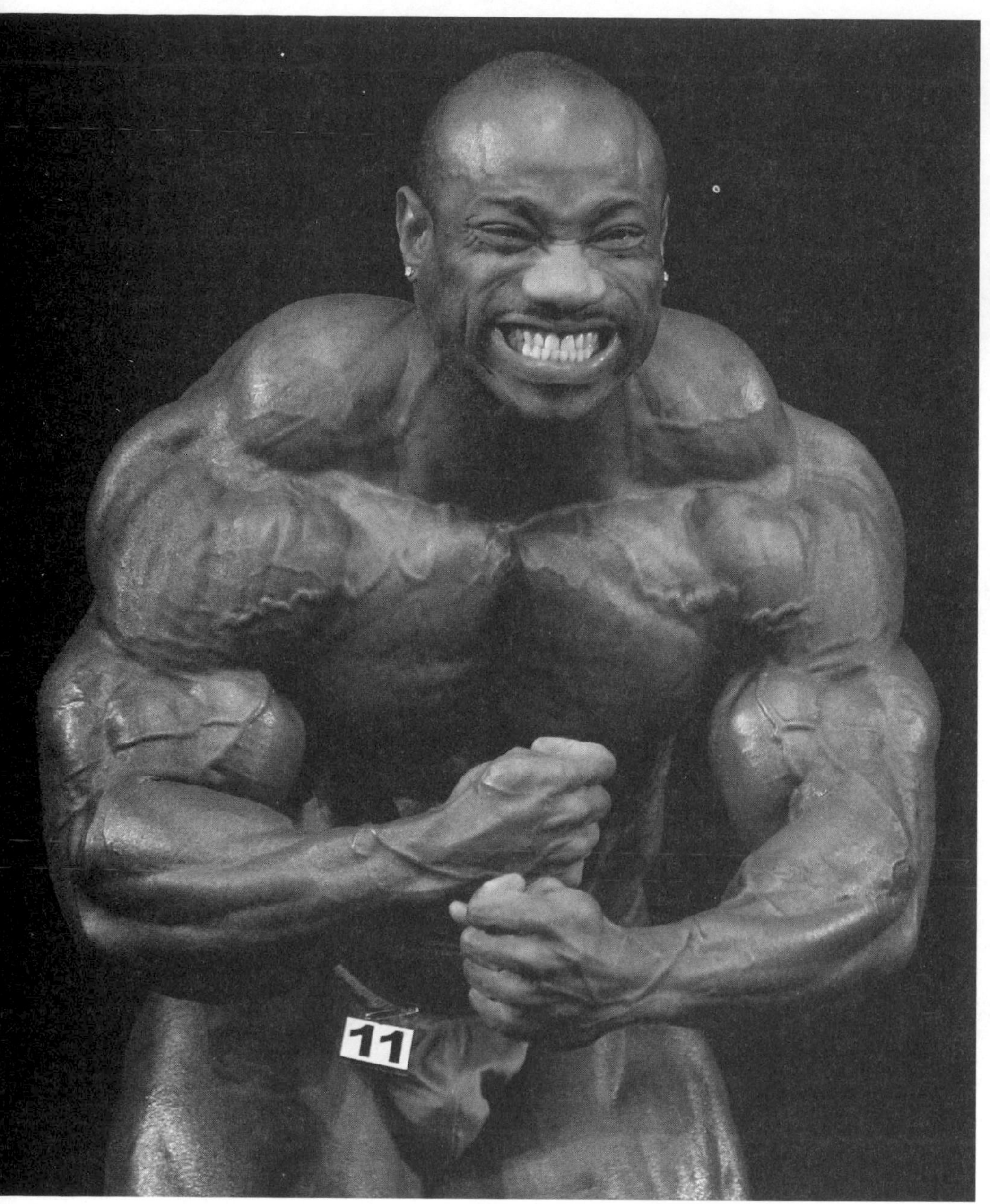

Mass Appeal. Dexter "The Blade" Jackson, a #3 ranked IFBB professional bodybuilder, won his fourth Arnold Classic Title in 2013. In 2008, he defeated Jay Cutler to become Mr. Olympia.

Steroid Culture and the Emergence of the Natural Bodybuilder

During the early '60s and '70s bodybuilders began to experiment with performance-enhancing drugs. As competitions became more prestigious and lucrative, competitors looked to every method possible to gain an edge.

The use of performance enhancers wasn't frowned upon or ever much of a discussion. It was widely known and accepted in bodybuilding circles, especially among the top-level international competitors. The regulatory committees that govern competitive sports today didn't exist back then, and drugs were easy to procure. During this time, steroids and performance enhancers were far less advanced than those used by today's nontested athletes.

Today the purity of the sport has been infiltrated and overshadowed, for the most part, by the kind of high-stakes modern bodybuilding competitions that are fueled by performance-enhancing drugs, a billion-dollar supplement industry, and unrealistic expectations that push people to do dangerous and unhealthy things to their bodies.

When you talk about bodybuilding today, most people think of juiced-up, wild-eyed Incredible Hulks packing steroid syringes. But there's another, purer side of bodybuilding—natural bodybuilding—that's growing in popularity primarily because it's all about, well, not using performance-enhancing drugs. And this side of the sport—natural bodybuilding—has become the vibrant competitive sport that I love.

What does it mean to be a natural bodybuilder? From a competitive stand-

From the late '70s through the '90s, bodybuilding was defined by names like Frank Zane, Boyer Coe, Roy Callender, and Chris Dickerson. Bodybuilders were growing bigger. In the '80s the sport saw a shift from balance and aesthetics to massive muscle—like 245-pound Lee Haney, one of the heaviest bodybuilders. Haney broke Schwarzenegger's record with a total of eight consecutive Mr. Olympia titles. In the 2000s Ronnie Coleman did the same, winning Mr. Olympia eight times. His top competition weight: 297 pounds.

point, it depends. "Natural" means you build and sculpt your muscles from nothing more than good nutrition and hard work in the gym. Your muscles are not the result of taking steroids, prohormones or other performance-enhancing drugs, or illegal supplements. However, you should know that some organizations that hold competitions require competitors to be "clean" for a period of 7 years, while others require bodybuilders to be natural for life. All natural bodybuilding competitions test for performance-enhancing drug use. Various protocols are used: lie-detector testing, urine analysis, or a combination of the two. The goal of natural bodybuilding testing is to create a level playing field for competitors.

There continues to be much debate in the bodybuilding world about what exactly equals "truly natural." For example, some people feel that a bodybuilder is not natural if he takes vitamin supplements versus consuming only whole foods.

For the fan of bodybuilding, like myself, steroid-assisted bodybuilding and natural bodybuilding are two entirely different sports. The physiques being judged are entirely different and that alone keeps these two sides of bodybuilding separate. In the bodybuilding world you will never find the world's best natural bodybuilders competing against the world's best steroid-enhanced physiques.

Natural bodybuilding has grown so rapidly in recent years because there is a new generation of lifter who is just as concerned with health and wellness as he or she is with sculpting an aesthetic physique. This new school of bodybuilders treats the body like a temple. Nothing goes inside that isn't pure and natural. This new breed is always looking for new ways to train and to consume high-quality food. When natural bodybuilders seek to increase performance, they turn to natural supplementation rather than performance enhancers. And now more than ever before there are terrific, safe supplements like whey protein, creatine, and branched-chain amino acids (BCAAs) that are available to those who want to avoid the aid of steroidal substances. (We'll discuss these supplements in Chapter 6.)

Natural bodybuilding itself is divided—separated into numerous organizations such as the World Natural Bodybuilding Federation (WNBF) and the International Federation of Physique Athletes (IFPA) that thrive on amateur and professional membership dues. For an amateur, these organizations provide numerous opportunities to compete. But the lack of one unifying body governing professional competitions makes it impossible to crown a single best natural bodybuilder. For example, although WNBF pros cannot participate in competitions held by any other organizations, IFPA, National Gym Association (NGA), and others allow their competitors to compete in other organizations' pro competitions. For this reason, top-level natural bodybuilders like WNBF world title holders Martin Daniels, Brian Whitacre, Richard Godzecki, and Jim Cordova will never have the opportunity to compete against the likes of top IFPA world title pros like Phillip Ricardo, Cleveland Thomas, and Doug Miller.

Contributing to the splintering of natural bodybuilding are smaller organizations that are being formed. The Drug Free Athletes Coalition (DFAC) has been formed with the hope of providing an environment built solely around the athlete. Alliances like the Natural Bodybuilders Association (NBA) have been formed in order to bring the leaders of each individual organization together to form a mega competition. So far preliminary meetings and talks have made only small strides toward this goal.

For natural bodybuilding to make a bigger splash in mainstream culture, it would be ideal for the two largest organizations for natural bodybuilders, the WNBF and IFPA, to come to an agreement that allows professional natural bodybuilders, like myself, to compete against the very best from both organizations by creating a truly unified natural bodybuilding championship. It's what the athletes and the fans want. Until that day comes, natural bodybuilders will continue to wonder when our sport will be recognized for its true growth potential.

PART 1

CHAPTER 3

Compete or Just Look Good?

There are a lot of motives for building muscle

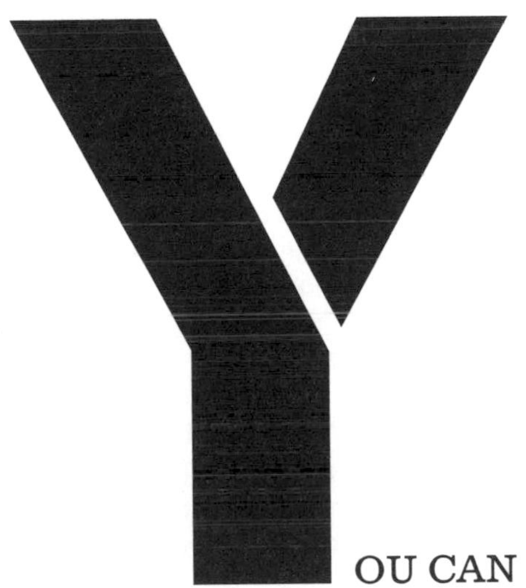

YOU CAN BE A BODYBUILDER and not go into competition. That's fine. Bodybuilding on the most basic level is about building up your body's muscles and getting into the best physical, mental, and aesthetic shape you can—and reaping all the physical and mental health benefits I outlined in the Introduction. You can get all that without ever slapping on the oil and posing on a stage. It's all good.

But if you are interested in taking bodybuilding to the next level—competition—you will want to explore exactly what preparing for a competition entails and to ask yourself some important questions:

- *Can I commit the time to prepare for competition?*
- *Do I have the time to do the required training?*
- *Can I afford it? (Not just entrance fees but the costs of a special diet, supplements, gym membership, and travel.)*
- *Should I train on my own or hire a coach?*

These are all legitimate questions that you should ask yourself before embarking on the journey to compete in a bodybuilding competition. Bodybuilding isn't only about the day of competition, it takes vast amounts of time to prepare yourself for that day, beginning months in advance.

The amount of time you'll need to train, prepare food, and practice the art of posing will be a big part of the journey. In addition, the costs associated with food, travel, and registration are many times overlooked by would-be bodybuilders.

Another potential cost that needs to be considered is hiring a prep coach. A big way to jump the learning curve is to have the guidance of coach.

Start with a realistic evaluation of your potential and ask

yourself, "Why do I want to compete?" Is this a personal journey or a challenge? Do you want to compete because you feel you have a physique that will win? If your sole purpose of competing is to win, I recommend that you reconsider your motives. A bodybuilding journey for the sole purpose of victory will keep you from being able to truly enjoy every step you take. By the time your competition arrives, you may have missed the grander rewards gained from all that preparation. Competing as a bodybuilder is more about the journey and about your personal commitment to bringing your physique to a level only a few achieve, than about any trophy or award you may take home.

Bodybuilding is a commitment. You must make a strong commitment to training, nutrition, meal preparation, and self-improvement, which all leads back to your strong commitment of time and money. See "The Cost of Competing" on page 32 for a general breakdown of the financial commitment you may need to make to succeed.

For many professional and elite level bodybuilders, a way to balance this all out is to hire a prep coach, someone who becomes a second set of eyes to evaluate your physique throughout the dieting and training process. This person can be someone who only evaluates your physique or someone who provides you with both training and nutrition coaching. This can be done personally by taking pictures week by week and reevaluating your progress or relying on the judgment of the coach you've hired. Of course, if you hire a coach, you are facing a bigger financial commitment.

The financial impact of preparing to compete in a bodybuilding competition is often overlooked by new competitors.

For one there is the jump in grocery costs for the duration of your contest preparation, and this cost can increase over time because food quantities may increase. Weekly grocery bills can run you anywhere from $150 to $300 per week.

Second, you have to look at the cost of the registration for a competition—and your membership dues to the organization holding the competition. This alone can run between $100 and close to $300.

For many who choose to compete, other surprising costs are the expenses of travel, hotel, tanning supplies, and perhaps even tickets for family to attend your competition. Each of these will add to your initial costs.

For example, in 2010 I won close to $3,000 by either winning or placing second or third in three competitions, and yet this didn't cover my costs during the contest prep season. But, as you can imagine, I'm not doing this to get rich or even to pay the bills. This is my avocation. I'm just fortunate that it meshes so closely with my day job.

Natural bodybuilding isn't about competing to win money or even about being awarded a trophy. Your decision to compete must be more about you challenging yourself, than it is about you beating any other competitor. Bodybuilding is a subjective sport: you're allowing a judging panel to decide whether they believe your physique is better than your fellow competitors'.

The Noncompetitive Bodybuilder

For some the idea of competing in a bodybuilding competition just isn't appealing. That doesn't mean they don't aspire to build the physique of a bodybuilder; that's still a very attainable goal. And it requires a similar commitment of time and resources. You are the person who will take the nutrition component, training program, and tools from this book and expand your training style while taking your physique to a new level. Bodybuilding isn't only about stepping onstage, and, in fact, for those who don't aspire to competition, training like a bodybuilder can provide amazing health benefits as well as tremendous personal satisfaction. If you can dedicate yourself to doing what it takes to bring your physique to the level of a bodybuilder, then competing onstage is only a bonus. There is nothing more rewarding than presenting a head-turning physique.

The Competitive Bodybuilder

The first step toward the stage is to select a competition. This allows you to set your short-term and long-term goals during the entire contest preparation process. Start with a local competition that supports a novice division for first-time bodybuilders. (If you are a teenager, choose a contest with a junior division.) Ideally, you'll want to look for one several months away to give yourself enough time to prepare. See the guidelines that follow on how many weeks of dieting are required for your body type.

Select a governing body.

The following is a list of the most popular organizations that put on competitions and what makes each unique.

WNBF/INBF

World Natural Bodybuilding Federation (WNBF), professional organization; International Natural Bodybuilding & Fitness Federation (INBF), amateur affiliate organization

- Founded in 1989, the WNBF is a leading organization for qualifying professional natural bodybuilders through the INBF amateur divisions. The INBF provides amateur natural bodybuilders the opportunity to compete year round in INBF amateur competitions, where bodybuilders can qualify into the WNBF professional ranks.

IFPA/OCB

International Federation of Physique Athletes (IFPA), professional organization; Organization of Competitive Bodybuilders (OCB), amateur affiliate organization

- The IFPA is a leading professional-level natural bodybuilding organization. IFPA professionals have qualified through competing and winning in the amateur OCB competitions.

National Gym Association (NGA)

- The NGA is an organization that promotes and sanctions natural bodybuilding contests nationwide.

North American Natural Bodybuilding Federation (NANBF)

- Founded in the early 1980s, the NANBF is now a professional affiliate with the IFPA and amateur ranks of the OCB.

Amateur Bodybuilding Association (ABA)

- The Amateur Bodybuilding Association was formed in 1989 and follows the motto "Serving the Athletes" by providing competitors an enjoyable and competitive forum with a quality reputation.

International Natural Bodybuilding Association (INBA)

- The INBA was formed by more than 15 countries to provide competitors the opportunity to compete in international contests.

Professional Natural Bodybuilding Association (PNBA)

- A worldwide natural bodybuilding organization and home to the Natural Olympia event.

Drug Free Athletes Coalition (DFAC)

- Founded in 2011, the DFAC was formed

to provide natural bodybuilding athletes the opportunity to compete in an organization that strengthens the relationship between organization, athlete, and promoter.

Choose your weight division.

Most bodybuilding competitions are set up by weight division. Here's a look at the typical breakdown for men and women:

Men
Bantamweight: up to 142 pounds
Lightweight: 143–156 pounds
Middleweight: 157–176 pounds
Light Heavyweight: 177–198 pounds
Heavyweight: over 198 pounds

Women
Lightweight: less than 114 pounds
Middleweight: 115–125 pounds
Heavyweight: over 125 pounds

Develop your strategy.

Compete at the weight class that allows you to bring your leanest, fullest physique. The judges prefer to see a light heavyweight who is ripped more than a middleweight with smooth bulked-up muscles.

Find a competition that allows enough time to diet. The dieting period is the most crucial part of your journey. For a bodybuilder the key is to give yourself enough time to get lean. It's vital to your success that you don't rush the process. How long you need to diet depends in large part on your specific body type and overall metabolism. Here are some general guidelines:

Body Type	Optimal Dieting Range
Ectomorph	10–16 weeks
Mesomorph	16–22 weeks
Endomorph	22–28 weeks

The program described in this book runs 24 weeks. Depending upon your body type and natural metabolism, you may need less or more time to prepare. But, as a general guide, 24 weeks will be a solid time frame for beginner contest prep. Remember: It is critical to be very lean for competition.

THE COST OF COMPETING

Here's a look at what's required for preparing to enter a local bodybuilding competition and how much it can set you back. These costs are based on the experience of a number of amateur and professional bodybuilders and can vary widely. You may be able to find ways to keep your costs much lower and achieve the results you want.

THE BASICS	THE $$$$
Training facility	$0–$200 per month
Special food and meal prep	$150–$300 per week
Supplements	$200 per month
Tanning	$30–$80
Posing suit	$30–$60
Posing music	$25–$100
Photography	$100–$500 per shoot
Posing coaching	$50–$100 per session
Posing choreography	$50–$100 per session
Competition registration	$100–$200 per competition
Travel and lodging	$150–$300 per night

OPTIONAL

Coaching	$1,000–$2,400 per year
Seminars	$200–$400 per year

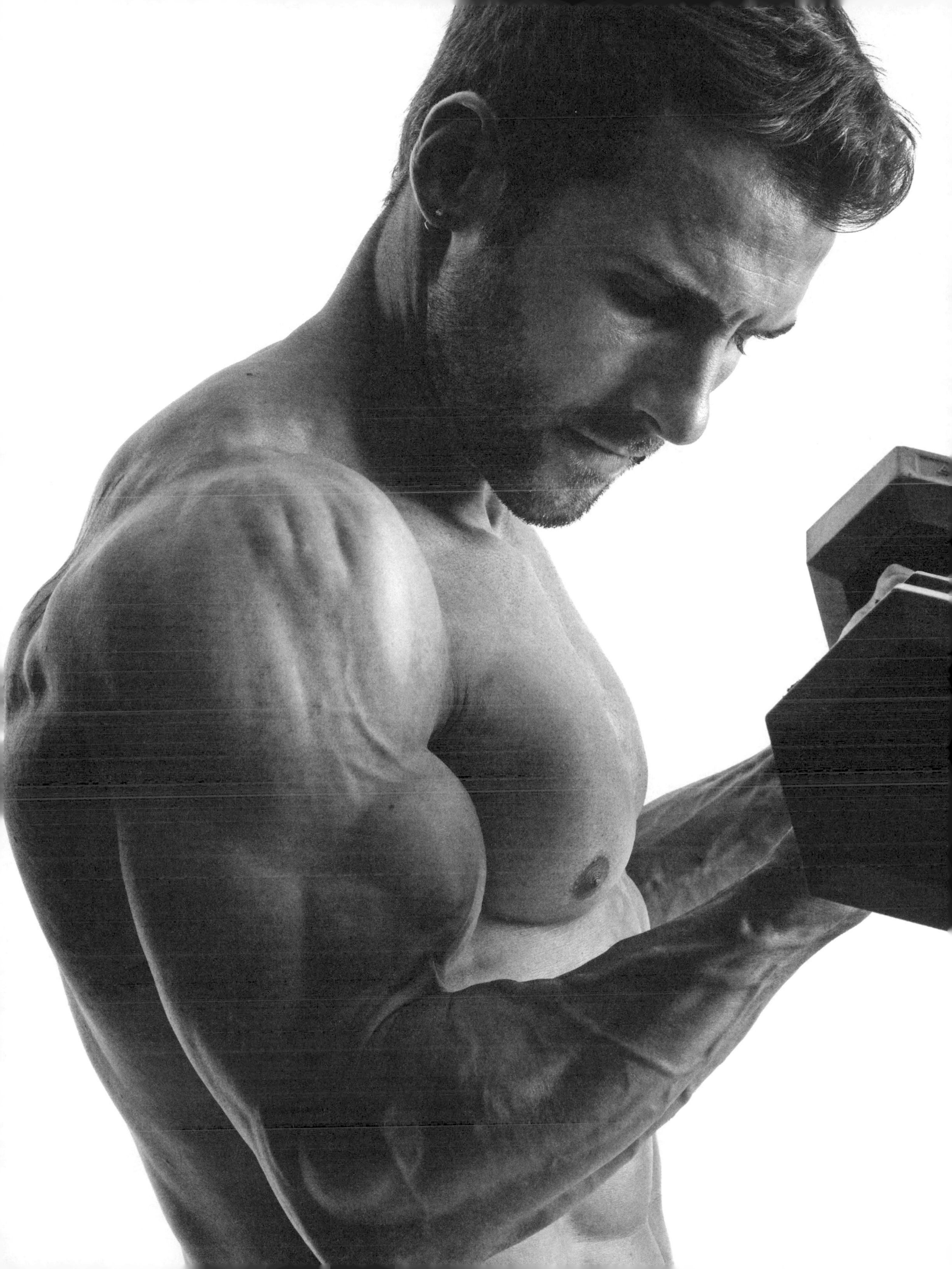

PART 2

Nutrition for Bodybuilders

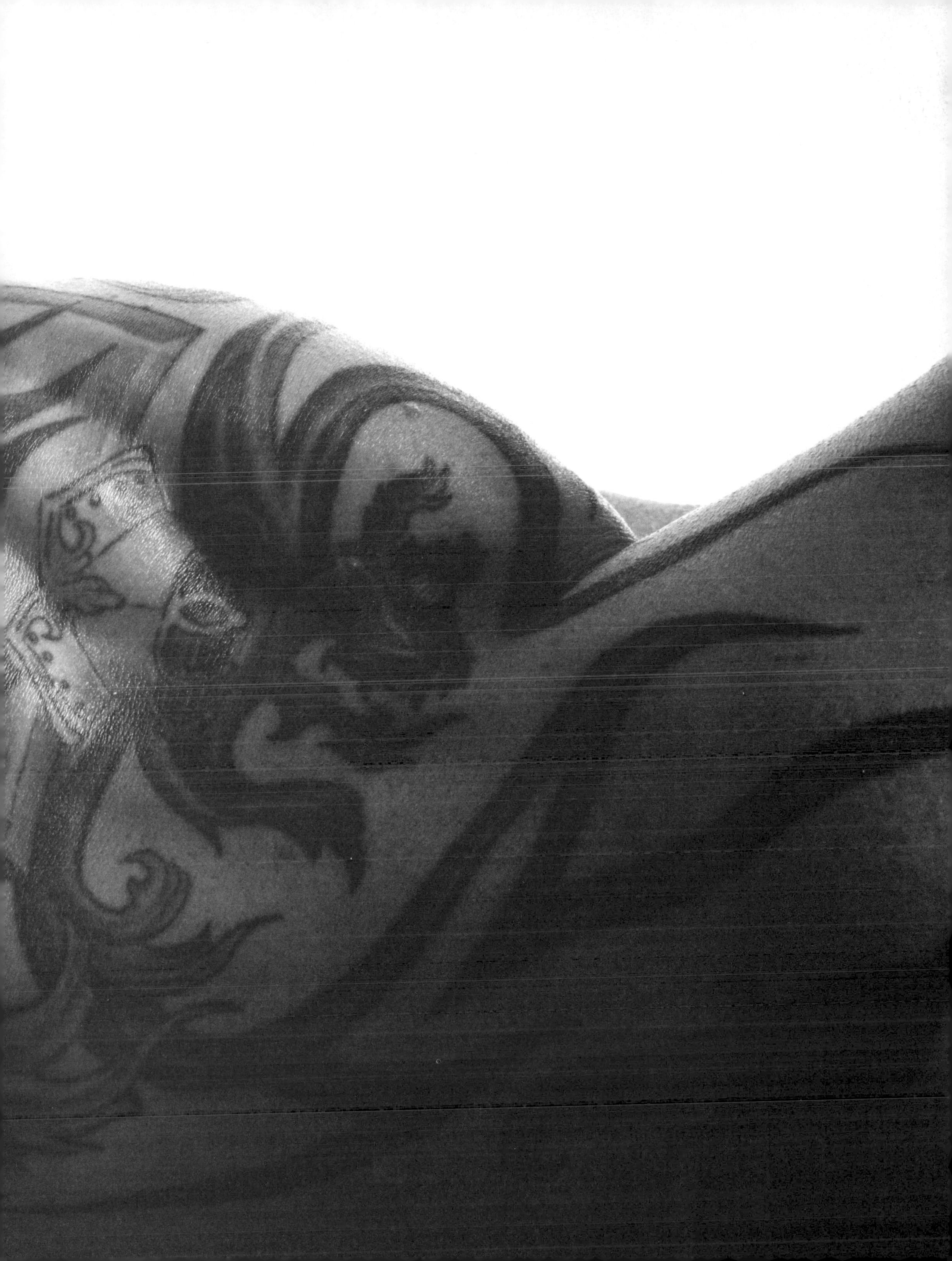

PART 2

CHAPTER 4

The New Rules of Getting Lean

To lose body fat, put time and science on your side

OUR SOCIETY IS QUICK TO explain body size with a word that most of us don't understand—*metabolism*.

You've probably heard statements like, "I have a slow metabolism so it's hard for me to lose weight," or "I have a naturally fast metabolism so I burn off anything I eat." No two people will lose body fat at the same rate for an extended period of time. Some will have an easier time losing body fat and preparing for a bodybuilding competition; others will grind it out week after week and see very minimal changes. But no matter what kind of natural resting metabolism you have, you can dramatically affect it through your diet, exercise, and other lifestyle choices.

The dieting bodybuilder will soon learn that what he or she eats, when he or she chows it down, how much is eaten, and the total calories consumed will all have a profound effect on the ability to burn fat at an advanced rate—the ultimate goal. The successful bodybuilder is in control of the metabolism because of a control of diet. In the dieting section of this book you will learn to use your diet to manipulate how fast you transform your physique.

The more aware you are of the effect of food and exercise on the landscape of your body, the greater ability you will have to make the necessary changes from week to week to elevate your metabolism to new levels, even when dieting. Undergoing a bodybuilding diet is a slow, grueling process that when done correctly will shed body fat and bring your metabolism to peak levels.

How Dieting Affects Metabolic Rate

Eating fewer calories than your body needs is the first step to losing weight. Everyone knows that. However, if it's not done correctly, calorie restriction can cause the body to do exactly what you don't want it to do—store fat. That's something you certainly cannot have when you are preparing your physique to be judged on stage.

As a bodybuilder, it is essential to maintain lean muscle mass and avoid muscle loss. This is a crucial balancing act that you must master in order to bring your best physique to the competition. The danger in dieting is that your body is capable of burning calories through catabolizing other tissues, even your muscle tissue. For a dieting bodybuilder, retaining muscle is not only important to enabling you to build your best-looking physique, but it's paramount to increasing metabolism, strength, and energy levels throughout the process of getting lean. And, frankly, that goes for anyone who is trying to build a lean, healthy body. Finding that balance will be the key to success. These rules will help guide you.

Rule 1. Find Your Body Type

The first step in creating the proper nutrition plan for you is determining how many calories your body needs to maintain muscle while burning body fat. And you need to determine the optimum combination of the macronutrients protein, carbohydrate, and fat.

The number of fat cells we are genetically dealt play a significant role in how much fat we carry on our bodies, and this varies greatly from person to person. Although anyone can lose or gain weight with the right plan, genetics can make one bodybuilder's journey to get lean easier, and another's much more difficult. That's why it's important for a bodybuilder transitioning into a contest prep diet to know his or her body type.

Humans typically fall into one of three body types, or somatotypes: ectomorph, mesomorph, and endomorph. Determining yours will allow you to understand how efficiently your body processes carbohydrates, a key component to losing body fat. In addition, this will allow you to determine the optimum way to structure your diet in terms of protein, carbohydrate, and fat; meal frequency; meal spacing; and cardio training. Find your body type below.

MAN IN THE MIRROR: WHICH SOMATOTYPE ARE YOU?

Ectomorph

An ectomorphic somatotype is naturally thin with skinny limbs with stringy muscles. Think of a person whose body type resembles that of an endurance athlete. These are the people whose body is thyroid dominant—meaning they have a fast metabolism and a higher carbohydrate tolerance. Growing up I found myself in this category but knew nothing about it. For me it would have been easier to eat more carbohydrates, but instead I found myself consuming all things protein.

Characteristics:

- Small frame and bone structure
- Thin
- Long and stringy muscles
- Flat chest
- Thin shoulders with little width
- Difficult to gain weight
- Fast metabolism

Usually ectomorphs find it very difficult to gain weight because of their fast metabolisms. Ectomorphs can usually lose body fat easily with small changes to diet though, making it extra difficult to hold on to valuable lean muscle mass.

Mesomorph

The mesomorphic body is naturally muscular. The people with an athletic frame find it easier to build muscle because they tend to be testosterone and growth-hormone dominant—meaning they tend to hold on to lean muscle although they gain fat more easily than ectomorphs.

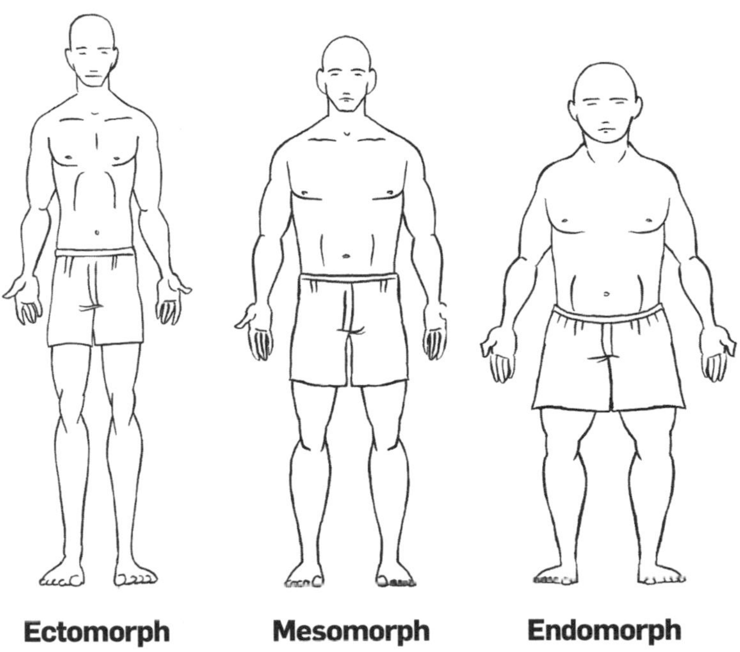

Characteristics:

- Naturally muscular
- Athletic
- Strong
- Well-defined muscles
- Rectangular-shaped physique
- Easy to gain muscle
- Easier to gain body fat than ectomorphs

The mesomorph body type is a great platform for a bodybuilder or physique competitor. Mesomorphs naturally have larger muscle that can easily be built upon.

Endomorph

A endomorphic somatotype is naturally broad and thick. The main characteristics are being insulin dominant, having a slow metabolic rate, and low carbohydrate tolerance. Their body structure is one of a wider waist and larger bone structure. They are heavily muscled yet carry extra body fat around the midsection.

Characteristics:

- Soft round body
- Shorter "stocky" build
- Round physique
- Thick arms and legs
- Difficult to lose body fat
- Slow metabolism

Because of the endomorph's low carbohydrate tolerance and insulin-dominant characteristics, they often find it very difficult to lose body fat, especially in the central region (abdominal and lower back).

The Body Type Hybrid

Have you figured out your basic body type? Good. Now, keep this in mind: Your body type may change as you get further along in the dieting process. There will be periods of time when you may feel like you could classify your body type as something different. A person's lifestyle can alter what may have been their natural body type and create a hybrid body type.

That's what happened to me. I grew up as a true ectomorph, but through strength training I increased my muscle mass, so my body resembles more of an ecto-mesomorph today. This hybrid body type presents some challenges and opportunities when it comes to my diet.

During the early stages of my contest preparation, I consume much lower levels of carbohydrates than when I'm further along in the dieting process. I do this to speed my way to becoming lean because I'm closer to the true mesomorph body type at that point. I'll eat closer to the way I do during "off-season" from competition prep. I consume fewer but larger meals spaced further apart. Later on, when I'm in the heat of competition training, my body's true genetic makeup peaks, and I find myself transformed into more of an ecto-mesomorph (athletic and muscular, yet still on the thin side). As such, I'll alter my diet toward smaller, more frequent meals, and more carbohydrates—nearly double the carbs I was originally eating.

You may be like me. Or you may find that midway through your contest preparation your body has shifted into endo-mesomorph mode (someone who is heavily muscled and carries extra body fat around the midsection).

This commingling of body types is a natural course of your journey. Where I became a hybrid of an ectomorph and mesomorph through my eating and exercise habits, someone can also be a natural ectomorph who due to years of inactivity and poor food choices might have developed poor insulin sensitivity and carbohydrate tolerance resulting in a mixture of an ectomorph and a mesomorph.

Rule 2. Know Yourself

Two endomorphs can have significantly different fat cells. This makes a competition between two bodybuilders of the same weight all that more interesting because both of these athletes have most likely taken entirely different diet and cardio exercise paths to prepare for their competition.

Although knowing your body type is important, so is understanding how your body metabolizes food. You can gain that understanding by looking at your past history of weight loss and weight gain. Just because your body is shaped more like an endomorph, doesn't mean you should eat like an endomorph. Get to know how your body responds to various stages of dieting and strength training to be able to tweak both in your quest for a lean bodybuilder's body.

Rule 3. Manage Your Carbs

Probably the most effective law of getting lean is controlling your carbohydrate intake. Do it right, and you will lose body fat faster, spare your hard-earned muscle, and control your energy levels—the hat trick of bodybuilding prep. In order to do this, it helps to understand how your body processes carbohydrates. While limiting calories is the first step toward losing body fat, it only will come with a decrease in carbohydrates.

Through the digestion process, carbohydrates are converted into glucose. How long this takes depends on the complexity of the carbohydrates consumed. High-glycemic carbs (simple carbs) are metabolized quickly; low-glycemic carbs (complex carbs) are metabolized slowly. When you eat too many of either type of carbohydrate or even a small bit of high-glycemic carbs, your blood sugar rises rapidly. This leads to insulin being released, so that the level of insulin in the body spikes above normal levels. Excess insulin causes glucose that isn't used by your body for energy to be stored as body fat. If you dramatically reduce your carbohydrate intake, your blood sugar levels will drop considerably, causing fatigue, hunger, cravings, low energy, and a crashing feeling. Since your body is retrieving or storing energy meal by meal, carbohydrate management is critically important for the bodybuilder.

In this program, I'll show you how to plan your meals to properly manage your carbohydrate intake throughout the dieting process and to increase your body's metabolic rate.

Rule 4. Give Yourself Enough Time

The perfect diet doesn't exist. What works for one person may not work for another. As a bodybuilder you will be constantly tweaking your diet from week to week to get lean and stage ready; you will be a work in progress. To be successful, the best thing you can do is start earlier, rather than later. Many bodybuilders rush to get their bodies ready for "game day," failing to give themselves enough time, specifically enough weeks, to be prepared and lean enough early on. By planning ahead to allow adequate time to lose weight, you will be dieting safely and that will lead to having your best physique ready on competition day.

As a general guide, a safe amount of time for any bodybuilder is 16 to 24 weeks. Your body type will determine your optimum time frame, but remember, the more time you have the better, because sufficient time allows room for error and for setbacks. Here are the optimal time frames for each body type:

Ectomorph: 10–16 weeks
Mesomorph: 16–22 weeks
Endomorph: 22–28 weeks

Most bodybuilders associate dieting with minimal carbohydrates, tons of cardio, and low energy. These elements may indeed come into play. The key here is to give yourself more than enough time to transform your body in the early stages. As your body approaches the final weeks of the dieting process—if you prepared early enough—you will be able to gradually increase carbohydrate intake, allowing your metabolic rate to increase. As any avid iron pumper will tell you, more food means more strength and energy during training, which is crucial right before competition.

How Much Fat Should You Expect to Lose?

Most men should count on losing 1 to 1.5 pounds of body weight per week during the dieting process. A longer dieting program provides you with the opportunity to increase calories later in the contest preparation, leading to more muscle fullness and increased body-fat loss.

I learned this trick as an amateur bodybuilder by reading old issues of *Natural Bodybuilding and Fitness* magazine and comparing my physique to pictures of WNBF pros. I noticed that those pros would give themselves several more weeks of preparation time than the 12 weeks that most bodybuilders (including me at the time) allotted for dieting.

If you are currently 15 to 20 pounds away from your anticipated competition weight, you may want to start to clean up your diet before giving yourself a certain number of allocated weeks of contest preparation. The goal for many competitive professional natural bodybuilders is to stay within 10 to 15 pounds of their contest weight in the off-season. For those of you sitting outside that range, a bodybuilding competition is not out of the question, you just need to give yourself more time to be ready. I'd love to tell you that you can consistently lose 2 to 3 pounds a week during the dieting process, but you won't. Make time your friend in the bodybuilding process.

Rule 5. Track Calories to Lower Body-Fat Percentage

A bodybuilder's end goal is to take body-fat percentage to the lowest possible level, while maintaining muscle mass. Tracking your overall calorie intake and your consumption of the proper amounts of macronutrients is a critical step toward reducing your body fat.

Before you can monitor your food intake, you need determine your caloric baseline, that is, the approximate amount of energy (calories) you require to maintain your current weight, assuming you do no exercise. To find that number you must know your current body-fat percentage (BFP) and lean body mass (LBM). Your BFP is a good measure of your fitness, and it's determined by dividing your total body weight by the total weight of the fat on your frame. Lean body mass (or weight) is the weight of your bones, muscles, and organs—everything that isn't fat. There are various ways to figure out these values.

Body-fat percentage is difficult to determine because it requires some technology. Underwater weighing, in which the volume of water displaced by your body is subtracted from the weight of the displaced water, is one of the most accurate. A newer method is a DEXA (dual-energy X-ray absorptiometry) scan, which measures body composition and bone-mineral density. Both are expensive procedures. More affordable and accessible are the body-fat measurements offered at many gyms using body-fat scales, or calipers, that measure the folds of fat at several points on your body. These are not highly accurate but can give you a usable ballpark figure. If you don't have calipers and you're itching to know your body-fat percentage right now, here's a simple, low-tech (albeit not very accurate) test:

- Sit in a chair with your knees bent and your feet flat on the floor.
- Using your thumb and index finger, gently pinch the skin on top of your right thigh.
- Measure the thickness of the pinched skin with a ruler.

Results:
- If it's about ¾ inch, you have about 14 percent body fat.
- If it's 1 inch, you're probably closer to 18 percent fat.
- If you pinch more than an inch, you have a lot of work ahead of you. But more important, BFPs over 20 may put you at increased risk for diabetes and heart disease.

You won't start seeing your abs until your body fat dips under 12 percent. Bodybuilders typically have a body-fat percentage in the 3 to 6 percent range just before competition.

Once you have your BFP, you can calculate your lean body mass (LBM) by using this formula:

Body weight – (body weight x body-fat percent) = lean body mass

Or just use an online LBM calculator.

Example:
Here's how to figure the lean body mass of a 180-pound man with 15 percent body fat

180 – (180 x 15 percent)
180 x 0.15 = 27
180 – 27 = 153 pounds (lean body mass)

Use the chart below to determine caloric baseline. Again, this is the minimum amount of calories you need to consume per day to maintain your current weight if you do no exercise. You will use your caloric baseline to help figure out how many calories to trim from your diet, taking into consideration your activity level, to lose weight.

DETERMINING CALORIC BASELINE BY YOUR LEAN BODY MASS

Current Body Fat	Daily Calorie Intake
6–12 percent	17 calories per pound of LBM
12.1–15 percent	16 calories per pound of LBM
15.1–19 percent	15 calories per pound of LBM
19.1–22 percent	14 calories per pound of LBM
22.1 percent or above	13 calories per pound of LBM

As the chart above shows, a man with a body fat percentage of 15 would determine his caloric baseline by multiplying 16 calories per pound of lean body mass.

A 180-pound man with 15 percent body fat, as we calculated earlier, has a LBM of 153 pounds. So he would multiply 16 calories by 153 to get a daily caloric baseline of 2,448 calories.

Don't be confused: The figure 2,448 is not the man's daily calorie consumption if he has a desire to either gain or lose weight. Instead it is the base number of calories required to maintain that 180-pound weight. If the man wishes to drop 1 pound of body weight per week, this individual would have to create a daily caloric deficit of 500 calories either through diet, calorie burn through exercise, or some combination of both. Why 500? Because 500 calories x 7 days = 3,500 calories, or 1 pound of body weight. To lose more than 1 pound per week, he will need to create a bigger daily calorie deficit.

Determining Daily Caloric Intake for Your Diet

Remember, a caloric baseline of 2,700 calories is not the number of calories that this mesomorph will eat daily if he wants to lose weight. To lose weight, he will have to create a calorie deficit below his caloric baseline. The easiest way to create a calorie deficit is through a combination of calorie restriction and calorie burning via cardio exercise.

For a dieting bodybuilder the ultimate goal is to lose 1.5 pounds per week. As a general rule, you can expect 80 percent of that weight to come from calorie restriction and 20 percent from exercise—1.2 pounds from dieting; 0.3 pound from cardiovascular workout. (A typical cardio session will burn about 350 calories.) Since cardio is very catabolic, you want to lose most of your weight from dieting to spare the expense of your muscle.

Caloric Intake Equation:

Caloric baseline total – 600 = caloric intake

In order to lose the 1.2 pounds of body fat per week (our 80 percent goal), we would create a caloric deficit of 600 calories. Using our calorie baseline, we would get 2,700 - 600 = 2,100 calories as a starting point for our daily calorie goal. This number would be monitored and adjusted as necessary during the dieting phases. The overall goal during the diet is to increase the quantity of food as the bodybuilder becomes further entrenched in the contest preparation process, but this is where that 180-pound mesomorph needs to start in order to reduce his body-fat percentage.

This may sound like a lot to calculate and to monitor, but it's really not. Once you begin, it will become second nature. Also, remember that you will be tweaking your calorie intake according to how your body feels, looks in the mirror, how your weight moves, and how your energy levels are affected. Your body will change, some weeks in small amounts, and significantly over time; it's your job as bodybuilder to evaluate this every step of the way. Your progress will hinge on your ability to be consistent and honest through the entire process. The next chapter will help you relearn how to eat. It will show you how to build your daily calorie goal using the macronutrients protein, fat, and carbohydrates according to your body type.

PART 2

CHAPTER 5

Relearning How to Eat

Understanding the balance of macro-nutrients and how much of each you need

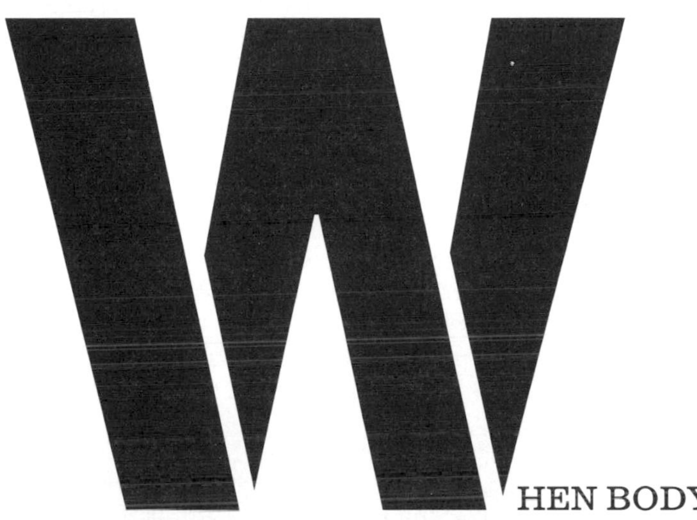

WHEN BODYBUILDERS step onstage, they bring their very best physiques against their competition. This very best starts with their discipline in monitoring everything they consume—from total calories to how many grams of protein, carbohydrates, and fats. If you want to become a champion bodybuilder, you need to be as detail oriented about your food as you are about your exercises and reps. To fuel your training, promote body-fat loss, and grow and maintain muscle, you will need to plan out every meal based on the proper mix of macronutrients. Invest in a food scale and measuring spoons and cups. You'll need them!

The first step in your contest preparation diet is to determine your starting macronutrient amounts. These amounts will not remain exactly the same throughout the entire diet and will be changed to promote greater fat loss and muscle sparing as the dieting process grows.

In order to help you get started I'll outline how to calculate your protein, carbohydrates, and fats based upon your body type, body weight, and overall caloric needs.

Protein

Muscle is primarily protein and water. In order to maintain your muscle mass, adequate dietary protein intake is required. Your rates of muscle protein degradation and synthesis increase in response to the high intensity of resistance training. In order to spare muscle it is vital that a bodybuilder consume the proper amounts of protein. Natural bodybuilders, especially, are more reliant on protein to increase metabolism, promote satiety, muscle growth, lose body fat, maintain nitrogen balance, and promote a natural increase of testosterone in the body.

The "gold standard" for protein intake for a male bodybuilder is around 1 gram per pound of body weight, but that can vary based on your body type as you'll see below. Also, most bodybuilders will need to increase this number slightly while dieting since protein is a key thermogenic macronutrient for sparing muscle tissue when in a caloric deficit.

When starting out, you want to set your protein levels high enough but not excessively high. Protein builds muscle, but protein in excess can be used as energy or converted to body fat. If you ingest too much protein and it is subsequently used as energy, then this means less body fat is being used as energy. The goal during the dieting process it to give your body enough protein to maintain muscle but not enough to hamper body-fat loss.

Protein Ranges Depending on Body Type

Ectomorph: 1.3g/lb–1.6g/lb
Mesomorph: 1.2g/lb–1.5g/lb
Endomorph: 1.4g/lb–1.7g/lb

Sample Subject

Let's take a man with a mesomorph body type and a body weight of 180 pounds whose daily calorie goal is 2,100 calories. To find the optimum grams of protein, multiply body weight by 1.2 grams and 1.5 grams and take the average.

180 x 1.2 = 216
180 x 1.5 = 270

For our sample bodybuilder this gives us a protein range of 216 to 270 grams per day, and so to start he will consume the average 243, which we will round off to 240 grams per day to make things easier. If he is someone who considers himself to be carb sensitive, we could set his protein intake higher, leaving fewer calories dedicated to carbohydrates, once fat intake is determined.

Average = 243 grams per day
(Round this to 240, for the sake of easier tracking.)
Protein = 240 grams per day

Those 240 grams would take up 960 calories of his 2,100-calorie daily goal because there are 4 calories to every 1 gram of protein. The subject is left with 1,140 calories for his remaining fat and carbohydrate intake.

Fat

Dietary fat is still the most misunderstood macronutrient. Some lifters still believe that it's to be avoided, fearing that it will increase body fat. Others believe they can eat as much fat as they want and that eliminating carbs is the key to losing body fat. Both are wrong. Carbs are important and fat is necessary. The trick is to strategically manage intake of both, and to do that it's critical that a bodybuilder understands how his body metabolizes fat.

Any fat intake discussion in the bodybuilding world needs to include the discussion of ketogenic diets, that is, diets in which one consumes super-high amounts of protein and fat while eliminating the carbohydrates. If we eliminate all carbohydrates, then our stored body fat will be released at a rapid rate, but this process can cause problems. You need some carbohydrate; it's the body's preferred fuel source! Not too much; not too little. Your body also uses fat for energy. Your adipose cells release fat in the form of glycerol and fatty acids. The body's cells then metabolize them to use as fuel. Ketogenic dieting phases of dieting can be effective when fat intake isn't too excessive. But it can be a slippery slope as your adipose cells are waiting to bring in new triglycerides to store after your meals, and if your carbohydrate levels are too low for too long, you'll eventually lower your testosterone levels and lose valuable muscle, regardless of how much protein you consume.

Look at reducing fat intake enough to decrease calories and keep testosterone production humming. Is there a optimal number or standard? Not specifically. Generally, a bodybuilder wants to keep his diet low in carbohydrates without increasing fat intake too much. A typical bodybuilder can take in anywhere between 15 to 30 percent of his total calories from fat depending on overall caloric intake and body composition.

As a general guide, here's the percentage of total calories that you should designate to fat intake when starting your dieting process.

Ectomorph: 15–20 percent
Mesomorph: 16–21 percent
Endomorph: 18–23 percent

SAMPLE SUBJECT:
Again, using our 180-pound mesomorph as an example with a 2,100-calorie daily goal, we would multiply 2,100 calories by 16 percent and 21 percent to arrive at an average.

2,100 x .16 = 336 calories from fat
2,100 x .21 = 441 calories from fat

336 + 441 ÷ 2 = 388.5

Since there are 9 calories in every gram of fat, we would divide total calories from fat by 9 to get total grams.

388.5 calories ÷ 9 calories = 43 grams fat per day
(Round this to 45 grams for easier tracking)

Fat: 45 grams (405 calories per day)
Protein: 240 grams (960 calories per day)

Carbohydrates

Figuring out the optimal carbohydrate intake for bodybuilders is about as easy as getting Congress to agree on how to balance the budget. And like a congress member's opinion, your carb needs can change day to day, hour to hour during the dieting process.

As I've said many times before, a major goal of any dieting bodybuilder is to maintain muscle mass while trimming body fat. Retaining muscle is ultra important to your long-term metabolic function and to maintaining strength levels and energy levels. Carbohydrates after all are a very anabolic macronutrient and have been shown to be protein sparing. That's important because dieting and training with weights breaks down tissue and puts you at greater risk of catabolism. Proper management of your carb intake will maximize fat loss by keeping your metabolic rate high and spare your muscle.

Your body burns calories in two ways, through glucose metabolism (using carbs for energy) and ketogenic metabolism (using dietary or stored fat for energy). The balancing act is to keep your fat intake low enough to allow you to eat more carbohydrates and benefit from their muscle-sparing properties.

To start you off in the right direction I've suggested percentages of calories from carbohydrates according to body type:

Ectomorph: 30–45 percent
Mesomorph: 25–40 percent
Endomorph: 20–35 percent

Again, using the example of the mesomorph weighing 180 pounds and consuming 2,100 calories per day, you can determine specific calories from carbs by adding the calories from fat and protein (calculated in those sections above and subtracting from the daily calorie goal):

388 (protein calories)
+ 960 (fat calories) = 1,348 calories

Measuring Your Food

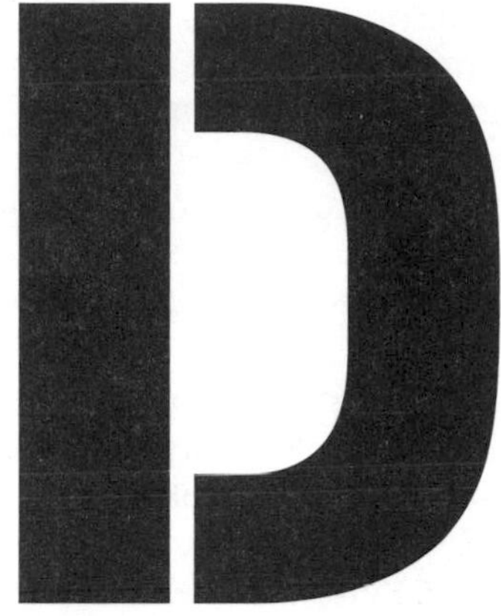

Dramatically reducing your body fat takes some sacrifice. One sacrifice that really pays off is taking the time to consistently measure your food before consuming it.

Measuring your food will allow you to truly understand the quantity you are consuming and allow for necessary tweaks in regard to macronutrients as your diet advances and your physique continues to progress. Once you've determined your required macronutrient consumption, this becomes the staple of your measurements during food preparation. Your ability to consistently track your caloric and macronutrient intake will allow for a smoother transition throughout each phase of the dieting process. So, buy a food scale and measuring spoons and cups and learn how to use them. Also use a journal, Excel spreadsheet, or online tracking application to keep yourself accountable.

2,100 – 1,348 = 752 calories from carbohydrates, or, because there are 4 calories per gram of carbohydrate, 188 grams. (Round this down to 185 for easier tracking.)

Here's the full macronutrient breakdown by grams and calories:
Protein: 240 grams (960 calories from protein per day)
Carbs: 185 grams (740 calories from carbohydrate per day)
Fat: 45 grams (405 calories from fat per day)

These are broad guidelines. Carbohydrate tolerance can differ from one person to the next. I once trained two bodybuilders of roughly the same weight, height, and age, and one dieted on 55 grams of carbs while the other was able to consume 350 grams of carbs and still lose body fat.

High Carbohydrate or Re-Feed Days

As you progress in your dieting, your leptin levels will naturally start to drop as your body attempts to hold on to body fat. Leptin is a hormone that regulates energy and suppresses food intake. When leptin goes down, so does the fat-burning process. An effective way to kick-start fat burn is with "re-feed days," when you switch your diet to high carbohydrate. These carb days raise leptin and boost the fat burn and can be quite anabolic. Incorporate re-feeds into your contest diet every 7 to 10 days for best results. Some pointers for getting the most from your re-feed days:

- Schedule high-carbohydrate days around days off or days on where the extra glucose will be used during workouts focused on large muscle groups like legs or back.
- Keep fat intake as low as possible—5 to 10 grams leaner on these days.
- Reduce protein intake to 1 gram to 1.3 grams per pound of body weight or slightly lower than what you are consuming at that point in your diet. This will help balance out overall calorie intake.
- Consume as little fructose (fruit) as possible. It won't increase your leptin levels.

Carb-Cycling Strategies

During the dieting phase, you might need to use carbohydrate cycling. On different days you will consume high, medium, or low amounts of carbohydrates, which will vary based on your body type. Below are some guidelines.

Ectomorph

Carbohydrate Recommendations for Carb Cycling
High Carb Days: 1.75–2.5 grams of carbs per pound of body weight
Medium Carb Days: 1–1.5 grams of carbs per pound of body weight
Low Carb Days: 0.5–1.25 grams of carbs per pound of body weight

Mesomorph

Carbohydrates Recommendations for Carb Cycling
High Carb Days: 1.25–1.75 grams of carbs per pound of body weight
Medium Carb Days: 0.75–1.25 grams of carbs per pound of body weight
Low Carb Days: 0.5–1 grams of carbs per pound of body weight

Endomorph

Carbohydrate Recommendations for Carb Cycling
High Carb Days: 1–1.5 grams of carbs per pound of body weight
Medium Carb Days: 0.75–1.25 grams of carbs per pound of body weight
Low Carb Days: 0.25–1 grams of carbs per pound of body weight

CARB-CYCLING FORMATS

•3 Days, 1 Day
3 baseline carbohydrate days would be combined with a high carbohydrate day every 4th day.
•6 Days, 1 Day
3 low carb days, followed by 2 medium and 1 high. This is a popular re-feeding format for bodybuilders when starting their contest preparation. It gives the body enough time to access more body fat by limiting carbohydrate intake, but consistently adds the benefits associated with the high-carb day.

I have had great success using the carb cycles above with clients. In some instances I have seen clients' metabolisms increase to where they were consuming upwards of 3 grams of carbohydrates per pound of body weight on a high carb day. It just goes to show how activity and fuel impact metabolic rates.

Planning Your Meals

A failure to plan is a plan to fail. Becoming successful means more than spending time in the gym. It requires organization. You will quickly learn to be more deliberate in your life than you ever have before. Making decisions about food, workouts, and rest on the fly won't work. You need to think and plan. Meal planning and prep are the largest and toughest parts of the dieting process. Consumption is easy.

Meal frequency is an important part of planning. Here's a general guideline for how often you should eat a meal based on your body type.

Ectomorph: every 2–3 hours
Mesomorph: every 2.5–3.5 hours
Endomorph: every 3.5–5 hours

How carefully you stick to this plan will depend on your personal work/life schedule, but no matter how often you eat, you must track those meals carefully.

Start by thinking about the proper balance of your meals. Including protein, carbohydrates, and fat in every meal is crucial for satiety. The three macronutrients work together in helping the bodybuilder deal with feelings of hunger during the time between meals. Having each macronutrient represented in each meal allows your body to absorb them and use them properly and efficiently. As you've learned earlier in this chapter, most meals will be protein dominant with carbohydrates coming in second and fat being the least important per meal.

Aim to include a lean protein, complex carbohydrate, and fibrous carbohydrate in every meal. This combination will allow you to balance your predetermined macronutrient levels throughout the day.

Food Preparation

Every bodybuilder has a formula that works for their weekly food preparation. For some it's daily, for others it's weekly. When I was starting out in bodybuilding, I would prepare a week's worth of meals in a day and be good to go. That isn't the case today. Now I can succeed with just as much precision by preparing 1 to 3 days ahead of time.

Preparation, any way we look at it, is a crucial step to any bodybuilder's success while following a contest preparation diet. Our lives are hectic and if you are going to consume the amount of food required by your diet, food preparation is key.

Preparing your food the night before is probably the easiest because it can be done quickly. Place your meals in containers including everything you need. If the meal consists of a protein, a vegetable, and a starch, make sure it's measured out to your needs and go a step further and label the meal.

Protein powders, fruits, and even raw vegetables can be stored in similar containers or even zipper-lock bags.

I've never met a successful bodybuilder who doesn't bring prepared meals wherever he travels. If you're going to a friend's party or relative's house, bring your own food or you'll end up sabotaging your diet.

Water

Water is essential to fat loss and body function. Figure on targeting your intake to between 1 and 2 gallons per day. As you begin to lose more body fat, you may feel the need to increase your daily intake. Again, it is crucial to track your water consumption to assess your body's performance and weight. Keep your water as clear as possible; the addition of sweeteners like Crystal Light can be used, but in moderation. Coffee and tea can be consumed, but the water content of those beverages does not count towards your water total because the caffeine in them is a diuretic. Not drinking enough water can lead to water retention and affect your weight and your physique.

PART 2

CHAPTER 6

How Macronutrients Work in Your Body

Choose the best sources of protein, carbohydrates, and fats to maximize fat loss and muscle building

EVERYTHING YOU EAT causes metabolic and physiological responses in your body. Each of the three macronutrients—Protein, Carbohydrate, and Fat—plays its role in altering the shape and size of your physique. As a bodybuilder, you will become an expert at eliciting the changes you desire, mainly body fat loss and muscle gain, by manipulating your intake of the macronutrients.

Understanding the basics of how different macronutrients work will allow you to tweak your diet according to your body's needs throughout your physique transformation. Let's take an in-depth look at each macronutrient.

Protein

There has always been debate over the protein requirements of bodybuilders. Muscle contains about 40 percent of the protein in the human body, which has led people to believe that eating dietary protein correlates directly to large muscles.

Yes, dietary protein is crucial in the rebuilding and recovery process, but in and of itself, protein does not build muscle. This misguided belief is particularly common among bodybuilders, who regularly consume an abundance of protein supplements, amino acids, and dietary protein in an attempt to gain an edge.

The truth is that eating protein does not build muscle alone; it is the stimulus of exercise (resistance training) that ultimately starts the muscle-building process. Muscle growth can occur only if muscle protein synthesis exceeds muscle protein breakdown, so there must be a positive muscle protein balance. Strength training improves muscle protein balance, but, in the absence of food, the balance will remain negative, or catabolic.

There are more reasons protein is important for bodybuilders beyond muscle. Protein also helps in the construction and repair of bone, organs, and connective tissues. It helps your muscles contract, and it regulates the balance of water in your tissues and fosters oxygen and energy transportation. Protein produces enzymes that are essential for digestion and it's found in antibodies that resist disease.

The exact protein requirements for bodybuilders can be debated for days on end, with some bodybuilders saying their protein requirements are no higher than those of the general population and others believing that they must eat beef every day in order to grow muscle.

Whole Foods versus Supplemental Protein

When dieting for a competition, you need to take into consideration whole food options versus protein supplementation. Whole food provides a distinct benefit, thanks to the "thermic effect of food," which is the amount of calories (energy) your body expends above your resting metabolic rate simply digesting and processing the food that you eat. In fact, a study from the Department of Nutrition at Arizona State University East found that people who ate a high-protein diet burned twice as many calories as subjects who ate less protein. The extra protein resulted in about an extra 30 calories burned per meal. But it's important to know that compared to a protein supplement like a whey protein drink, whole food protein contributes a far greater increase to your metabolic rate. Whole food protein sources provide slower absorption and a complete micronutrient profile (vitamins and minerals). What's more, whole food protein makes your stomach feel full quicker and longer. Research shows that digestion of whole food protein takes about 2 hours longer than digestion of carbohydrates. This is important for the dieting bodybuilder since slower digestion and absorption will allow the person on a calorie-restricted diet to maintain satiety for a longer period of time. For that reason, whole food protein should form the basis for the majority of your meals. Use protein supplements as they are intended, as supplementation.

Understanding Essential Amino Acids

Growing muscle is the recurring process of damage and repair, more damage and more repair. Essential amino acids are vital in the repairing of tissue and the growth of muscle, so they must be included in your diet.

Your body has the ability to make 12 amino acids, known as non-essential amino acids; however, the nine essential amino acids can only be supplied by the diet. Some of these amino acids are lost each day through activity and must be replaced from sources outside your body. The best way to repair this damage is to maintain an adequate intake of complete protein sources. What are complete protein sources?

A protein is considered complete if it contains an adequate amount of *all* of the essential amino acids needed to build new proteins. But my favorite definition of complete protein sources is . . .

"A complete protein source at some point in their life had a face, a mother, could swim, or could fly."

Aside from providing your body with the muscle-building compounds of essential amino acids, protein aids in satiety and thermogenesis (your body's inner calorie-burning mechanism).

One of the best sources of complete protein is the hen's egg. Eggs have a biological value (BV) of 93.7 on a scale of 100. BV is a scientific measurement of the amount of protein in a food that is able to be digested and used by the body. Eggs are one of the most easily digestible forms of protein and have a BV higher than milk, chicken, beans, or beef. But all complete proteins are the building blocks of muscle.

Complete Protein Sources

TUNA
SALMON
COTTAGE CHEESE
EGGS—MORE PROTEIN IN THE WHITES
CHICKEN BREAST—BONELESS AND SKINLESS
TURKEY BREAST—BONELESS AND SKINLESS
LEAN BEEF —FLANK STEAK, BISON, SIRLOIN, LEAN GROUND BEEF
LOW-FAT PORK
MILK PROTEIN ISOLATE
WHEY PROTEIN
SOY PROTEIN

Keep your diet full of many of these complete protein sources to improve muscle repair following intense strength-training sessions throughout the dieting process.

An incomplete protein source is a protein that lacks or is too low in one or more of the essential amino acids. Incomplete proteins are also called partial proteins. Some examples include:

GRAINS, SEEDS, NUTS, BEANS, CORN, PEAS

You can turn incomplete proteins into complete proteins by combining them in your meals. These complementary protein sources are two or more incomplete proteins that when combined provide adequate amounts of all nine essential amino acids. A meal of rice and beans, for example, provides adequate amounts of essential amino acids because each contains certain amino acids that the other lacks enough of.

Complementary Proteins

NATURAL NUT BUTTERS (ALMOND AND PEANUT BUTTER)
WHOLE RAW NUTS (ALMONDS, CASHEWS, PEANUTS, MACADAMIA NUTS, PISTACHIOS, WALNUTS)
LEGUMES (LENTILS, BEANS)
CHEESES
YOGURT (GREEK YOGURT PROVIDES TWICE THE PROTEIN OF REGULAR YOGURT)

Bottom line: When you want muscle, think meat. A study in the *British Journal of Nutrition,* for example, showed that women who ate a diet rich in chicken and other complete protein sources from meat gained significantly more muscle mass than another group of women that ate only vegetarian sources of protein, such as beans and tofu.

Protein Measurements

	AMOUNT	PROTEIN (G)	CARBS (G)	FAT (G)	TOTAL CALORIES
beef, flank steak	3 oz	22	0	13	205
	4 oz	29	0	17	269
	5 oz	37	0	22	346
	6 oz	44	0	26	410
beef, ground	3 oz	22	0	6	142
	4 oz	23	0	8	164
	5 oz	29	0	10	206
	6 oz	35	0	12	248
beef, top round	3 oz	27	0	4.8	151.2
	4 oz	36	0	6.4	201.6
	5 oz	45	0	8	252
	6 oz	54	0	9.6	302.4
beef. top sirloin	3 oz	16.6	0	12	174.4
	4 oz	22	0	16	232
	5 oz	27.6	0	20.1	291.3
	6 oz	33.1	0	24.1	349.3
chicken	3 oz	21	0	2.3	104.7
	4 oz	28	0	3	139
	5 oz	35	0	3.8	174.2
	6 oz	42	0	4.5	208.5
dairy, cottage cheese (1% fat)	½ c	13	6	1	85
	¾ c	20	9	1.5	129.5
	1 c	26	12	2	170
dairy, milk (fat-free, 0%)	8 oz	8	11	0	76
dairy, milk (low-fat, 2%)	8 oz	8.1	11.4	4.8	121.2
dairy, milk (whole)	8 oz	7.9	11	7.9	146.7
egg, whole (large)	1	6.3	0.4	4.8	70
fish, cod	4 oz	25	0	1	109
	5 oz	33	0	1.3	143.7
	6 oz	39	0	1.5	169.5

	AMOUNT	PROTEIN (G)	CARBS (G)	FAT (G)	TOTAL CALORIES
fish, haddock	4 oz	28	0	1.1	121.9
	5 oz	34	0	1.4	148.6
	6 oz	41	0	1.7	179.3
fish, salmon	3 oz	19	0	11	175
	4 oz	25	0	15	235
	5 oz	31	0	19	295
	6 oz	37	0	26	382
fish, swordfish	3 oz	22	0	4.4	127.6
	4 oz	29	0	5.8	168.2
	5 oz	36	0	7.3	209.7
	6 oz	43	0	8.7	250.3
fish, tuna	3 oz	13.8	0	2.3	75.9
	4 oz	18.5	0	3.1	101.9
	5 oz	23.1	0	3.8	126.6
	6 oz	27.7	0	4.6	152.2
shellfish, scallops	3 oz	19	2.7	1	95.8
shellfish, shrimp	3 oz	18	0	0.9	80.1
	4 oz	24	0	1.2	106.8
	5 oz	30	0	1.5	133.5
	6 oz	36	0	1.8	160.2
turkey, breast	3 oz	25	0	3	127
	4 oz	34	0	4	172
	5 oz	42	0	5	213
	6 oz	51	0	6	258
veggie cheese	1 oz	6	2	3	59
veggie shred	0.5 oz	3	1	1.5	29.5
veggie slice	1	4	0.5	2	36

Protein and Amino Acid Supplements

Beyond whole-food-based protein intake, protein and amino acid supplements are another way to ensure you get enough protein. These nutritional supplements have grown exponentially in popularity in the bodybuilding world over the past decade. They can be helpful in situations where whole-food protein is limited, inaccessible, or undesired. But I want to stress that lean, whole-food options should be preferred over supplements due to the food's slower absorption and more complete micronutrient (vitamins and minerals) profile. Due to the thermic effect and the feeling of satiety it delivers, I've become a fan of a whole food–based post-workout meal.

You will want to find out what works best for your body and your lifestyle. We live our lives on the go, and many people find that they just cannot always find the time in their fast-paced lives to prepare a whole food protein meal. In such situations, a protein supplement or an amino acid supplement can be a big aid in helping to reach a daily protein goal and to get enough of the essential amino acids needed to preserve valuable lean muscle. What's more, a liquid nutritional supplement meal can offer a strategic benefit for weight lifters when used immediately after a workout. It fosters recovery and rebuilding correctly and at a much more effective rate.

There are numerous ways you can consume a protein supplement. I recommend using milk, egg, and rice proteins that have a complete amino acid profile and are "non-GMO" (genetically modified organism), meaning that the protein comes from a naturally occurring source in nature and has not been created through genetic engineering. Look for "non-GMO" on the label of the protein supplements and make sure they do not include bovine growth hormone. The market has recently become flooded with low-grade protein supplements that can do your body more harm than good.

A protein supplement like a whey, rice, or egg protein can be mixed into snacks such as yogurt, oatmeal, or cottage cheese, or used as a baking ingredient to increase the overall protein value in a recipe. A popular use for powdered protein supplements is in smoothie recipes that can be consumed post-workout, as midday snacks, or as meal replacements. Experiment with various combinations of fruit, yogurt, and almond or rice milk to create your own favorite muscle smoothies. Here are some different types of protein supplements.

Whey protein: This is considered a "fast-acting protein" because it breaks down into amino acids and absorbs into your bloodstream within 15 minutes after consumption. A dairy protein, whey consists of 10 percent of the amino acid leucine—other animal-based proteins consist of only 5 percent. Whey protein has long been considered a building block of muscle because of its ability to activate protein synthesis. It has become the number-one choice of bodybuilders for post-workout consumption.

Casein protein: A slower-digesting protein and another dairy protein, casein protein has become a top protein to consume before bed to maintain a positive nitrogen balance and anabolic state during sleep.

Egg protein: Found in whole eggs, egg protein is an excellent source of high-quality protein. Egg protein helps with satiety over longer periods of time and includes a high concentration of leucine.

Another great source of protein supplementation is premade protein and carbohydrate workout drinks. They should contain a mixture of quickly digested and well-tolerated carbohydrates and proteins—in a carbohydrate-to-protein ratio of two to one or three to one. These drinks should be consumed following all high-intensity exercise when increases in muscle strength and size and athletic performance are desired. For fat loss and muscle preservation, try a branched-chain amino acid (BCAA) supplement, which contains the three BCAAs: leucine, isoleucine, and valine. Drink these during and after all high-intensity exercise sessions.

Protein and Nitrogen Balance: Staying Anabolic

Taking in the proper amounts of protein on a consistent basis allows your body to remain in a positive nitrogen balance, which is important for remaining in an anabolic state.

The body's nitrogen balance can be classified in three basic states—positive, negative, and equilibrium. Positive nitrogen balance is your state for muscle growth. A positive nitrogen balance occurs when the total nitrogen excreted is less than the total nitrogen ingested or your nitrogen intake is greater than your nitrogen output. Positive nitrogen balance must exist for new tissue to be synthesized. Recent research has made it clear that athletes and bodybuilders need to consume more protein than the current US recommended daily intake (USRDA) of 0.8 gram per kilogram of bodyweight per day in order to maintain a positive nitrogen balance. The key here is to supply your body with the proper amount of dietary protein throughout the contest preparation diet.

A bodybuilder wants to avoid the state of negative nitrogen balance, which will occur if nitrogen loss is greater than nitrogen intake. A negative nitrogen balance will lead to muscle loss and eventually to a catabolic state. For some bodybuilders on strict caloric diets during periods of dieting an equal nitrogen balance may be maintained. In this state the bodybuilders are not losing muscle, but neither are they in a state to build much muscle.

Achieving a positive nitrogen balance is much easier than most lifters think. By consuming lean protein sources with each and every meal and by using protein supplements strategically, a bodybuilder can maintain this positive nitrogen balance and ultimately remain anabolic throughout the day.

Tips for maintaining a positive nitrogen balance

- Eat protein with every meal, aiming for 25 to 50 grams, depending on your personal macronutrient needs.
- Consume a whole food-based meal or liquid meal containing protein and carbohydrates 60 minutes before a training session.
- Follow your training session with a liquid protein and carbohydrate drink to fill the muscles with amino acids and promote protein synthesis.
- Before going to sleep, consume a liquid drink with a combination of whey and micellar casein (a slow-releasing protein), to avoid a catabolic state overnight.
- Give your muscles adequate rest and recovery time. Training too frequently can use protein stores for fuel during workouts instead of helping to create a positive nitrogen balance.
- Train when your body is fully recovered from your past exercise sessions.
- Train in an anabolic state.
- Keep workouts short and intense. Train for a maximum of 45 minutes and limit workouts to two to three exercises per body part.
- Allow muscle groups enough time to recover before exercising them again.

Protein and Hormones

Insulin is the body's storage hormone. Glucagon is the body's retrieval hormone. Categorized as a catabolic hormone, glucagon promotes the use of glucose for energy. Glucagon is released when we eat protein, much like insulin is released when we consume carbohydrates. When you limit your carbohydrates during the dieting process, your body may not have enough glucose for energy. When that happens glucagon works overtime, helping to mobilize body fat to be used for energy. This is even more reason for a dieting bodybuilder to include protein with each and every meal.

High Protein and Its Effect on Kidneys

A constant question raised regarding protein intake revolves around the safety of higher protein consumption on the kidneys. While high-protein diets may increase loss of kidney function in people with early kidney disease, studies suggest that they won't harm people with normal kidney function.

The amounts of protein a bodybuilder will consume, when properly calculated will not negatively affect his kidneys. During a bodybuilder's dieting process there will be times when protein amounts can be as high as 1.7 grams per pound per day, and sometimes even higher. I can speak for my own dieting history when I say that there have been periods of time when I've consumed as much as 350 to 375 grams per day, and I have had no problems.

While high-protein diets seem to have no negative consequences for healthy individuals, it is wise to inform your doctor about your diet and to be monitored for normal kidney function as part of your annual physical exam.

Carbohydrates

New bodybuilders tend to follow the advice they hear from seasoned veterans:

"Stay away from all carbs during the dieting process." "Never eat fruit because it contains too many carbohydrates." "You can eat as much protein and fat as you like as long as you avoid carbs like the plague."

So what is the truth? The truth is that carbohydrates are great for you. That's right. I'll even go so far as to say they are essential to the bodybuilder. Instead, it is the type and amount of carbohydrates you consume that should be of concern to you, rather than avoiding carbohydrates altogether.

The key with carbohydrates is to always, always, always think "fiber," not "carbohydrates." High-fiber carbohydrates are fantastic for you; they will not only aid in the dieting process to fuel your workouts, but they provide loads of nutrients you can't get from other foods. If you look to high-fiber carbs, you will automatically avoid simple carbohydrates. These are the carbs made up of one or two sugar molecules, which break apart during digestion and are quickly absorbed into the bloodstream through the small intestine. These are the sugars that spike your blood sugar and trigger an influx of insulin. Although sugars are used to fuel your body and brain, any excess that isn't needed is converted to fat for storage.

Some of the more common simple sugars are:

Cortisol: The Muscle-Eating Hormone

When your body is put under stress, whether by an angry dog chasing you during a run or an intense lifting session, it naturally produces a stress hormone called cortisol.

Cortisol is a lifesaver in certain situations, keeping your body from going into shock when traumatized. It also helps energize protein synthesis following exercise. But in high chronic levels, cortisol is catabolic. It breaks down muscle and contributes to increased belly fat. Studies have shown that obese people have significantly higher levels of this hormone than thin people. Unfit people typically have more cortisol than fit people do. More cortisol means less of the anabolic hormones like testosterone and growth hormone.

The body releases cortisol in response to any type of stress, including exercise. Overtraining is a type of body stress that triggers a great amount of cortisol to be released. This is why adequate rest and recovery are so important to the training bodybuilder. To control levels of cortisol, the dieting bodybuilder should (1) consume enough protein, including branched-chain amino acids to enhance recovery and (2) get good sleep, at least 8 hours, and carefully plan workouts to ensure adequate rest to avoid overtraining.

- Raw sugar
- Brown sugar
- Corn syrup
- Fructose
- Dextrose
- High fructose corn syrup
- Glucose
- Honey

The only time simple carbohydrates should be part of your diet when you are preparing for a bodybuilding competition is in your post-workout nutrition. Simple carbohydrates will aid insulin's ability to increase the absorption into the muscles and begin the recovery process.

The primary carbs anyone, especially bodybuilders, should consume are complex carbohydrates commonly found in vegetables, legumes, and whole grains. Complex carbs are better for you because they are high in fiber, vitamins, and minerals.

They are called complex because they have a chemical structure made up of three or more sugars, so they take longer to digest, won't raise blood sugar as quickly, and provide the body with a steady source of fuel. Carbohydrates play a number of roles in the body. Two of the primary functions of carbohydrates are to provide glucose for the brain and energy for working muscles. Carbohydrates are stored in the muscles and liver as glycogen. Glycogen allows individuals to perform exercise for a sustained period of time.

While there are no essential carbohydrates per se (meaning the body can make its own glucose during extreme situations, such as fasting), carbohydrates play a crucial role during your training. Energy levels will decrease if carbohydrate intake is limited or carbohydrate stores in the body are low. As a bodybuilder you will feel periods of low energy, so structuring a majority of your carbohydrate intake around your workout will benefit your performance during training. Some individuals need higher levels of carbohydrates than others, but no bodybuilder should eliminate carbohydrates from their diet entirely.

Avoiding the Ketogenic Diet

Eliminating carbohydrates from your bodybuilding diet while boosting protein and fat would categorize the diet as a ketogenic. If your body is provided with little to no glucose, the brain will not be able to provide the body with energy, and your body will begin to produce ketones. Ketone production is a by-product of fat oxidation and will be used for energy. A ketogenic diet will severely reduce your insulin levels, leading to a high rate of fat loss, but not without catabolizing important lean muscle tissue in the process. Doing so will hurt mental and physical performance and undermine your goal of building muscle.

Carbohydrates to Select Most Often:

- Sweet potatoes
- Oatmeal, oat bran, oat bran cereal
- Brown rice
- Wild rice
- Quinoa
- Whole wheat pasta (minimal)
- Whole wheat tortillas (minimal)
- Wheat bread (minimal)
- Beans
- Fruits (two to three servings per day)
- Maltodextrin (during or after workouts)
- Dextrose (during or after workouts)
- Vegetables

Note: This is not a complete list of all food choices.

Carbohydrates and Hormones

Carbohydrates cause insulin to release, which is muscle sparing, but which also keeps the body from burning fat. It is therefore important that we construct a diet that intermingles long periods of low insulin levels (in order to maximize fat burning) with short periods of high insulin levels (to protect muscle when it is at the greatest risk of catabolism). The periods of low insulin levels can be created by extending the amount of time between meals; the amount of time will depend on your body type.

Your body is at its greatest risk of catabolism during your workout. Intense exercise is in fact highly catabolic. As your body remains in a calorie deficit, the catabolic effect of training will be enhanced. During this process the body will attempt to raise low glucose levels by using amino acids from your muscle and converting them to glucose. In effect, your body is feeding upon itself. As a bodybuilder in training, you can combat this and spare your muscles by consuming a whole-food meal or a protein–carbohydrate blend liquid meal replacement 60 minutes before training.

Carbohydrates and Leptin

Leptin is a hormone produced mostly by the fat cells and is a regulatory hormone for our hunger and satiety. Understanding leptin's role in your body will allow you to understand the importance of "re-feed" days, or high carbohydrate days.

Leptin is the hormone that signals to your brain that you've had enough to eat. Unlike insulin, leptin does not increase when we consume one single meal, like insulin, instead leptin rises by increasing our overall carbohydrate and caloric intake over a period of time, usually 12 to 24 hours.

Leptin also helps signal your body to begin burning body fat and increase energy expenditure. The lesson here is to work in your higher carbohydrate days every 7 to 10 days or as needed during a carbohydrate cycling period of dieting.

Fruits and Vegetables

Remember, too, that fruits and vegetables are carbohydrates; make sure each of these categories is covered on a daily basis because they are rich in nutrients a bodybuilder needs.

That's right, you can and should eat fruit. It won't make you fat. Surprised? For as long as I can remember bodybuilders have been afraid to eat fruit. Most bodybuilders, when they start their contest prep diet, eliminate all fruit. In my early years in bodybuilding, I did just that. I avoided fruit, and for no other reason than because fructose was said to stall fat loss. What the studies on fructose really pointed toward was avoiding high-fructose corn syrup, not whole fruit. Fructose restores the liver glycogen, and depending on what study you look at, your liver can only store about 50 grams of fructose. If we talk about whole fruit, fruit and fructose aren't exactly the same thing. Many people and bodybuilders for that matter believe that all the sugars in fruit are fructose. The typical piece of fruit contains about 6 to 7 grams of fructose. Berries, on the other hand, are very high in fiber and contain only 2 to 3 grams of fructose. You'd have to eat a large banana to consume close to 10 grams of fructose in one piece of fruit. So a dieting bodybuilder or anyone who is in a caloric deficit would be hard pressed to consume close to that amount and cause any fat storage.

Fruit is high in vital nutrients, fiber, and water content. The high fiber and high water content is a great combination to help reduce hunger and make the dieting bodybuilder feel full. Fruit is vital and its nutritional value is too high to eliminate it in a contest prep diet. Timing fruit consumption around pre- and post-workout snacks is a good strategy because that's when your body can use the extra sugars.

Cruciferous vegetables, such as broccoli, kale, Brussels sprouts, cauliflower, and cabbage, contain cancer-fighting compounds called indoles and glucosinolates. Tomatoes are high in lycopene, which may help prevent prostate cancer and breast cancer. Dark, leafy green vegetables have a pigment called carotenoids that enhances the body's immune response. The pigment protects skin cells against dangerous ultraviolet rays. These foods are rich in vitamin A and antioxidants. Their anti-inflammatory powers also help block pain.

A good strategy when it comes to eating fruits and vegetables is to choose a rainbow of colors for your diet each week to ensure that you consume a broad range of vitamins and other nutrients. (See "Eat the Rainbow.")

EAT THE RAINBOW

Color	Fruits and vegetables	Some of the benefits
Blue and Purple	Blackberries, blueberries, eggplant, figs, grapes, plums, purple cabbage, raisins	High in vitamin C and other antioxidants, calcium, and fiber. May reduce risk of heart disease and stroke and some cancers.
Green	Artichokes, asparagus, avocados, broccoli, celery, cucumbers, kiwi, green apples, green beans, green cabbage, green grapes, lettuce, limes, okra, peas, spinach	High in iron; fiber; calcium; magnesium; vitamins C, E, K; and many of the B vitamins. Green foods help eyesight, digestion, and boost the immune system.
Yellow and Orange	Apricots, cantaloupes, carrots, corn, lemons, mangoes, nectarines, oranges, papayas, peaches, pineapple, pumpkin, sweet potatoes, yellow peppers	High in vitamin C and beta-carotene. They help keep your heart healthy, are good for eyesight, and build healthy bones.
Red	Beets, cherries, cranberries, radishes, raspberries, red apples, red peppers, rhubarb, tomatoes, watermelon	High in antioxidants and fiber, red foods help fight cancers, lower blood pressure, lower cholesterol, and keep your heart healthy. Lycopene in tomatoes and watermelon has been linked to lower prostate cancer and greater heart health.
White	Bananas, cauliflower, garlic, ginger, mushrooms, onions, parsnips, potatoes, turnips	These foods help strengthen and improve the immune system, balance hormones, and may reduce cancer risk.

Fat

In the early 1990s, dietary fat received the same bad rap that carbohydrates are now receiving. It was thought that fat would be detrimental to performance, health, and cause weight gain when eaten in excess. Fats were said to cause heart disease and strokes. Dietary fat was demonized in the press, and it spawned an entire industry devoted to creating nonfat and low-fat food products. But without fats, foods don't taste good, so manufacturers added more simple sugars, especially the sweetener high-fructose corn syrup.

Today, the tide is turning: Scientific research now suggests that it is not dietary fat and cholesterol that cause heart disease, diabetes, and other metabolic diseases but too many carbohydrates. Scientists are realizing that fats play a crucial role in the body's performance and health. The key is to focus on the quality of the fat—maybe even more so than the quantity. Aside from protein, fat is the only other essential macronutrient; dietary fat provides essential fatty acids (like essential amino acids) that cannot be produced by the body and must be consumed.

The dietary fat theory continues to be discussed in dieting circles and among bodybuilders. Low-fat diets, balanced diets, and high-fat diets have all made their way into the mainstream and have been used by bodybuilders to achieve low body-fat percentages for game day. After a bodybuilder has taken the initial step to bring his caloric intake low enough to

Fruit Measurements

FOOD	AMOUNT	PROTEIN (G)	CARBS (G)	FAT (G)	TOTAL CALORIES
apple	1 medium	0	21	1	93
banana	1 medium	2	40	1	177
blueberries	½ cup	0	12	0	48
cantaloupe	1 cup	2	13	0	60
grapes	10 medium	0	9	0	36
honeydew	1 cup	0	13	0	52
kiwifruit	1 medium	1	11	0	48
mandarin oranges	½ cup	0	13	0	52
papaya	½ cup	0	7	0	28
pineapple	½ cup	0	17	0	68
raisins	1 oz	1	23	0	96
raspberries	½ cup	0	7	0	28
strawberries	½ cup	1	5	0	24

support the best rate of fat loss, he can then determine what best fits his needs for dietary fat intake.

For an aspiring bodybuilder it is important to understand how the body metabolizes body fat and dietary fat. The body is constantly storing triglycerides in adipose, or fat, cells and then releasing them as it needs energy between meals. Since your body will easily store excess carbs as body fat and lead to that lethargic feeling, it is crucial to keep carb levels low enough to not meet all your body's energy requirements but high enough to access adequate body fat. Therefore monitoring dietary fat intake is also crucial as it too can be stored as body fat if you allow overall caloric intake to fall lower than what your metabolic rate requires.

Lowering dietary fat levels below 15 to 20 percent of your total caloric intake can cause a drop in testosterone production. There can be periods of time during later stages of dieting when, in order to access the last few pounds of body fat, dropping dietary fat below 15 percent may be required, but for the bulk of your diet program, you should eat enough fat.

For a dieting bodybuilder, the goal is to have less fat available for storage after your meals and to have a smaller amount of stored fat for use between your meals for energy. This can be achieved by implementing periods of time when your fat intake is limited to 10 to 15 percent of your total calories. It is also key to manage your carbohydrate intake when planning meal strategies.

Vegetable Measurements

FOOD	AMOUNT	PROTEIN (G)	CARBS (G)	FAT (G)	TOTAL CALORIES
asparagus	10 spears	5	7	1	57
broccoli	1 cup	5	9	0	56
cabbage, raw	1 cup	1	4	0	20
carrots	1 cup	1	11	0	48
cauliflower	1 cup	2	5	0	28
cucumber	¼ cup	1	2	0	12
green beans	1 cup	2	10	0	48
pea pods	½ cup	2	5	0	28
romaine lettuce	1 cup	0.6	1.5	0.1	9.3
spinach	1 cup	0.9	1.1	0	8
summer squash	1 cup	2	8	1	49
tomatoes	½ cup	1	3	0	16
zucchini	1 cup	1	4	0	20

Types of Fats

All fatty acids have the same basic structure; they are a chain of carbon atoms with varying amounts of hydrogen atoms attached to each carbon. One simple way of describing the various types of fats is to think of the structure of fats as a school bus; the bus itself is the carbon atom chain and all the seats are the hydrogen atoms. Here are the main types of fats:

1. Saturated fat (SFA): All the carbon atoms are full of hydrogen atoms, making the "seats on the bus" full. No other atoms can fit onto the structure because there are no "empty seats." Saturated fats are easy to identify because they are solid at room temperature (butter, shortening, animal fats, etc.).
2. Monounsaturated fat (MUFA): By mono, we mean there is one "empty seat" on the bus and the rest are full. There is room to fit more hydrogen because of the one "empty seat." Monounsaturated fats are liquid at room temperature (vegetable oils, olive oil, canola oil, etc.).
3. Polyunsaturated fat (PUFA): As poly, meaning "many," suggests, several of the "seats" on the bus are empty. Polyunsaturated fats are also liquid at room temperature (flax oil, fish oil, etc.).
4. Trans fats: Trans fats are basically vegetable fats that have been changed chemically by a process known as hydrogenation. Remember the unsaturated fats from above had empty "seats" without a hydrogen atom. The process of hydrogenation or partial hydrogenation is when food manufacturers artificially add hydrogen to liquid unsaturated fats to provide greater stability and, ultimately, longer shelf life. Hydrogenation makes liquid fats solid at room temperature. Trans fats should be avoided as much as possible because they raise levels of low-density lipoprotein (LDL), the so-called "bad" cholesterol, and lower levels of high-density lipoprotein (HDL), the good stuff. Trans fats have been connected to increased risk of heart disease and type 2 diabetes. There is no need for trans fats in the diet. Foods such as hard margarines, shortenings, and most commercially fried foods and bakery items usually contain trans fats.

Essential Fatty Acids

These fats are called essential because they cannot be synthesized in the body and they must be consumed from dietary sources. Omega-3 and omega-6 fatty acids are crucial to normal function of all tissues in the body, and adequate amounts offer many health benefits, including reducing heart disease, depression, dry skin, and joint pain.

The three omega-3 acids are alpha-linoleic acid (ALA), eicosapentaenoic acid (EPA), and docosahexaenoic acid (DHA).

ALA is found in the plant sources of omega-3s such as flaxseeds and nuts, while DHA and EPA are both found in highest concentrations in such cold-water fish as salmon, mackerel, lake trout, tuna (both fresh and canned), anchovies, and sardines. ALA can convert to the more useful EPA and DHA, but the conversion rate is low (5 to 15 percent).

The major omega-6 fatty acid is known as linoleic acid and is found primarily in vegetable oils such as canola and corn oils. Although these are essential fatty acids, the typical American diet is already very high in omega-6 fats; it is recommended instead to boost the intake of omega-3s. The goal with essential fatty acids is to shoot for a few grams each day. In addition to making sure to include fish in the diet, omega-3 supplements are recommended for optimal health.

Good Fat Measurements

	AMOUNT	PROTEIN (G)	CARBS (G)	FAT (G)	TOTAL CALORIES
avocado	¼ large	1	4.3	7.4	87.8
	½ large	2	8.6	14.7	174.7
	¾ large	3	12.9	22.1	262.5
	1 large	7	17.1	29.5	361.9
cheese (Cheddar)	½ oz	3.5	0.5	4.5	56.5
	1 oz	7	1	9	113
cheese (mozzarella)	½ oz	3.2	0	3	39.8
	1 oz	6.3	0	6	79.2
cheese (Parmesan)	½ oz	5.1	0.5	3.7	55.7
	1 oz	10.1	0.9	7.3	109.7
cheese (pepper jack)	½ oz	3.5	0.5	4.5	56.5
	1 oz	7	1	9	113
cheese (Swiss)	½ oz	4	0	4.5	56.5
	1 oz	8	0	9	113
extra-virgin olive oil	½ tbsp	0	0	7	63
	1 tbsp	0	0	14	126
flaxseed oil	½ tbsp	0	0	5.5	49.5
	1 tbsp	0	0	11	99
fish oil	1 g	0	0	1	9
	2 g	0	0	2	18
	3 g	0	0	3	27
	4 g	0	0	4	36
	5 g	0	0	5	45
	6 g	0	0	6	54

(continued)

Good Fat Measurements (cont.)

FOOD	AMOUNT	PROTEIN (G)	CARBS (G)	FAT (G)	TOTAL CALORIES
natural almond butter	8 g	1.2	1.7	4.8	54.8
	16 g	2.4	3.4	9.5	108.7
	32 g	4.8	6.8	19	217.4
natural cashew butter	8 g	1	2.2	3.8	47
	16 g	2	4.5	7.5	93.5
	32 g	4	9	15	187
natural peanut butter	8 g	2	2	4	52
	16 g	4	3	8	100
	32 g	8	6	16	200
nuts (almonds)	½ oz	3	3	7.5	91.5
	1 oz	6	6	15	183
nuts (brazil nuts)	1/2 oz	2	1.5	9.5	99.5
	1 oz	4	3	19	199
nuts (peanuts)	½ oz	3.35	3.05	7	88.6
	1 oz	6.7	6.1	14.1	178.1
nuts (pecans)	½ oz	1.3	1.9	10.5	107.3
	1 oz	2.7	3.8	21	215
nuts (walnuts)	½ oz	2	2	9	97
	1 oz	4	4	18	194

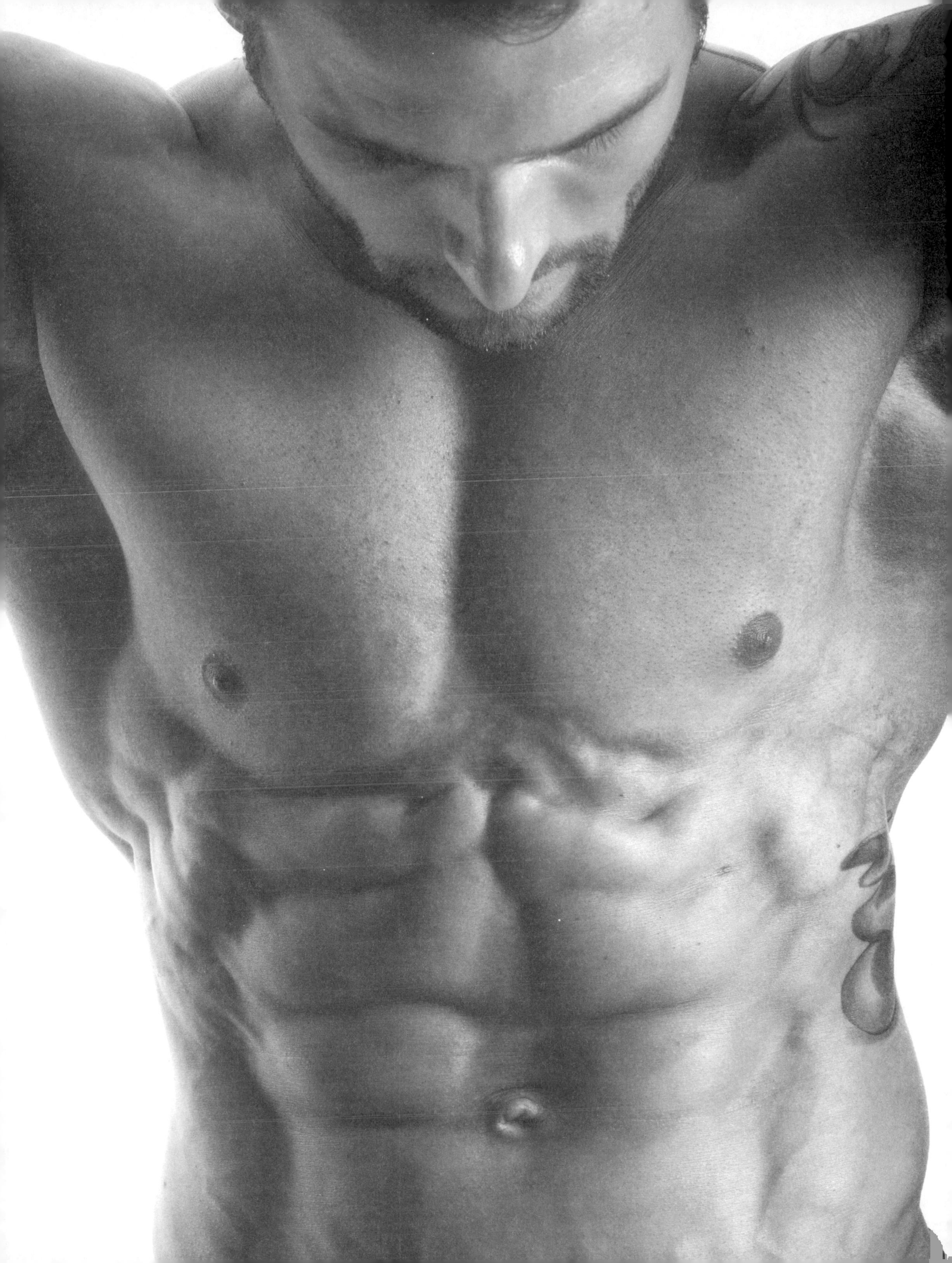

PART 2

CHAPTER 7

Nutrient Timing and the Phases of Dieting

Eat strategically for better, faster results

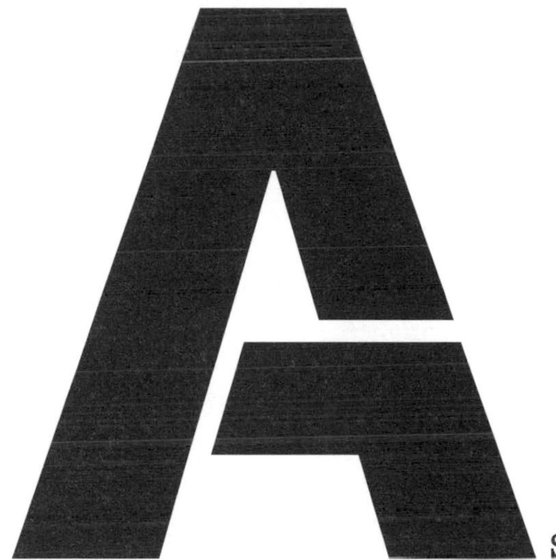

S BODYBUILDERS we have to pay close attention to the food we consume and, more important, when we consume it. By scheduling our meals around our strength training, cardio workouts, and recovery, we can maximize the fat-loss process and stimulate new muscle growth.

Our bodies naturally produce both anabolic and catabolic hormones that can either work with us or against us in the dieting process. Anabolic hormones stimulate rebuilding and repair reactions in your muscles. Catabolic hormones stimulate the breakdown of carbohydrate, fat, and protein for energy.

Through the proper nutrient timing we can allow our bodies to utilize more naturally occurring anabolic hormones and avoid the breakdown of tissue and, more specifically, muscle associated with catabolic hormones.

Meal Timing

Bodybuilders of the past ate three or four meals a day, never the five or six that are common today. But we now know much more about nutrition than those early musclemen did.

As a bodybuilder training for competition, you will become keenly attuned to how your body feels and when you need to eat. You will learn how to plan your meals around your work and your workouts and when to fit in the all-important meal preparation. Much of this will come through trial and error. Your routine will become easier and more finely honed with each competition you train for.

Many bodybuilders find that the biggest lifestyle change to get used to is meal preparation. Shopping for the right ingredients, planning the ideal macronutrient mix, preparing and cooking the meals, measuring and weighing out the portions, and packing meals can be very time-consuming and a lot more involved than what you are used to. But it is one of the big keys to your success.

Once your preparation is complete the next steps are to plan out the times of your food consumption based upon your body type and meal-spacing needs.

Pre-Workout Nutrition

The most important meals in a bodybuilder's day revolve around his training sessions, with the meal before the workout being crucial.

Many bodybuilders underestimate the importance of timing a pre-workout meal properly and making sure it contains adequate carbohydrates. Properly timed, your carbohydrate intake will allow an increase in muscle glycogen levels to improve your performance and decrease muscular fatigue. It will provide your body fuel for the anaerobic pathway and allow your body to spare muscle from being converted to glucose for fuel. This pre-workout meal balanced with carbohydrates should be eaten no fewer than 90 minutes and no more than 2 hours before a training session.

Post-Workout Nutrition

Your post-workout refueling is critical, too. You should consume carbohydrates in liquid form to speed the sugar delivery into your bloodstream and to your muscles. Make sure you drink it within 30 minutes of finishing your workout.

A post-workout shake containing a simple carbohydrate like dextrose will resupply muscle glycogen that has been depleted during training and spare muscle tissue by absorbing into the bloodstream at a much faster rate than a low-glycemic carb would. A high-glycemic carb will cause a very large insulin spike. As the insulin ushers the glucose into muscle tissue, you can experience a hypoglycemic (low-blood sugar) feeling.

To combat this feeling, follow your post-workout shake with a post-workout meal within another hour. This meal should include some low-glycemic complex carbohydrates that will counteract this negative effect by helping stabilize your blood sugar levels. The complex carbohydrates will also encourage protein synthesis, retard the release of catabolic hormones, and spare muscle tissue.

Raise Your Anabolic Hormones

No, I have not gone performance enhancing on you. Instead I'm talking about boosting the naturally occurring anabolic hormones in your body that stimulate rebuilding and repair reactions in your muscles. Your body also produces catabolic hormones that stimulate the breakdown of carbohydrate, fat, and protein for energy. We as bodybuilders often associate the word *catabolic* with bad news for muscle building, though these catabolic hormones can also work with us in our pursuit of a perfect physique for competition day.

Our anabolic hormones include testosterone, growth hormone, IGF-1, and insulin. Through diet and exercise we can release these anabolic hormones to spur on muscle growth and make the dieting process easier. Let's take a look at these helpful hormones.

Spark Protein Synthesis with Insulin

Insulin might very well be the most misunderstood hormone among men due to its association with carbohydrates and type 2 diabetes. When insulin levels are high and there are also high levels of carbohydrate intake, studies have shown a resulting increase in fat synthesis and a decrease in fat breakdown. But even with its association with fat synthesis, insulin is highly effective in promoting carbohydrate fuel storage and muscle–protein synthesis.

Your muscle cells are especially insulin sensitive right after exercise. This is important because the more insulin sensitive your muscle cells, the more insulin will act to promote muscle glycogen storage and protein synthesis, exactly what we want occurring after an intense training session. Making glucose and amino acids available at this time is important to allowing insulin to work with your body to synthesize muscle proteins and muscle glycogen at a high rate. At the same time very little fat will be synthesized or stored away.

You can take advantage of insulin, through timed carbohydrate consumption following strength training. Studies have shown that insulin not only increases protein synthesis but increases amino acid uptake into your muscle and reduces protein degradation.

Insulin can be classified as the most anabolic hormone and the most important hormone in relation to muscle growth. Insulin may not be friendly to sedentary individuals or to those on an unbalanced high-carbohydrate diet, but to a bodybuilder who trains and diets intelligently, insulin can lead to muscle and strength gains and very low body-fat percentages.

Insulin's Benefits to a Bodybuilder:

- Increases protein synthesis
- Increases glucose transport into the muscle
- Increases amino acid transport into the muscle
- Increases blood flow into the muscle
- Increases muscle glycogen storage
- Suppresses the release of cortisol
- Reduces protein degradation

Tap Your Natural Testosterone

Testosterone is a bodybuilder's natural ally. In bodybuilding we associate the main male hormone with the term *anabolic* or building up. Testosterone has a number of effects that can classify it as anabolic, the major effect for a bodybuilder is its ability to accelerate the growth of muscle. Testosterone is believed to be anticatabolic because it can block cortisol (the stress hormone associated with belly fat). It's because of this characteristic that increased testosterone in the body leads to an increase in muscle recovery. This alone is a major reason why drug-using bodybuilders use anabolic steroids to help them train harder, recover faster, and ultimately grow muscle faster. These effects can be short-lived because as cortisol release is blocked, even higher levels of cortisol are produced shortly thereafter. So when a drug-using bodybuilder stops taking an anabolic steroid, the catabolic effects of cortisol increase lead to a rapid loss of muscle strength and size.

Natural testosterone production can be increased through proper protein intake, intense strength training, adequate rest and recovery, and increased consumption of cruciferous vegetables such as broccoli and cauliflower.

Build Muscle with Your Body's Growth Hormone

The role of growth hormone in the sports world is highly controversial. Athletes have been using synthetic growth hormone to get ahead for years. But to natural bodybuilders, that's cheating big-time. They know that they can naturally trigger their bodies to secrete more growth hormone through strength training.

Growth hormone stimulates muscle growth, increases the breakdown of fat, and inhibits carbohydrate metabolism. To a male, growth hormone is the body's natural liposuction. Growth hormone's role in exercise is not well understood, but we do know that it rises during exercise and drops following exercise. Because it rises during exercise, growth hormone can play a role in maintaining muscle throughout the dieting process.

Squeeze out More IGF-1

IGF-1 stands for insulin-like growth factor, and its primary effect is to stimulate protein synthesis in bone, cartilage, and muscle. IGF is responsible for the muscle growth that occurs during puberty. It boosts amino acid and glucose transport into cells. It also makes muscles more sensitive to insulin's effects and increases the number of muscle cells in your tissue, which can grow larger and stronger through weight lifting. IGF-1 is controlled by the intensity of muscle contraction, leading to an increase during exercise and a decrease afterward.

The Phases of Dieting

Getting lean for a bodybuilding competition can seem overwhelming. But there's an effective way to approach the task: Break it up into manageable chunks, as I did when I wrote this book. If I look at the book as a collection of parts rather than a complete volume, and then I attack the writing one chapter at a time, it seems much less intimidating. The same goes for contest preparation dieting. If you build a step-by-step plan, a course of action that is well defined and manageable and achievable, hell, you can do anything. And dropping body fat while sparing muscle will be a goal for which you can see a clear path.

I learned this valuable lesson from my mentor in contest preparation coaching, Joe Klemczewski, PhD, a World Natural Bodybuilding Federation (WNBF) professional bodybuilder and nutritionist. Dr. Joe specializes in intensive nutritional consulting and works with the highest-level professional bodybuilders, models, and members of the general public through his nutritional program and Web site TheDietDoc.com. Before Dr. Klemczewski organized the contest prep dieting process into well-defined phases, bodybuilders had no clear structure to contest prep nutrition or understanding of the changes in body and diet that bodybuilders endure as they train.

Dr. Klemczewski's "phases of dieting" have made the contest preparation journey of many bodybuilders, including myself, much easier to follow by providing an understanding of the physical changes the body endures—including the way the metabolism changes—and the need to be patient as the process moves along.

TRANSITIONING PHASE (2 TO 4 WEEKS)

This is your starting point in the journey. You are beginning to transition from an off-season diet surplus of calories and carbohydrates to dieting mode when you have to get serious about caloric and carbohydrate restriction. Although dieting to lose body fat can be fairly easy, dieting to lose body fat while retaining your muscle can be a challenge. Begin by creating a good diet plan based on what you learned in the previous chapters. Map out your macronutrient intake for every day in a solid meal plan. If you try to eat right on the fly, that is, without a plan, you will without a doubt fall into a pattern of eating the wrong foods at the wrong times. Planning is one of the key tools in breaking down this monumental task of contest prep into achievable pieces.

Thanks to your preseason indulgences, your metabolism is jacked up and ready to start your total body transformation. Your time spent with a surplus of calories and carbohydrates has you primed to lose body fat fast. During the first 2 weeks of training, glycogen and water will constitute a good amount of weight lost and you will continue to lose at a better-than-average rate. Do not be alarmed if you are one of those people who needs to drop your caloric deficit lower than initially projected in order to lose the weight you are targeting.

CORE PHASE (8 TO 12 WEEKS)

The core phase is the longest period of dieting and when the real work begins. The program is taken to a new level. Weight training is ramped up, and your cardio program increases, too. You may need to work in different types of carbohydrate cycling to keep your body losing 1 to 2 pounds of body fat per week. During the core phase a bodybuilder may notice the greatest amount of fat loss, but it feels like the slowest, most drawn-out process of his life. How long it lasts really depends on the length of your dieting, how much your metabolic rate slows, and your energy levels before entering the grind of the set point phase.

SET POINT PHASE

During the set point phase, your body begins to resist you. At this time your body is approaching a level of body fat where cells have lost enough volume so that you body feels as if it's starving. You're really not starving at all; instead, your body has become more efficient. It is smaller now, lacking all that fat, and therefore it doesn't need as many calories as it once did. It is during this phase that many competitors become frustrated with their bodies. The once noticeable and consistent scale change has ground to a halt, and it's time to once again change things up. During this phase, the diet must become tighter. You will likely need to further reduce the amount of food you eat, lower carbohydrate intake even more, and increase your cardio. You will begin to recognize an overall hardening of your physique.

Often enough, many bodybuilders will stay within the set point phase right up to the show, whether they find their physique ready or needing more time. When a bodybuilder reaches the level of conditioning that's contest ready, with time remaining in the dieting process, they can enter a step neglected by bodybuilders for years—the metabolic building phase.

You'll be able to increase the level of food consumption, and your body will react not by gaining weight but by losing it, while hunger increases. This is when you enter the metabolic building phase.

METABOLIC BUILDING PHASE

During the metabolic building phase you'll begin to increase your food quantity by small amounts—10 grams of protein here, 10 grams of carbohydrates there. This will boost your metabolic rate, which is exactly what you want to happen during this last phase of the dieting process. As food begins to be added, you'll notice changes in your body. You will notice changes in your body temperature as it will become warmer more often, and you'll keep losing body fat and seeing the weight loss on the scale.

As you keep losing weight, you'll continue to eat more food (usually an increase in carbs) to balance the increases in your metabolic rate. In turn your body will become less catabolic and far less carb sensitive.

The small increases in food will not only result in higher energy levels, strength increases, muscle fullness, and slight increases in body weight, but body-fat levels will also continue to decrease. The metabolic building phase can continue into your off-season as you return your intake back to maintenance levels of consumption.

FINE-TUNING PHASE

At this point you've been dieting longer and have given your body plenty of time to build your food intake. This allows your skin to become thinner and has your body ready for a show.

Since muscle is roughly 70 percent water, being well hydrated during peak week is critical for show preparation. If you're dehydrated, your muscles will look smaller and your skin may look saggy. Drinking lots of water will fill your muscles up like air in a balloon, making them fuller and harder. What's more, full, well-hydrated muscle tissue results in better definition by increasing the separation between muscles.

Don't make the mistake of many bodybuilders who still adhere to the old strategy of carb depletion during peak week. What did we learn in the previous chapters? It is crucial that you eat carbohydrates after your training sessions. So, why would you stop doing this during the week before competition? It's crazy. Your body needs the glycogen, otherwise catabolism sets in, exactly what you don't want to happen. A better strategy is to take in higher amounts of carbs during the beginning of peak week training and gradually reduce carb intake as contest day nears.

What about protein and fat? I typically keep my protein intake constant to maintain lean body mass. It's the fat I'll reduce, keeping it low so the carbs can do the heavy lifting. Of course, as I've said numerous times, every bodybuilder is different. You need to know your body and how it metabolizes these macronutrients so you can tweak your intake appropriately for best results on "game day."

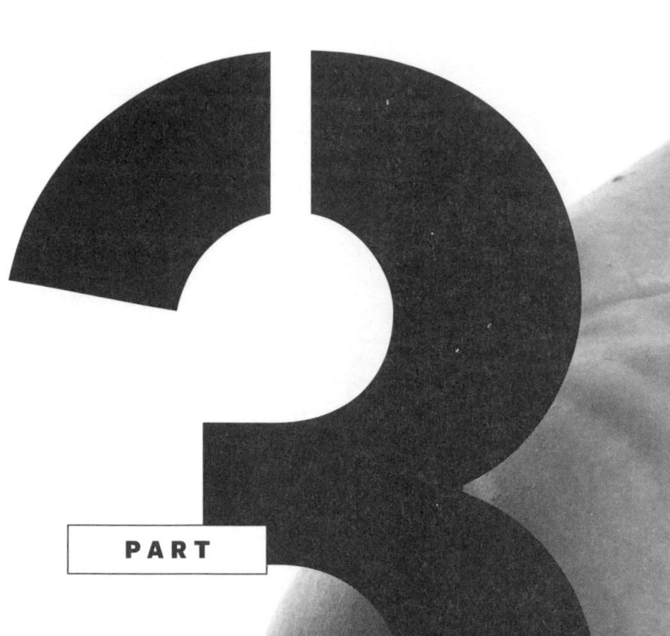

PART 3

The Bodybuilder's Workout

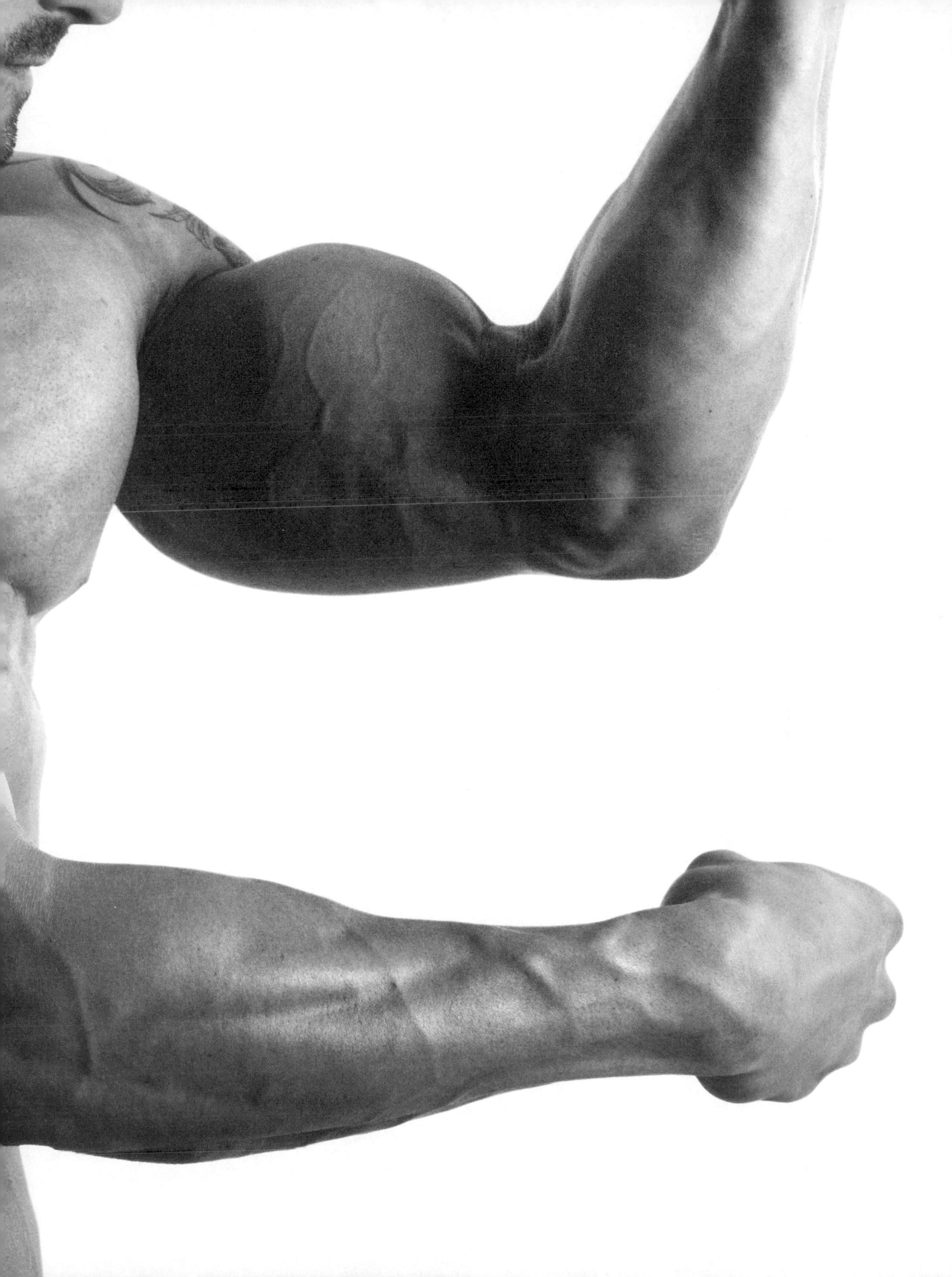

PART 3

CHAPTER 8

Growing and Sculpting Muscle

Using the tools of the trade to create a new physique

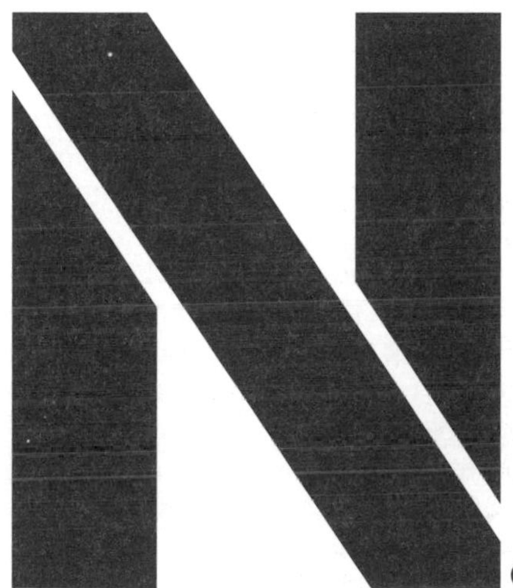

O TWO BODYBUILDERS' physiques are exactly the same, but even two people with completely different bodies can use the same exact workout and achieve what they've individually set out to accomplish. That's the nature and the beauty of weight training.

Of course, these two very different bodybuilders probably need to diet differently: One may be an ectomorph consuming 350 grams of carbs a day while his training partner, an endomorph, may only be consuming 175 grams of carbs per day. The amount of cardio they need will differ, too. But in the weight room, the same program will help them achieve what every lifter wants: muscularity and strength.

Bodybuilders have long been strength athletes. The bodybuilding workout program on the following pages and the 24-week program in the next chapter are grounded in that tradition.

And that's what makes them so useful and effective, even if you have no intention of competing in a bodybuilding event. I don't know many guys who step into the gym and don't want to get stronger. These workouts will do that for you.

In Chapter 9, I've outlined a specific full 24-week weight training program that I've followed successfully and recommended to the people I've trained. It's a terrific program to follow. But it's not the only one with merit. There are many paths you can take to reach the same destination, each with advantages and disadvantages that you should consider as you search for the best plan for you.

How many times you train during the week and which exercises you do on one day versus another are important decisions to make but your choice won't make or break the end result. What's more important is that whatever program you use, it allows you to progress at a strategic pace by increasing intensity, volume and density throughout the weeks of the plan.

Starting on page 82, you'll find sample splits for 3-, 4-, 5-, and 6-day-per-week training sessions—with advantages and disadvantages listed for each. This demonstrates the great potential for flexibility in personalizing a training program to your individual needs.

As I mentioned, no two bodybuilders are alike. One might be in better shape than the other and require less time to prepare for competition. Another may not have the luxury of 6 months to prepare for an upcoming competition. This lifter will need to alter his starting point and endpoint in the workout. Still another bodybuilder may have only enough free time to work out 3 days a week, while another may want to train 5 days a week. For these reasons, I designed bodybuilding workouts for three different training splits: 3, 4, and 5 days. All are built into the 24-week program of 4-week cycles, which will be detailed in the next chapter.

How Often Should a Bodybuilder Train?

If I had a container of whey protein for every time I heard that question, I could open a supplement store.

"What is the best training split to use?" It's the most popular question in bodybuilding. I often laugh when I hear this, because any training schedule can work if you are committed and you work hard. It truly comes down to one thing: Finding the one that works best for you.

If you want to know how many work days per week to build into your training program, ask yourself: "How many days do I have available to train?"

The fact is different training programs benefit different people. And there isn't one single best program. Any of them can work the best for you if it fits into your schedule and you follow it consistently. Besides, the training program you choose isn't all that important. It's not going to make or break your effort.

Some people may be surprised to hear this, but the bodybuilder's journey begins with his contest preparation diet. That's the most important part of the whole process and why I devoted a large chunk of the beginning of this book to nutrition. Training falls a distant second place to strategic dieting. This fact is probably why there is a big difference between those who call themselves bodybuilders, yet never will compete, and those who are bodybuilders.

My strong advice to you is this: Put your greatest effort into following the nutrition program to a T. Then, for your workout, examine your life and figure out which of the training splits best fits with your schedule.

In the 24-week training splits that I will outline for you on the following pages I've described three weekly training splits to accommodate different lifestyles and schedules. Each uses a traditional bodybuilding format and traditional training methods. I've used all three different splits and even a 6-day schedule with success. Find the program that works for you and put all your intensity and effort into every workout.

Building Materials

Equipment needed for an effective bodybuilding program

I'm a firm believer in training with equipment that allows you to utilize your body more efficiently. This pretty much eliminates most exercise machines. The only exercise machine we have in my gym is a chest-supported row. Machines limit the lifter's range of motion. Your muscles don't work like a robot's limbs in real life and they shouldn't in the gym. Free weights are best, but there are other tools of the trade that can help you achieve the body you're looking for. Here's my list of essential gear.

Dumbbells—preferably a set of 20-pound to 100-pound weights
The dumbbell is the most versatile training tool, and most gyms carry weights up to 100 pounds. If you train at home, you may want to consider buying a set of PowerBlocks or looking to local "for sale" lists online to find an inexpensive set of used dumbbells.

Barbells—45-pound barbell with 300 to 400 pounds
You can get a standard Olympic barbell at most fitness equipment stores that will come with a 300-pound weight set of plates. I've had major success finding extra weights on craigslist, but shop around and you'll find what you are looking for. A company like gopherperformance.com offers many options for weight plates and barbells.

Exercise Bench
An adjustable bench is best. A flat bench will work, but in order to hit both incline and decline exercises, you'll need one that is more versatile. Look to performbetter.com for good options.

Squat Rack
A squat rack can act as the foundation for all your barbell movements. Pressing, rowing, chins, deadlifts, and squats all need a home. The squat rack will provide this. If you are willing to spend the money on a solid squat rack for your home, look into roguefitness.com, but most gyms will have you covered.

Blast Strap
A great bodyweight tool for pushing and pulling movements, the blast strap is available at elitefts.net.

TRX
This suspension trainer is a versatile tool for bodyweight movements that you can take anywhere. TRX straps are a bit more expensive but a valuable tool to take on the road. You can pick one up at trxtraining.com.

Track, Hill, or Stadium Steps
Use these options during high-intensity cardio days.

High-Density Foam Roller
For warmup and self-massage, foam rollers come in various sizes. A good versatile size is a 36-inch round model available in fitness supply stores and at power-systems.com.

Bike, Treadmill, Track
These can be used for other cardio options or high-intensity interval training (HIIT).

SAMPLE TRAINING SPLITS

You can configure your workouts dozens of ways to hit every muscle in your body. On the following pages are just a few samples of how you can fill 3-, 4-, 5-, or 6-day training splits with exercises by major muscle groups. (Note: These samples are different from the 24-week plan I'm recommending in Chapter 9. Choose what works best for you.)

THE 3-DAYS-PER-WEEK WORKOUT

Day 1: Back, Rear Deltoids, Biceps
Day 2: Chest, Shoulders, Triceps
Day 3: Quadriceps, Hamstrings, Calves

ADVANTAGES

- Overall muscle stimulation
- Greater frequency to major muscles
- Greater strength gains
- More recovery
- Less central nervous system fatigue
- Ideal for ectomorphs

DISADVANTAGES

- Less muscle specialization
- Less isolation
- Elimination of weak point training
- Less volume per body part
- Less frequency to the "show muscles"
- Not for all endomorphs
- Less "pump"

SAMPLE 3-DAY BODYBUILDING TRAINING SPLIT

WORKOUT 1—BACK, REAR DELTOIDS, BICEPS

EXERCISE TYPE	EXERCISE	SETS X REPETITIONS
Horizontal Pull	A) Barbell Pronated Row	4 x 8
Back/Lat Superset*	B1) Sternum Chinup B2) Dumbbell Single-Arm Row	3 x 10 3 x 15 each arm
Vertical Pull	C) Wide-Grip Pullup	3 x 8
Horizontal Pull	D) TRX Face Pull	3 x 15
Biceps Superset	E1) Dumbbell Standing Hammer Curl E2) Barbell Reverse-Grip Curl	3 x 10 3 x 12

* In a superset, you complete all sets of the pair of exercises before moving to the next pair of lifts.

WORKOUT 2—CHEST, SHOULDERS, TRICEPS

EXERCISE TYPE	EXERCISE	SETS X REPETITIONS
Vertical Push	A) Barbell Military Press	5 x 8 to 10
Chest/Shoulder Superset	B1) Dumbbell Bench Press B2) Single-Arm Dumbbell Rear Lateral Raise	4 x 12 4 x 8 to 12 each arm
Chest/Triceps Superset	C1) Parallel Dip C2) Feet-Elevated Pushup	3 x 15 to 20 3 x 15 to 20
Triceps Superset	D1) Lying Pronated Triceps Extension D2) Bench Dip	3 x 15 to 20 3 x 15 to 20

WORKOUT 3—QUADRICEPS, HAMSTRINGS, CALVES

EXERCISE TYPE	EXERCISE	SETS X REPETITIONS
Bilateral Push/Knee—Quad Dominant	A) Barbell Squat	4 x 20
Bilateral Pull/Hip—Hamstring Dominant	B) Barbell Romanian Deadlift	4 x 8 to 10
Quadriceps/Hamstring Superset	C1) Dumbbell Bulgarian Split Squat C2) Glute Ham Raise	3 x 12 each leg forward 3 x 10
Unilateral/Quad Dominant	D) Dumbbell Walking Lunge	3 x 20 each leg forward
Bilateral/Specialization	E) Barbell Standing Calf Raise	5 x 25

There are numerous ways to work the 3-day split into your week.
(Note: The cardio workouts will be described in Chapter 11.)

ALTERNATING WORK/REST DAYS

Monday: Workout 1, High-Intensity Cardio
Tuesday: Rest
Wednesday: Workout 2, Cardio
Thursday: Rest
Friday: Workout 3, High-Intensity Cardio
Saturday: Rest
Sunday: Rest

3 DAYS ON, 1 DAY OFF, REPEAT

Monday: Workout 1, High-Intensity Cardio
Tuesday: Workout 2, Cardio
Wednesday: Workout 3, High-Intensity Cardio
Thursday: Rest
Friday: Workout 1, Cardio
Saturday: Workout 2, High-Intensity Cardio
Sunday: Workout 3, Cardio

3 DAYS ON, 2 DAYS OFF, REPEAT

Monday: Workout 1, High-Intensity Cardio
Tuesday: Workout 2, Cardio
Wednesday: Workout 3, Cardio
Thursday: Rest
Friday: Rest
Saturday: Workout 1, High-Intensity Cardio
Sunday: Workout 2, Cardio
Monday: Workout 3, Cardio

THE 4-DAYS-PER-WEEK WORKOUT

Day 1: Chest, Back, Traps, and Abs
Day 2: Quads and Calves
Day 3: Shoulders and Triceps
Day 4: Hamstrings, Back, and Biceps

ADVANTAGES
- Greater volume
- Greater overall "pump"
- More muscle specialization
- More isolation exercises
- Greater structure for hypertrophy
- Favorite of endomorph and mesomorph body types

DISADVANTAGES
- Average strength gains
- Less recovery
- More central nervous system fatigue
- Not preferred method for ectomorphs
- Higher volume
- Greater chance of overtraining

SAMPLE 4-DAY BODYBUILDING TRAINING SPLIT

WORKOUT 1—CHEST, BACK, TRAPS, ABS

EXERCISE TYPE	EXERCISE	SETS X REPETITIONS
Chest Superset*	A1) Barbell Bench Press A2) Dumbbell Incline Fly	4 x 6 4 x 15
Back Superset	B1) Barbell Supine Row B2) Eccentric Pullup† †Take 3 seconds to lower.	4 x 8 4 x 10
Chest Exercise	C) Dumbbell Bench Press	3 x 10
Back/Traps Superset	D1) Dumbbell Single-Arm Row D2) Barbell Shrug	3 x 15 to 20 each arm 3 x 20
Abs Superset	E1) Hanging Leg Raise E2) Supine Floor Reverse Crunch	5 x 15 to 20 5 x 15 to 20

WORKOUT 2—QUADS AND CALVES

EXERCISE TYPE	EXERCISE	SETS X REPETITIONS
Calf Superset	A1) Donkey Calf Raise A2) Jump Rope	4 x 20 4 x 30 seconds
Bilateral Exercise	B) Barbell Squat	4 x 15, 12, 10, 8
Quads Superset	C1) Barbell Front Squat C2) Dumbbell Split Squat	3 x 8, 6, 4 3 x 5 each leg forward (3 seconds eccentric)
Quads Finisher	D) Dumbbell Walking Lunge	2 x 20 steps

* In a superset, you complete all sets of the pair of exercises before moving to the next pair of lifts.

WORKOUT 3—SHOULDERS AND TRICEPS

EXERCISE TYPE	EXERCISE	SETS X REPETITIONS
Shoulder Exercise	A) Barbell Standing Military Press	4 x 6
Shoulder Exercise	B) Dumbbell Arnold Press	3 x 8
Shoulder Giant Set	C1) Dumbbell Seated Press C2) Dumbbell Front Raise C3) Dumbbell Rear Delt Raise C4) Exercise Band Pull Apart	3 x 8 3 x 10 3 x 12 3 x 15 to 20
Triceps Superset	D1) Barbell Close-Grip Bench Press D2) Lying EZ Bar Overhead Extension Skullcrusher	4 x 6 4 x 10 to 12
Triceps Finisher	E) Parallel Dip	3 x 30

WORKOUT 4—HAMSTRINGS, BACK, AND BICEPS

EXERCISE TYPE	EXERCISE	SETS X REPETITIONS
Total Body	A) Trap Bar Deadlift	4 x 6
Back/Hamstring Superset	B1) Barbell Stiff-Legged Deadlift B2) Chinup	3 x 12 3 x 4
Back/Hamstring Superset	C1) Barbell Romanian Deadlift C2) Glute Ham Raise	3 x 15 3 x 8
Biceps Superset	E1) Dumbbell Standing Hammer Curl E2) Barbell Reverse-Grip Curl	4 x 10 4 x 12

Sample Configurations for 4-Day Bodybuilding Training Split

ALTERNATE WORK/REST DAYS (Allows for a greater volume of training)

Monday: Workout 1, Cardio
Tuesday: Rest
Wednesday: Workout 2, High-Intensity Cardio
Thursday: Rest
Friday: Workout 3
Saturday: Workout 4, High-Intensity Cardio
Sunday: Rest

4 DAYS ON, 2 DAY OFF, REPEAT (Allows for a greater balance of training and recovery)

Monday: Workout 1, High-Intensity Cardio
Tuesday: Workout 2, Cardio
Wednesday: Workout 3
Thursday: Workout 4, High-Intensity Cardio
Friday: Rest
Saturday: Rest
Sunday: Workout 1 (start rotation again)

2 DAYS ON, 2 DAYS OFF, REPEAT (Allows for greater recovery)

Monday: Workout 1, Cardio
Tuesday: Workout 2, High-Intensity Cardio
Wednesday: Rest
Thursday: Rest
Friday: Workout 3, Cardio
Saturday: Workout 4, High-Intensity Cardio
Sunday: Rest
Monday: Rest
Tuesday: Workout 1 (start rotation over)

THE 5- AND 6-DAYS-PER-WEEK WORKOUT

The typical bodybuilding training program calls for training 5 to 6 days per week. I have used all six splits successfully. Recently, I have found that a 3- or 4-day split fits nicely into my schedule in the off-season. However, when I'm preparing for an upcoming bodybuilding competition, I will incorporate training cycles where I train 5 days per week. I know plenty of successful bodybuilders who follow a 6-day split schedule even for off-season training. Again, it really depends on how much time you can devote to your training.

There isn't much of a difference between a 5- or 6-day split. But they are quite different from 3- and 4-day splits.

ADVANTAGES

- Greater training frequency
- Greater muscle isolation
- More muscle specialization
- Ability to shorten training time
- Favorite of most bodybuilders

DISADVANTAGES

- Less recovery
- Average strength gains
- High volume
- Central nervous system fatigue

SAMPLE "BODY PART" WORKOUTS FOR USE ON 5- OR 6-DAY PROGRAMS

DAY 1: CHEST WORKOUT

EXERCISE	SETS X REPETITIONS
A) Barbell Bench Press	5 x 10
B1) Dumbbell Incline Fly B2) Suspended Blast Strap Pushup	4 x 12 4 x 10
C) Dumbbell Bench Press	4 x 8
D) Exercise Band Pushup	3 x 20

DAY 2: ARM WORKOUT

EXERCISE	SETS X REPETITIONS
A1) Dumbbell Standing Hammer Curl A2) Exercise Band Pushdown	4 x 8 4 x 15
B1) Barbell Wide-Grip Curl B2) EZ Bar Skullcrusher	4 x 10 4 x 12
C1) EZ Bar Preacher Curl C2) Parallel Dip	4 x 10 4 x 15 each

DAY 3: LEG WORKOUT

EXERCISE	SETS X REPETITIONS
A) Barbell Squat	5 x 5
B1) Barbell Reverse Lunge B2) Glute Ham Raise	4 x 6 each leg 4 x 8
C1) Dumbbell Goblet Squat C2) Barbell Romanian Deadlift (RDL)	3 x 15 3 x 15
D) Dumbbell Walking Lunge	3 x 30 yards
E) Standing Calf Raise	1 x 100 (minimal rest as needed)

Note: For the 6-day split, break the leg workout into 2 days: Quads and Hamstrings/Calves.

DAY 4: SHOULDER WORKOUT

EXERCISE	SETS X REPETITIONS
A) Barbell Standing Military Press	4 x 6
B1) Dumbbell Arnold Press B2) Lying Incline Internal Rear Raise	4 x 8 to 12 4 x 15
C1) Dumbbell Lateral Raise C2) Dumbbell Incline Press	3 x 15 to 20 3 x 10

DAY 5: BACK WORKOUT

EXERCISE	SETS X REPETITIONS
A) Trap Bar Deadlift	5 x 5
B1) Overhand-Grip Barbell Row B2) Eccentric Chinup	4 x 8 4 x 6 (3-second negative)
C1) Barbell Shrug C2) Dumbbell Farmer's Walk	3 x 10 3 x 30 yards

SAMPLE FREQUENCY FOR 5-DAY SPLIT

Sunday: Rest
Monday: Legs (Quads, Hamstrings, Calves)
Tuesday: Shoulders
Wednesday: Back
Thursday: Chest
Friday: Arms (Biceps, Triceps)
Saturday: Rest

SAMPLE FREQUENCY FOR 6-DAY SPLIT

Sunday: Rest
Monday: Quads
Tuesday: Back
Wednesday: Chest
Thursday: Hamstrings, Calves
Friday: Shoulders
Saturday: Arms

THE BEST DEFENSE FROM INJURY IS A GREAT WARMUP

COLD MUSCLES ARE TIGHT MUSCLES. Tight muscles often lead to fatigue, soreness, injury, lack of mobility, and even a reduction in the muscle symmetry you are trying to achieve. Warm, flexible muscles are muscles ready for work. Good flexibility allows a muscle to lengthen and the joints to operate through a full range of motion. When muscles are elastic, your posture improves and you breathe deeper, sending more oxygen-rich blood to your muscles and brain. That's everything a bodybuilder in training needs. So, never jump into a workout without doing a proper warmup. You'll get a better workout if you do, and you'll significantly reduce your risk of injury.

No matter which workout split you choose, begin each workout by preparing your muscles. On the following page are three of my favorite warmup routines. In addition to common dynamic stretches, I always incorporate some myofascial release moves into my warmup using a high-density closed-cell foam roller, so I've built roller exercises into the three sample warmups. A foam roller is an amazing tool for bodybuilders because the self-massage quickly forces warming blood to the muscle tissues and helps to elongate muscles. You can also use the foam roller whenever you feel tight and sore. Here are the warmup exercise lists. Detailed instructions on how to do each move start on page 281.

SAMPLE WARMUP 1

EXERCISE	TIME OR REPETITIONS
Foam Roller Calves	30 seconds
Foam Roller Iliotibial Band	30 seconds
Foam Roller Glutes	30 seconds
Foam Roller Lats	30 seconds
Foam Roller Pecs	30 seconds
Supine Hip Internal Rotation	10 repetitions
Inchworm	10 repetitions
Sumo Squat to Stand	10 repetitions
Walking Heel to Butt	10 repetitions each leg

SAMPLE WARMUP 2

EXERCISE	TIME OR REPETITIONS
Foam Roller Iliotibial Band	30 seconds
Foam Roller Adductor	30 seconds
Foam Roller Glutes	30 seconds
Foam Roller Lats	30 seconds
Foam Roller T-Spine	30 seconds
Prone Hip External Rotation	10 repetitions
Sumo Squat to Stand	10 repetitions
Walking Knee Hug	10 repetitions each leg
Forearm to Instep Lunge	10 repetitions each leg
Lateral Lunge	10 repetitions each leg
Scapular Wall Slide	10 repetitions

SAMPLE WARMUP 3

EXERCISE	TIME OR REPETITIONS
Foam Roller Calves	30 seconds
Foam Roller Hips/Quads	30 seconds
Foam Roller Glutes	30 seconds
Foam Roller Lats	30 seconds
Foam Roller Pecs	30 seconds
Prone Hip External Rotation	10 repetitions
Side-Lying Thoracic Rotation	10 repetitions each side
Quadruped Thoracic Rotation	10 repetitions each
Sumo Squat to Stand	10 repetitions
Inchworm	10 repetitions
Bent-Over T-Spine Mobility	10 repetitions each side

PART 3

CHAPTER 9

The Bodybuilder's Workout 24-Week Plans

Take your pick of the 3- to 5-day splits and start your first of six workout cycles for total-body transformation

THE 24-WEEK WORKOUT PROGRAM IS BROKEN DOWN into six 4-week cycles, which are designed with exercise and set/rep changes to keep your muscles challenged and growing. The charts that follow show these cycles for 3-, 4-, and 5-day training splits indicating which muscle groups you will target on each day. Choose the split that fits best into your personal schedule and create a workout log allowing room to record sets, reps, and weight amounts. Photos and descriptions of the exercises are found in Chapter 10.

Remember to warm up and cool down before and after each workout to reduce soreness and risk of injury. Good warmups were given at the end of the last chapter, along with an effective myofascial release routine using a closed-cell foam roller. Team these splits with the cardio workout suggested in Chapter 11.

3-Days-Per-Week Schedule · Cycle 1 · Weeks 1 to 4

WORKOUT 1: QUADS, HAMSTRINGS, CALVES

EXERCISE	SETS X REPETITIONS
A) Barbell Squat	4 x 10 Rest 90 seconds
B1) Dumbbell Romanian Deadlift	3 x 12 Rest 30 seconds
B2) Dumbbell Split Squat	3 x 8 each leg forward Rest 60 seconds
C1) Barbell Front Squat	3 x 12 Rest 30 seconds
C2) Glute Ham Raise	3 x 8 Rest 30 seconds
C3) Dumbbell Walking Lunge	3 x 15 alternating steps Rest 60 seconds
D) Barbell Standing Calf Raise	4 x 20 (constant tension) Rest 30 seconds

WORKOUT 2: CHEST, SHOULDERS, TRICEPS

EXERCISE	SETS X REPETITIONS
A) Barbell Bench Press	4 x 8 Rest 90 seconds
B1) Dumbbell Standing Press	3 x 10 Rest 60 seconds
B2) Dumbbell Incline Bench Press	3 x 10 Rest 60 seconds
C1) Barbell Close-Grip Bench Press	3 x 12 Rest 30 seconds
C2) Dumbbell Arnold Press	3 x 12 Rest 30 seconds
C3) Dumbbell Bent-Over Rear Deltoid Raise (Standing)	3 x 15 Rest 30 seconds
D1) Dumbbell Decline Skull Crusher	3 x 8 Rest 30 seconds
D2) Weighted Pushup	3 x 20 Rest 60 seconds

WORKOUT 3: BACK, TRAPS, BICEPS, FOREARMS, ABS

EXERCISE	SETS X REPETITIONS
A) Barbell Deadlift	4 x 6 Rest 90 seconds
B1) Chinup	4 x 8 Rest 60 seconds
B2) Dumbbell Single-Arm Row	4 x 20 Rest 60 seconds
C1) Dumbbell Standing Hammer Curl	4 x 15 Rest 30 seconds
C2) Barbell Reverse-Grip Curl	4 x 10 Rest 30 seconds
C3) Barbell Behind-the-Back Shrug	4 x 12 Rest 30 seconds
D) Hanging Knee Raise	4 x 20 Rest 30 seconds

3-Days-Per-Week Schedule • Cycle 2 • Weeks 5 to 8

WORKOUT 1: QUADS, HAMSTRINGS, CALVES

EXERCISE	SETS X REPETITIONS
A) Barbell Front Squat	4 x 15 Rest 60 seconds
B1) Barbell Stiff-Legged Romanian Deadlift	4 x 10 Rest 60 seconds
B2) Dumbbell Walking Lunge	4 x 15 steps Rest 60 seconds
C1) Barbell Reverse Lunge	4 x 8 each leg No rest
C2) Glute Ham Raise with Stability Ball	4 x 15 Rest 60 seconds
D1) Jump Rope	4 x 20 (constant tension) Rest 30 seconds
D2) Seated Plate Calf Raise	4 x 10

WORKOUT 2: CHEST, SHOULDERS, TRICEPS

EXERCISE	SETS X REPETITIONS
A) Standing Barbell Military Press	4 x 6 Rest 90 seconds
B1) Dumbbell Bench Press	4 x 8 Rest 60 seconds
B2) Dumbbell Incline Fly	4 x 12 Rest 60 seconds
C1) Barbell Reverse-Grip Bench Press	4 x 8 Rest 30 seconds
C2) Parallel Dip	4 x 10 Rest 30 seconds
D1) Dumbbell Standing Front and Lateral Raise Combo	4 x 8 each side Rest 30 seconds
D2) Dumbbell Seesaw Press	4 x 10 each arm Rest 60 seconds

WORKOUT 3: BACK, TRAPS, BICEPS, FOREARMS, ABS

EXERCISE	SETS X REPETITIONS
A) Barbell Sumo Deadlift	4 x 8 Rest 90 seconds
B1) Barbell Supine Row	4 x 10 Rest 60 seconds
B2) Wide-Grip Pullup	4 x 8 (emphasize concentric) Rest 60 seconds
C) Dumbbell Shrug	4 x 12 Rest 30 seconds
D1) Dumbbell Incline Hammer Curl	4 x 10 each arm Rest 30 seconds
D2) Dumbbell Zottman Preacher Curl	4 x 8 each arm Rest 60 seconds
E) Barbell Rollout	4 x 10

3-Days-Per-Week Schedule • Cycle 3 • Weeks 9 to 12

WORKOUT 1: QUADS, HAMSTRINGS, CALVES

EXERCISE	SETS X REPETITIONS
A) Barbell Squat	5 x 20 Rest 2 minutes
B1) Dumbbell Bulgarian Split Squat	5 x 10 each leg Rest 90 seconds
B2) Barbell Split-Stance Romanian Deadlift	5 x 12 each foot forward Rest 90 seconds
C1) Dumbbell Reverse Lunge	5 x 15 each leg
C2) Dumbbell Romanian Deadlift	5 x 12 Rest 60 seconds
D) Donkey Calf Raise	5 x 25 Rest 15–30 seconds

WORKOUT 2: CHEST, SHOULDERS, TRICEPS

EXERCISE	SETS X REPETITIONS
A) Barbell Incline Bench Press	5 x 8 Rest 90 seconds
B1) Dumbbell Neutral-Grip Incline Bench Press	5 x 10 Rest 60 seconds
B2) Dumbbell Flat Chest Fly	5 x 15 Rest 60 seconds
C1) Parallel Dip	5 x 12 Rest 30 seconds
C2) Weighted Pushup	5 x 10 Rest 30 seconds
D1) Dumbbell Neutral-Grip Press	5 x 8 Rest 30 seconds
D2) Bent-Over Dumbbell Rear Deltoid Raise (head on bench)	5 x 15 Rest 60 seconds

WORKOUT 3: BACK, TRAPS, BICEPS, FOREARMS, ABS

EXERCISE	SETS X REPETITIONS
A) Barbell Deadlift	5 x 5 Rest 90 seconds
B1) Pullup	5 x 5 Rest 60 seconds
B2) Dumbbell Elbow-Out Row	5 x 10 each arm Rest 60 seconds
B3) Barbell Snatch Shrug	5 x 10 Rest 30 seconds
C1) Dumbbell Cross-Body Hammer Curl	5 x 15 each arm Rest 30 seconds
C2) Barbell Drag Curl	5 x 10 Rest 60 seconds
D) Supine Floor Reverse Crunch	5 x 20 Rest 30 seconds
E) Dumbbell Seated Palms-Up Wrist Curl	5 x 10 Rest 30 seconds

3-Days-Per-Week Schedule • Cycle 4 • Weeks 13 to 16

WORKOUT 1: QUADS, HAMSTRINGS, CALVES

EXERCISE	SETS X REPETITIONS
A) Barbell Front Squat (with crossed arms)	4 x 6 Rest 45 seconds
B1) Barbell Walking Lunge	4 x 10 steps Rest 45 seconds
B2) Glute Ham Raise	4 x 10
B3) Dumbbell Stiff-Legged Deadlift	4 x 12 Rest 45 seconds
C1) Dumbbell Split Squat	4 x 8 each leg forward Rest 45 seconds
C2) Dumbbell Single-Leg Romanian Deadlift	4 x 10 each leg Rest 45 seconds
C3) Dumbbell Walking Lunge	4 x 20 steps Rest 2 minutes

WORKOUT 2: CHEST, SHOULDERS, TRICEPS

EXERCISE	SETS X REPETITIONS
A) Barbell Close-Grip Bench Press	4 x 6 Rest 60 seconds
B1) Dumbbell Bench Press	4 x 10 Rest 45 seconds
B2) Standing Dumbbell Single-Arm Press	4 x 12 each arm Rest 45 seconds
B3) Parallel Dip	4 x 20 Rest 45 seconds
C) Weighted Pushup	4 x 10 Rest 45 seconds
D1) Dumbbell Neutral-Grip Seated Press	5 x 8 Rest 45 seconds
D2) Bent-Over Dumbbell Rear Deltoid Raise (head on bench)	5 x 15 Rest 45 seconds

WORKOUT 3: BACK, TRICEPS, BICEPS, FOREARMS, ABS

EXERCISE	SETS X REPETITIONS
A) Barbell Deadlift	4 x 6 Rest 90 seconds
B1) Barbell Overhand-Grip Row	4 x 12 Rest 60 seconds
B2) Pullup	4 x 6 Rest 60 seconds
B3) Barbell Behind-the-Back Shrug	4 x 15 Rest 30 seconds
C1) Dumbbell Standing Hammer Curl	5 x 10 each Rest 30 seconds
C2) EZ Bar Preacher Curl	5 x 8 Rest 60 seconds
C3) Dumbbell Concentration Curl	5 x 8 Rest 60 seconds
D) Supine Floor Reverse Crunch	5 x 20

3-Days-Per-Week Schedule • Cycle 5 • Weeks 17 to 20

WORKOUT 1: QUADS, HAMSTRINGS, CALVES

EXERCISE	SETS X REPETITIONS
A1) Barbell Squat	3 x 20 Rest 60 seconds
A2) Barbell Romanian Deadlift	3 x 15 Rest 60 seconds
B1) Dumbbell Reverse Lunge	4 x 12 each leg Rest 60 seconds
B2) Barbell Front Squat	4 x 8 Rest 60 seconds
B3) Dumbbell Walking Lunge	4 x 20 steps Rest 60 seconds
B4) Glute Ham Raise with Stability Ball	4 x 15 Rest 2 minutes
C1) Barbell Stiff-Legged Deadlift	4 x 10
C2) Dumbbell Bulgarian Split Squat	4 x 6 each leg forward Rest 60 seconds
D) Seated Calf Raise	1 x 100 Rest as needed

WORKOUT 2: CHEST, SHOULDERS, TRICEPS

EXERCISE	SETS X REPETITIONS
A1) Barbell Incline Bench Press	3 x 10 Rest 60 seconds
A2) Dumbbell Standing Press	3 x 8 Rest 60 seconds
B1) Dumbbell Incline Fly	4 x 15 Rest 30 seconds
B2) Dumbbell Incline Bench Press	4 x 12 Rest 30 seconds
C1) Dumbbell One-Arm Incline Lateral Raise	4 x 10 each arm Rest 30 seconds
C2) Dumbbell Arnold Press	4 x 8 Rest 30 seconds
D1) Barbell Decline Close-Grip Skull Crusher	5 x 10 Rest 30 seconds
D2) Parallel Dip (weighted)	5 x 8

WORKOUT 3: BACK, TRAPS, BICEPS, FOREARMS, ABS

EXERCISE	SETS X REPETITIONS
A1) Chinup	6 x 6 Rest 90 seconds
A2) Barbell Supine Row	6 x 6
B1) Dumbbell Single-Arm Row	4 x 20 each arm Rest 30 seconds
B2) Dumbbell Pullover	4 x 10 Rest 30 seconds
B3) Barbell Behind-the-Back Shrug	4 x 15 Rest 30 seconds
C1) Standing Zottman Curl	4 x 8 Rest 30 seconds
C2) Dumbbell Spider Curl	4 x 10 each arm Rest 60 seconds
D) Barbell Seated Wrist Palms-Down Curl	4 x 15
E) Hanging Leg Raise	4 x 10

3-Days-Per-Week Schedule · Cycle 6 · Weeks 21 to 24

WORKOUT 1: QUADS, HAMSTRINGS, CALVES

EXERCISE	SETS X REPETITIONS
A) Barbell Squat	10 x 10 Rest 60 seconds
B) Barbell Romanian Deadlift	1 x 6, 1 x 12, 1 x 25 Rest 60 seconds
C) Barbell Front Squat	1 x 6, 1 x 12, 1 x 25 Rest 60 seconds
D) Dumbbell Walking Lunge *Choose dumbbells 5 to 10 pounds less in weight than the amount with which you would achieve muscle failure at 10 repetitions or steps.	3 x 10 steps (*drop set) Minimal rest
E1) Glute Ham Raise with Stability Ball	3 x 20 Rest 30 seconds
E2) Dumbbell Stiff-Legged Romanian Deadlift	3 x 10 Rest 30 seconds
F) Barbell Rocking Standing Calf Raise	1 x 100 (rest/pause)

WORKOUT 2: CHEST, SHOULDERS, TRICEPS

EXERCISE	SETS X REPETITIONS
A) Barbell Close Grip Bench Press	10 x 10 Rest 60 seconds
B1) Dumbbell Arnold Press	3 x 6, 3 x 12, 3 x 25 Rest 45 seconds
B2) Standing Barbell Front Raise	3 x 8 Rest 45 seconds
C) Dumbbell Neutral-Grip Incline Bench Press	3 x 8 (drop set) Minimal rest
D1) Barbell Neck Bench Press	3 x 6 Rest 60 seconds
D2) Standing Dumbbell Triceps Kickback	3 x 10 Rest 60 seconds
E1) Dumbbell Iron Cross	3 x 10 Rest 30 seconds
E2) Suspended Pushup (with Blast Strap)	3 x 15 Rest 30 seconds
E3) Dumbbell Side-Lying One-Arm Lateral Raise	3 x 10 each Rest 30 seconds

WORKOUT 3: BACK, TRAPS, BICEPS, FOREARMS, ABS

EXERCISE	SETS X REPETITIONS
A) Barbell Sumo Deadlift	10 x 10 Rest 90 seconds
B1) Trap Bar Deadlift	3 x 6 Rest 30 seconds
B2) Sternum Chinups	3 x 6 Rest 30 seconds
B3) Barbell Landmine Row	3 x 8 each Rest 30 seconds
C1) Dumbbell Chest-Supported Row	3 x 12 Rest 30 seconds
C2) Barbell Chest-Supported Spider Curl	3 x 8 Rest 30 seconds
D1) Dumbbell Shrug	3 x 15 Rest 30 seconds
D2) Seated Palms-Down Dumbbell Wrist Curl	3 x 15 Rest 30 seconds
E) Hanging Knee Raise	5 x 20

4-Days-Per-Week Schedule • Cycle 1 • Weeks 1 to 4

WORKOUT 1: QUADS AND CALVES

EXERCISE	SETS X REPETITIONS
A) Barbell Squat	4 x 10 Rest 90 seconds
B1) Dumbbell Bulgarian Split Squat	3 x 12 each leg Rest 30 seconds
B2) Dumbbell Reverse Lunge	3 x 8 each leg Rest 60 seconds
C1) Barbell Front Squat (with crossed arms)	3 x 12 Rest 30 seconds
C2) Dumbbell Walking Lunge	3 x 15 steps Rest 60 seconds
D) Barbell Standing Calf Raise	4 x 20 (constant tension) Rest 15–30 seconds

WORKOUT 2: CHEST, SHOULDERS, ABS

EXERCISE	SETS X REPETITIONS
A) Barbell Bench Press	4 x 8 Rest 90 seconds
B1) Dumbbell Standing Press	3 x 10 Rest 60 seconds
B2) Dumbbell Incline Bench Press	3 x 10 Rest 60 seconds
C1) Barbell Incline Bench Press	3 x 12 Rest 30 seconds
C2) Dumbbell Arnold Press	3 x 12 Rest 30 seconds
C3) Bent-Over Dumbbell Rear Deltoid Raise (Standing)	3 x 15 Rest 30 seconds
D) Dumbbell Front and Lateral Raise Combo	3 x 10 Rest 30 seconds
E) Hanging Knee Raise	3 x 10 Rest 30 seconds

WORKOUT 3: BACK, HAMSTRINGS, TRAPS, CALVES

EXERCISE	SETS X REPETITIONS
A) Barbell Deadlift	4 x 6 Rest 90 seconds
B1) Chinup	3 x 8 Rest 60 seconds
B2) Dumbbell Romanian Deadlift	3 x 12 Rest 60 seconds
C1) Barbell Pronated Row	3 x 8 Rest 30 seconds
C2) Glute Ham Raise	3 x 10 Rest 30 seconds
C3) Barbell Behind-the-Back Shrug	3 x 12 Rest 30 seconds
D) Seated Plate Calf Raise	4 x 20 Rest 30 seconds

WORKOUT 4: BICEPS, TRICEPS, FOREARMS, ABS

EXERCISE	SETS X REPETITIONS
A1) Dumbbell Cross-Body Hammer Curl	4 x 10 Rest 30 seconds
A2) Close-Grip Bench Press	4 x 10 Rest 30 seconds
B1) EZ-Bar Standing Curl	3 x 12 Rest 30 seconds
B2) Parallel Dip (weighted)	3 x 8 – Heavy (3-second negative) Rest 30 seconds
C1) Barbell Wide-Grip Curl	3 x 8 Rest 30 seconds
C2) Bench Dip	3 x 15 Rest 30 seconds
D1) Seated Dumbbell Curl (3-second descent)	3 x 8 Rest 30 seconds
D2) Dumbbell Skull Crusher	3 x 15 Rest 30 seconds
E1) Barbell Rollout	3 x 15 Rest 30 seconds
E2) Dual Dumbbell Wrist Curl	3 x 8

4-Days-Per-Week Schedule • Cycle 2 • Weeks 5 to 8

WORKOUT 1: QUADS AND CALVES

EXERCISE	SETS X REPETITIONS
A) Barbell Front Squat (with crossed arms)	4 x 15 Rest 60 seconds
B1) Barbell Squat	4 x 10 (drop set) Minimal rest
B2) Dumbbell Reverse Lunge	4 x 8 each leg Rest 60 seconds
C) Barbell Walking Lunge	4 x 15 steps No rest
D1) Barbell Standing Calf Raise	4 x 20 (constant tension) Rest 15–30 seconds
D2) Seated Plate Calf Raise	4 x 10

WORKOUT 2: CHEST, SHOULDERS, ABS

EXERCISE	SETS X REPETITIONS
A) Barbell Military Press	4 x 6 Rest 90 seconds
B1) Dumbbell Bench Press	4 x 8 Rest 60 seconds
B2) Dumbbell Incline Fly	4 x 12 Rest 60 seconds
C1) Barbell Wide-Grip Bench Press	4 x 8 Rest 30 seconds
C2) Dumbbell Flat Chest Fly	4 x 10 Rest 30 seconds
D1) Dumbbell Seesaw Press	4 x 8 each arm Rest 30 seconds
D2) Dumbbell Single-Arm Rear Lateral Raise	4 x 10 each arm Rest 30 seconds
E) Supine Floor Reverse Crunch	4 x 25

WORKOUT 3: BACK, HAMSTRINGS, TRAPS, CALVES

EXERCISE	SETS X REPETITIONS
A) Barbell Sumo Deadlift	4 x 8 Rest 90 seconds
B1) Barbell Supine Row	4 x 10 Rest 60 seconds
B2) Wide-Grip Pullup	4 x 8 (emphasize concentric) Rest 60 seconds
B3) Back Extension (with hyperextension)	4 x 15 Rest 60 seconds
C1) Dumbbell Stiff-Legged Deadlift	4 x 12 Rest 60 seconds
C2) Dumbbell Shrug	4 x 12 Rest 30 seconds
D) Donkey Calf Raise	4 x 20 Rest 30 seconds

WORKOUT 4: BICEPS, TRICEPS, FOREARMS, ABS

EXERCISE	SETS X REPETITIONS
A1) Dumbbell Standing Hammer Curl	4 x 10 Rest 30 seconds
A2) Barbell Reverse-Grip Bench Press	4 x 10 Rest 30 seconds
B1) Dumbbell Incline Curl	4 x 12 Rest 30 seconds
B2) Barbell Triceps Extension	4 x 8 Rest 30 seconds
C1) Barbell Reverse-Grip Curl	4 x 8 Rest 30 seconds
C2) Dumbbell Skull Crusher	4 x 15 Rest 30 seconds
D1) Dumbbell Zottman Curl	4 x 8 (emphasize eccentric) Rest 30 seconds
D2) Standing Dumbbell Triceps Kickback	4 x 15 Rest 30 seconds
E) Hanging Leg Raise	4 x 10 Rest 30 seconds
F) Standing Palms-Up Behind-the-Back Wrist Curl	4 x 10

4-Days-Per-Week Schedule • Cycle 3 • Weeks 9 to 12

WORKOUT 1: QUADS AND CALVES

EXERCISE	SETS X REPETITIONS
A) Barbell Squat	5 x 20 Rest 2 minutes
B1) Dumbbell Bulgarian Split Squat	5 x 10 each leg Rest 90 seconds
B2) Barbell Zercher Squat	5 x 12 Rest 90 seconds
C1) Dumbbell Reverse Lunge	5 x 15 each leg
C2) Dumbbell Goblet Squat	5 x 12 Rest 60 seconds
D) Donkey Calf Raise	5 x 25 Rest 15–30 seconds

WORKOUT 2: CHEST, SHOULDERS, ABS

EXERCISE	SETS X REPETITIONS
A) Barbell Incline Bench Press	5 x 8 Rest 90 seconds
B1) Dumbbell Neutral-Grip Incline Bench Press	5 x 10 Rest 60 seconds
B2) Dumbbell Flat Chest Fly	5 x 15 Rest 60 seconds
C) Barbell Standing Military Press	4 x 8 Rest 30 seconds
D1) Weighted Pushup	5 x 10 Rest 30 seconds
D2) Bent-Over Dumbbell Rear Deltoid Raise (head on bench)	5 x 15 Rest 60 seconds
D3) Neutral-Grip Seated Press	5 x 8 Rest 30 seconds
E) Hanging X-Body Knee Raise (oblique raise)	5 x 10 each leg

WORKOUT 3: BACK, HAMSTRINGS, TRAPS, CALVES

EXERCISE	SETS X REPETITIONS
A) Barbell Deadlift	5 x 5 Rest 90 seconds
B1) Pullup (weighted)	5 x 5 Rest 60 seconds
B2) Barbell Split-Stance Romanian Deadlift	5 x 10 Rest 60 seconds
C) Barbell Good Morning	5 x 8 Rest 60 seconds
D1) Barbell Snatch Shrug	5 x 10 Rest 30 seconds
D2) Dumbbell Standing Calf Raise	5 x 12 (emphasize 3-second eccentric) Rest 30 seconds

WORKOUT 4: BICEPS, TRICEPS, FOREARMS, ABS

EXERCISE	SETS X REPETITIONS
A1) Standing Alternate Curl	5 x 8 each arm Rest 30 seconds
A2) Parallel Dip (weighted) Flat-Bench Curl	5 x 8 Rest 30 seconds
B1) Dumbbell Supine	5 x 10 Rest 30 seconds
B2) Barbell Close-Grip Bench Press	5 x 8 Rest 30 seconds
C1) Barbell Drag Curl	5 x 12 Rest 30 seconds
C2) Dumbbell Seated Kickback	5 x 10 Rest 30 seconds
D) Dumbbell Seated Palms-Up Wrist Curl	5 x 20 Rest 30 seconds
E) Barbell Rollout	5 x 15 Rest 30 seconds

4-Days-Per-Week Schedule • Cycle 4 • Weeks 13 to 16

WORKOUT 1: QUADS AND CALVES

EXERCISE	SETS X REPETITIONS
A) Barbell Front Squat (with crossed arms)	4 x 6 Rest 45 seconds
B) Barbell Walking Lunge	4 x 10 steps Minimal rest
C1) Dumbbell Bulgarian Split Squat	4 x 8 each leg Rest 45 seconds
C2) Dumbbell Goblet Squat	4 x 10 Rest 45 seconds
D) Dumbbell Walking Lunge	4 x 20 steps Rest 60 seconds
E) Barbell Seated Calf Raise	4 x 10 (emphasize eccentric)

WORKOUT 2: CHEST, SHOULDERS, ABS

EXERCISE	SETS X REPETITIONS
A) Barbell Close-Grip Bench Press	4 x 6 Rest 60 seconds
B1) Dumbbell Bench Press	4 x 10 Rest 45 seconds
B2) Dumbbell Standing Press	4 x 12 each arm Rest 45 seconds
B3) Pushup	4 x 20 Rest 45 seconds
C) Seated Barbell Military Press	4 x 6 Rest 30 seconds
D) Dumbbell Lying Incline Rear Lateral Raise	4 x 12 (drop set) Rest 30 seconds
E) Barbell Press Situp	4 x 8

WORKOUT 3: BACK, HAMSTRINGS, TRAPS, CALVES

EXERCISE	SETS X REPETITIONS
A) Barbell Deadlift	4 x 6 Rest 90 seconds
B1) Barbell Overhand-Grip Row	4 x 12 Rest 60 seconds
B2) Pullup (weighted)	4 x 6 Rest 60 seconds
C) Barbell Stiff-Legged Deadlift	4 x 10 Rest 60 seconds
D1) Barbell Behind-the-Back Shrug	4 x 15 Rest 30 seconds
D2) Barbell Standing Calf Raise	4 x 12 (emphasize 3-second eccentric) Rest 30 seconds

WORKOUT 4: BICEPS, TRICEPS, FOREARMS, ABS

EXERCISE	SETS X REPETITIONS
A1) Dumbbell Standing Hammer Curl	4 x 12 Rest 30 seconds
A2) Behind-the-Leg Barbell Triceps Kickback	4 x 10 Rest 30 seconds
B1) Seated Dumbbell Curl	4 x 8 each arm Rest 30 seconds
B2) Barbell Reverse-Grip Bench Press	4 x 6 Rest 30 seconds
C1) EZ Bar Preacher Curl	4 x 8 Rest 30 seconds
C2) Dumbbell Decline Skull Crusher	4 x 12 Rest 30 seconds
D) Seated Palms-Down Dumbbell Wrist Curl	4 x 20 Rest 30 seconds
E) Supine Floor Reverse Crunch	4 x 25

4-Days-Per-Week Schedule • Cycle 5 • Weeks 17 to 20

WORKOUT 1: QUADS AND CALVES

EXERCISE	SETS X REPETITIONS
A) Barbell Squat	4 x 20 Rest 60 seconds
B1) Dumbbell Reverse Lunge	4 x 12 each leg Rest 60 seconds
B2) Barbell Front Squat (with crossed arms)	4 x 8 Rest 60 seconds
B3) Dumbbell Walking Lunge	4 x 20 steps Rest 60 seconds
C1) Barbell Front Squat with Heels Elevated	4 x 6 (5-second eccentric) Rest 30 seconds
C2) Dumbbell Bulgarian Split Squat	4 x 6 each leg Rest 30 seconds
D) Seated Plate Calf Raise	1 x 100 (rest/pause)

WORKOUT 2: CHEST, SHOULDERS, ABS

EXERCISE	SETS X REPETITIONS
A1) Barbell Incline Bench Press	4 x 10 Rest 60 seconds
A2) Dumbbell Arnold Press	4 x 8 Rest 60 seconds
B1) Dumbbell Incline Fly	4 x 15 Rest 30 seconds
B2) Dumbbell Incline Bench Press	4 x 12 Rest 30 seconds
C1) Seated Dumbbell Side Raise	4 x 10 Rest 30 seconds
C2) Dumbbell Standing Press	4 x 8 Rest 30 seconds
D) One-Arm Incline Lateral Raise	4 x 10 each (drop set) Rest 30 seconds
E) Stability Ball Crunch	4 x 15

WORKOUT 3: BACK, HAMSTRINGS, TRAPS, CALVES

EXERCISE	SETS X REPETITIONS
A1) Chinup (weighted)	6 x 6 Rest 60 seconds
A2) Barbell Romanian Deadlift	6 x 6 Rest 60 seconds
B1) Barbell Supine Row	6 x 6 Rest 30 seconds
B2) Dumbbell Single-Arm Row	4 x 20 each arm Rest 30 seconds
B3) Glute Ham Raise with Stability Ball	4 x 15 Rest 30 seconds
B4) Barbell Inverted Row	4 x 20 Rest 2 minutes
C) Barbell Behind-the-Back Shrug	4 x 15 Rest 30 seconds
D) Seated Plate Calf Raise	1 x 100 (rest/pause)

WORKOUT 4: BICEPS, TRICEPS, FOREARMS, ABS

EXERCISE	SETS X REPETITIONS
A1) Dumbbell Zottman Preacher Curl	4 x 8 Rest 30 seconds
A2) Decline Close-Grip Skull Crusher	4 x 10 Rest 30 seconds
B1) Dumbbell Hammer Grip Spider Curl	4 x 10 each Rest 30 seconds
B2) Parallel Dip (weighted)	4 x 8 Rest 30 seconds
C1) EZ Bar Standing Curl	4 x 8 Rest 30 seconds
C2) Barbell Lying Triceps Extension	4 x 12 Rest 30 seconds
D) Seated Palms-Up Barbell Wrist Curl	1 x 100 (rest/pause)
E) Hanging Leg Raise	1 x 50 (rest/pause)

4-Days-Per-Week Schedule • Cycle 6 • Weeks 21 to 24

WORKOUT 1: QUADS AND CALVES

EXERCISE	SETS X REPETITIONS
A) Barbell Squat	10 x 10 Rest 90 seconds
B) Barbell Front Squat (with crossed arms)	8 x 8 Rest 90 seconds
C) Dumbbell Partial Romanian Deadlift	1 x 6, 1 x 12, 1 x 25 Rest 60 seconds
D) Dumbbell Walking Lunge	3 x 10 steps (drop set) Minimal rest
E) Dumbbell Bulgarian Split Squat	4 x 6 each leg
F) Barbell Rocking Standing Calf Raise	1 x 100 (rest/pause)

WORKOUT 2: CHEST, SHOULDERS, ABS

EXERCISE	SETS X REPETITIONS
A) Barbell Bench Press	10 x 10 Rest 60 seconds
B) Barbell Push Press	10 x 10 Rest 60 seconds
C1) Dumbbell Arnold Press	1 x 6, 1 x 12, 1 x 25 Rest 45 seconds
C2) Standing Barbell Front Raise	3 x 8 Rest 45 seconds
D1) Dumbbell Decline Fly	8 x 8 Rest 30 seconds
D2) Dumbbell Bench Press	8 x 8 Rest 30 seconds
E) Stability Ball Knee Tuck	5 x 20 Rest 30 seconds

WORKOUT 3: BACK, HAMSTRINGS, TRAPS, CALVES

EXERCISE	SETS X REPETITIONS
A) Barbell Sumo Deadlift	10 x 10 Rest 90 seconds
B1) Barbell Landmine Row	8 x 8 each arm Rest 60 seconds
B2) Dumbbell Chest-Supported Row	8 x 8 Rest 60 seconds
C) Dumbbell Shrug	4 x 12 Rest 30 seconds
D) Partial Romanian Deadlift	8 x 8 Rest 60 seconds
E) Seated Plate Calf Raise	1 x 100 (rest/pause)

WORKOUT 4: BICEPS, TRICEPS, FOREARMS, ABS

EXERCISE	SETS X REPETITIONS
A1) Barbell Curl	10 x 10 Rest 60 seconds
A2) Barbell Close-Grip Bench Press	10 x 10 Rest 60 seconds
B1) Dumbbell Standing Hammer Curl	8 x 8 Rest 60 seconds
B2) Parallel Dip (weighted)	8 x 8 Rest 60 seconds
C1) Barbell Drag Curl	4 x 10 Rest 30 seconds
C2) Suspended Prone Triceps Extension (blast strap/TRX)	4 x 10 Rest 30 seconds
D) Standing Palms-Up Behind-the-Back Barbell Wrist Curl	1 x 50 (rest/pause)
E) Supine Floor Reverse Crunch	1 x 100 (rest/pause)

5-Days-Per-Week Schedule • Cycle 1 • Weeks 1 to 4

WORKOUT 1: SHOULDERS, TRICEPS, ABS

EXERCISE	SETS X REPETITIONS
A) Barbell Military Press	4 x 8 Rest 90 seconds
B1) Barbell Reverse-Grip Bench Press	4 x 8 Rest 30 seconds
B2) Parallel Dip (weighted)	4 x 10 Rest 30 seconds
C1) Dumbbell Seesaw Press	3 x 10 each arm Rest 60 seconds
C2) Dumbbell Arnold Press	3 x 12 Rest 30 seconds
D1) Dumbbell Seated Triceps Kickback	4 x 8 Rest 30 seconds
D2) Dumbbell Reverse Fly	4 x 10 Rest 30 seconds
E) Supine Floor Reverse Crunch	4 x 20 Rest 30 seconds

WORKOUT 2: QUADS AND CALVES

EXERCISE	SETS X REPETITIONS
A) Barbell Squat	4 x 10 Rest 90 seconds
B1) Dumbbell Bulgarian Split Squat	3 x 12 each leg Rest 30 seconds
B2) Barbell Front Squat (with crossed arms)	3 x 10 Rest 60 seconds
C1) Dumbbell Split Squat	3 x 12 each leg forward Rest 30 seconds
C2) Dumbbell Walking Lunge	3 x 15 steps Rest 60 seconds
D) Barbell Standing Calf Raise	4 x 20 (constant tension) Rest 15–30 seconds

WORKOUT 3: BACK, TRAPS, ABS

EXERCISE	SETS X REPETITIONS
A) Barbell Deadlift	4 x 6 Rest 90 seconds
B1) Chinup	3 x 8 Rest 60 seconds
B2) Dumbbell Single-Arm Row	3 x 12 each arm Rest 60 seconds
C1) Barbell Seated Good Morning	3 x 8 Rest 30 seconds
C2) Barbell Behind-the-Back Shrug	3 x 12 Rest 30 seconds
D) Barbell Rollout	3 x 10 Rest 30 seconds

WORKOUT 4: CHEST, BICEPS, FOREARMS

EXERCISE	SETS X REPETITIONS
A) Barbell Bench Press	4 x 8 Rest 90 seconds
B1) Dumbbell Flat-Chest Fly	3 x 10 Rest 60 seconds
B2) Barbell Incline Bench Press	3 x 12 Rest 60 seconds
C1) Dumbbell Incline Bench Press	3 x 10 Rest 60 seconds
C2) Weighted Pushup	3 x 10 Rest 60 seconds
D) Barbell Curl	4 x 10 Rest 30 seconds
E1) Seated Dumbbell Reverse Curl	3 x 12 Rest 30 seconds
E2) EZ Bar Curl	3 x 10 Rest 30 seconds

WORKOUT 5: HAMSTRINGS AND CALVES

EXERCISE	SETS X REPETITIONS
A) Barbell Romanian Deadlift	4 x 10 Rest 60 seconds
B1) Glute Ham Raise	3 x 12 Rest 30 seconds
B2) Dumbbell Stiff-Legged Deadlift	3 x 10 Rest 30 seconds
C) Barbell Partial Romanian Deadlift	3 x 15 Rest 30 seconds
D) Barbell Standing Calf Raise	4 x 25

5-Days-Per-Week Schedule • Cycle 2 • Weeks 5 to 8

WORKOUT 1: SHOULDERS, TRICEPS, ABS

EXERCISE	SETS X REPETITIONS
A) Barbell Military Press	4 x 6 Rest 90 seconds
B1) Dumbbell Arnold Press	4 x 8 Rest 30 seconds
B2) Parallel Dip	4 x 12 Rest 30 seconds
C1) Dumbbell Seesaw Press	4 x 10 each arm Rest 60 seconds
C2) Barbell Close-Grip Bench Press	4 x 10
D1) Dumbbell Decline Skull Crusher	4 x 8 Rest 30 seconds
D2) Dumbbell Reverse Fly	4 x 10 Rest 30 seconds
E) Supine Floor Reverse Crunch	4 x 20 Rest 30 seconds

WORKOUT 2: QUADS AND CALVES

EXERCISE	SETS X REPETITIONS
A) Barbell Front Squat (with crossed arms)	4 x 15 Rest 60 seconds
B1) Barbell Squat	4 x 10 (drop set) Minimal rest
B2) Dumbbell Reverse Lunge	4 x 8 each leg Rest 60 seconds
C) Barbell Walking Lunge	4 x 15 steps No rest
D) Seated Plate Calf Raise	4 x 10 (emphasize eccentric)

WORKOUT 3: BACK, TRAPS, ABS

EXERCISE	SETS X REPETITIONS
A) Barbell Romanian Deadlift	4 x 8 Rest 90 seconds
B1) Barbell Supine Row	4 x 10 Rest 60 seconds
B2) Wide-Grip Pullup	4 x 8 (emphasize concentric) Rest 60 seconds
B3) Back Extension	4 x 15 Rest 60 seconds
C1) Barbell Snatch Shrug	4 x 12 Rest 60 seconds
C2) Dumbbell Farmer's Walk	4 x 12 Rest 30 seconds
D) Hanging Knee Raise	4 x 15 Rest 30 seconds

WORKOUT 4: CHEST, BICEPS, FOREARMS

EXERCISE	SETS X REPETITIONS
A1) Dumbbell Bench Press	4 x 8 Rest 60 seconds
A2) Dumbbell Incline Chest Fly	4 x 12 Rest 60 seconds
B1) Barbell Wide-Grip Bench Press	4 x 8 Rest 30 seconds
B2) Dumbbell Flat-Chest Fly	4 x 10 Rest 30 seconds
C) Weighted Pushup	4 x 12 Rest 30 seconds
D1) Flexor Incline Dumbbell Curl	4 x 10 Rest 30 seconds
D2) Barbell Reverse-Grip Curl	4 x 8 Rest 30 seconds

WORKOUT 5: HAMSTRINGS AND CALVES

EXERCISE	SETS X REPETITIONS
A) Barbell Stiff-Leg Deadlift	4 x 12 Rest 60 seconds
B1) Dumbbell Romanian Deadlift	4 x 10 Rest 30 seconds
B2) Barbell Split-Stance Romanian Deadlift	4 x 8 each leg Rest 30 seconds
C) Dumbbell Single-Leg Romanian Deadlift	3 x 20 each leg Rest 30 seconds
D) Barbell Seated Calf Raise	5 x 20 Rest 15 seconds
E) Barbell Standing Calf Raise	5 x 10 Rest 15 seconds

5-Days-Per-Week Schedule • Cycle 3 • Weeks 9 to 12

WORKOUT 1: SHOULDERS, TRICEPS, ABS

EXERCISE	SETS X REPETITIONS
A1) Dumbbell Neutral-Grip Seated Press	5 x 8 Rest 30 seconds
A2) Dumbbell Iron Cross	5 x 12 Rest 30 seconds
B1) Reverse-Grip Bench Press	5 x 5 Rest 30 seconds
B2) Bent-Over Dumbbell Rear Deltoid Raise (head on bench)	5 x 15 Rest 30 seconds
C1) Barbell Close-Grip Bench Press	5 x 8 Rest 30 seconds
C2) Dumbbell Seated Kickback	5 x 10 Rest 30 seconds
D) Bench Dip	5 x 10 (drop set) Minimal rest
E) Supine Floor Reverse Crunch	4 x 20

WORKOUT 2: QUADS AND CALVES

EXERCISE	SETS X REPETITIONS
A) Barbell Squat	5 x 20 Rest 2 minutes
B1) Dumbbell Bulgarian Split Squat	5 x 10 each leg Rest 90 seconds
B2) Barbell Zercher Squat	5 x 12 Rest 90 seconds
C) Dumbbell Walking Lunge	5 x 20 steps Rest 60 seconds
D) Donkey Calf Raise	5 x 25 Rest 15 seconds

WORKOUT 3: BACK, TRAPS, ABS

EXERCISE	SETS X REPETITIONS
A) Barbell High Pull	5 x 5 Rest 90 seconds
B1) Pullup	5 x 5 Rest 60 seconds
B2) Trap Bar Deadlift	5 x 10 Rest 60 seconds
C) Barbell Good Morning	5 x 8 Rest 60 seconds
D) Barbell Snatch Shrug	5 x 10 Rest 30 seconds
E) Hanging Leg Raise	5 x 10 Rest 30 seconds

WORKOUT 4: CHEST, BICEPS, FOREARMS

EXERCISE	SETS X REPETITIONS
A) Barbell Incline Bench Press	5 x 8 Rest 90 seconds
B1) Dumbbell Neutral-Grip Incline Bench Press	5 x 10 Rest 60 seconds
B2) Dumbbell Flat-Chest Fly	5 x 15 Rest 60 seconds
C) Weighted Pushup	5 x 10 (drop set) Minimal rest
D1) Dumbbell Zottman Curl	5 x 10 Rest 30 seconds
D2) Chest-Supported Spider Curl	5 x 10 Rest 30 seconds
E) EZ Bar Reverse-Grip Curl	5 x 10 Rest 30 seconds

WORKOUT 5: HAMSTRINGS AND CALVES

EXERCISE	SETS X REPETITIONS
A) Sumo Deadlift	5 x 10
B) Barbell Split-Stance Romanian Deadlift	5 x 10 Rest 60 seconds
C) Barbell Good Morning	5 x 8 Rest 60 seconds
D1) Barbell Wide-Stance Stiff-Legged Romanian Deadlift	5 x 10 Rest 30 seconds
D2) Glute-Ham Raise	5 x 8 (emphasize eccentric) No rest
E) Barbell Seated Calf Raise	5 x 20 Rest 15 seconds
F) Standing Dumbbell Calf Raise	1 x 50 (rest pause; emphasize eccentric) Rest 15 seconds

5-Days-Per-Week Schedule • Cycle 4 • Weeks 13 to 16

WORKOUT 1: SHOULDERS, TRICEPS, ABS

EXERCISE	SETS X REPETITIONS
A) Barbell Push Press	4 x 6 Rest 90 seconds
B) Incline Dumbbell Shoulder Press (75 degrees)	4 x 10 Rest 90 seconds
C1) Barbell Reverse-Grip Bench Press	4 x 10 Rest 60 seconds
C2) Bent-Over Dumbbell Rear Deltoid Raise (standing)	4 x 20 Rest 60 seconds
D) Barbell Decline Close-Grip Skull Crusher	4 x 10 (drop set) Minimal rest
E) Behind-the-Leg Barbell Triceps Kickback	4 x 10 (drop set) Minimal rest
F) Hanging Leg Raise	4 x 15 Rest 30 seconds

WORKOUT 2: QUADS AND CALVES

EXERCISE	SETS X REPETITIONS
A) Barbell Bulgarian Split Squat	4 x 6 each leg Rest 45 seconds
B) Barbell Lunge Combo (front/reverse)	4 x 6 each leg Minimal rest
C) Barbell Front Squat (heels elevated)	4 x 8 Rest 45 seconds
D) Dumbbell Walking Lunge	4 x 20 steps Rest 60 seconds
E) Barbell Seated Calf Raise	4 x 10 (emphasize eccentric)

WORKOUT 3: BACK, TRAPS, ABS

EXERCISE	SETS X REPETITIONS
A) Barbell Deadlift	4 x 6 Rest 90 seconds
B1) Barbell Inverted Row	4 x 12 Rest 60 seconds
B2) Pullup	4 x 6 Rest 60 seconds
C1) Face Pull (TRX)	4 x 10 Rest 60 seconds
C2) Power-Clean Shrug	4 x 6 Rest 60 seconds
D) Barbell Rollout	4 x 10 Rest 30 seconds

WORKOUT 4: CHEST, BICEPS, FOREARMS

EXERCISE	SETS X REPETITIONS
A) Barbell Bench Press	4 x 6 Rest 90 seconds
B1) Barbell Neck Bench Press	4 x 10 Rest 60 seconds
B2) Dumbbell Decline Bench Press	4 x 10 Rest 60 seconds
C) Feet-Elevated Pushup	4 x 10 (drop set) Minimal rest
D) Elbows-Out Parallel Dip	4 x 10 (drop set) Minimal rest
E1) Standing Alternate Dumbbell Biceps Curl	4 x 8 each arm Rest 30 seconds
E2) Dumbbell Cross-Body Hammer Curl	4 x 10 each arm Rest 30 seconds

WORKOUT 5: HAMSTRINGS AND CALVES

EXERCISE	SETS X REPETITIONS
A) Sumo Deadlift	4 x 8 Rest 90 seconds
B) Dumbbell Stiff-Legged Deadlift	4 x 8 Rest 60 seconds
C) Glute-Ham Raise	4 x 6 Rest 60 seconds
D) Barbell Romanian Deadlift	4 x 12 (emphasize eccentric) Rest 60 seconds
E) Barbell Standing Calf Raise	1 x 75 (rest/pause)

5-Days-Per-Week Schedule • Cycle 5 • Weeks 17 to 20

WORKOUT 1: SHOULDERS, TRICEPS, ABS

EXERCISE	SETS X REPETITIONS
A) Dumbbell Arnold Press	8 x 8 Rest 90 seconds
B) Barbell Push Press	8 x 8 Rest 60 seconds
C1) Incline Dumbbell Shoulder Press (75 degrees)	6 x 6 Rest 60 seconds
C2) Bent-Over Dumbbell Rear Deltoid Raise (standing)	3 x 20 Rest 60 seconds
D) Dumbbell Decline Skull Crusher	3 x 10 (drop set) Minimal rest
E) Bench Dip (weighted)	4 x 10 (drop set) Minimal rest
F) Hanging Leg Raise	4 x 15 Rest 30 seconds

WORKOUT 2: QUADS AND CALVES

EXERCISE	SETS X REPETITIONS
A) Barbell Front Squat (with crossed arms)	10 x 10 Rest 60 seconds
B) Barbell Reverse Lunge	8 x 8 each leg Rest 60 seconds
C) Dumbbell Bulgarian Split Squat	3 x 8 each leg Rest 30 seconds
D) Barbell Walking Lunge	3 x 15 steps Rest 60 seconds
E) Donkey Calf Raise	5 x 20 (emphasize eccentric)

WORKOUT 3: BACK, TRAPS, ABS

EXERCISE	SETS X REPETITIONS
A) Barbell Deadlift	8 x 8 Rest 90 seconds
B1) Chinup	3 x 6 Rest 60 seconds
B2) Dumbbell Single-Arm Row	3 x 10 each arm Rest 60 seconds
C1) Suspended Inverted Row with TRX	3 x 15 Rest 60 seconds
C2) Dumbbell Shrug	3 x 20 Rest 60 seconds
D) Stability Ball Crunch	5 x 10 Rest 30 seconds

WORKOUT 4: CHEST, BICEPS, FOREARMS

EXERCISE	SETS X REPETITIONS
A) Dumbbell Incline Bench Press	8 x 8 Rest 60 seconds
B) Seated Close-Grip Concentration Curl	8 x 8 Rest 60 seconds
C1) Dumbbell Flat-Chest Fly	3 x 12 Rest 30 seconds
C2) Dumbbell Bench Press	3 x 8 Rest 30 seconds
D1) Barbell Reverse-Grip Curl	4 x 10 Rest 30 seconds
D2) Standing Hammer Curl	4 x 12 Rest 30 seconds

WORKOUT 5: HAMSTRINGS AND CALVES

EXERCISE	SETS X REPETITIONS
A) Barbell Romanian Deadlift	8 x 8 Rest 90 seconds
B) Glute Ham Raise	3 x 8 Rest 60 seconds
C) Barbell Stiff-Legged Deadlift	3 x 15 Rest 60 seconds
D) Barbell Standing Calf Raise	1 x 75 (rest/pause) Minimal rest
E) Barbell Seated Calf Raise	1 x 75 (rest/pause) Minimal rest

5-Days-Per-Week Schedule • Cycle 6 • Weeks 21 to 24

WORKOUT 1: SHOULDERS, TRICEPS, ABS

EXERCISE	SETS X REPETITIONS
A) Standing Neutral-Grip Press	10 x 10 Rest 60 seconds
B) Parallel Dip (weighted)	10 x 10 Rest 60 seconds
C1) Dumbbell Arnold Press	1 x 6, 1 x 12, 1 x 25 Rest 45 seconds
C2) Barbell Standing Front Raise	3 x 8 Rest 45 seconds
D1) Barbell Close-Grip Bench Press	1 x 6, 1 x 12, 1 x 25 Rest 60 seconds
D2) Barbell Decline Close-Grip Skull Crusher	3 x 8 Rest 60 seconds
E) Bent-Over Dumbbell Rear Deltoid Raise (head on bench)	Rear 3 x 20 (drop set) Rest 60 seconds
F) Stability Ball Knee Tuck	3 x 20 Rest 30 seconds

WORKOUT 2: QUADS AND CALVES

EXERCISE	SETS X REPETITIONS
A) Barbell Squat	10 x 10 Rest 60 seconds
B) Barbell Zercher Squat	8 x 8 Rest 60 seconds
C1) Dumbbell Split Squat	1 x 6, 1 x 12, 1 x 25 Rest 30 seconds
C2) Dumbbell Reverse Lunge	1 x 6, 1 x 12, 1 x 25 Rest 30 seconds
D) Standing Bent-Knee One-legged Calf Raise	5 x 10 each leg (emphasize eccentric)

WORKOUT 3: BACK, TRAPS, ABS

EXERCISE	SETS X REPETITIONS
A) Barbell Romanian Deadlift	10 x 10 Rest 60 seconds
B) Pullup	10 x 10 Rest 60 seconds
C1) Supine Row	1 x 6, 1 x 12, 1 x 25 Rest 60 seconds
C2) Barbell Shrug	1 x 6, 1 x 12, 1 x 25 Rest 60 seconds
C3) Dumbbell Elbows-Out Row	1 x 6, 1 x 12, 1 x 25 Rest 60 seconds
D) Hanging Leg Raise	1 x 50 (rest/pause) Rest 30 seconds

WORKOUT 4: CHEST, BICEPS, FOREARMS

EXERCISE	SETS X REPETITIONS
A) Barbell Incline Bench Press	10 x 10 Rest 60 seconds
B) Dumbbell Bench Press	10 x 10 Rest 60 seconds
C) Dumbbell Standing Hammer Curl	10 x 10 Rest 30 seconds
D1) Dumbbell Incline Fly	1 x 6, 1 x 12, 1 x 25 Rest 30 seconds
D2) Dumbbell Incline Bench Press	1 x 6, 1 x 12, 1 x 25 Rest 30 seconds
E) Flexor Incline Dumbbell Curl	1 x 6, 1 x 12, 1 x 25 Rest 30 seconds
F) Dumbbell Zottman Preacher Curl	3 x 10 Rest 30 seconds

WORKOUT 5: HAMSTRINGS AND CALVES

EXERCISE	SETS X REPETITIONS
A) Barbell Romanian Deadlift	8 x 8 Rest 90 seconds
B) Glute Ham Raise	3 x 8 Rest 60 seconds
C) Barbell Stiff-Legged Deadlift	3 x 15 Rest 60 seconds
D) Barbell Standing Calf Raise	1 x 75 (rest/pause) Minimal rest
E) Barbell Seated Calf Raise	1 x 75 (rest/pause) Minimal rest

PART 3

CHAPTER 10

The Exercises

In this chapter, you'll find descriptions for all the exercises in the 24-week program organized according to main muscle worked and type of resistance used.

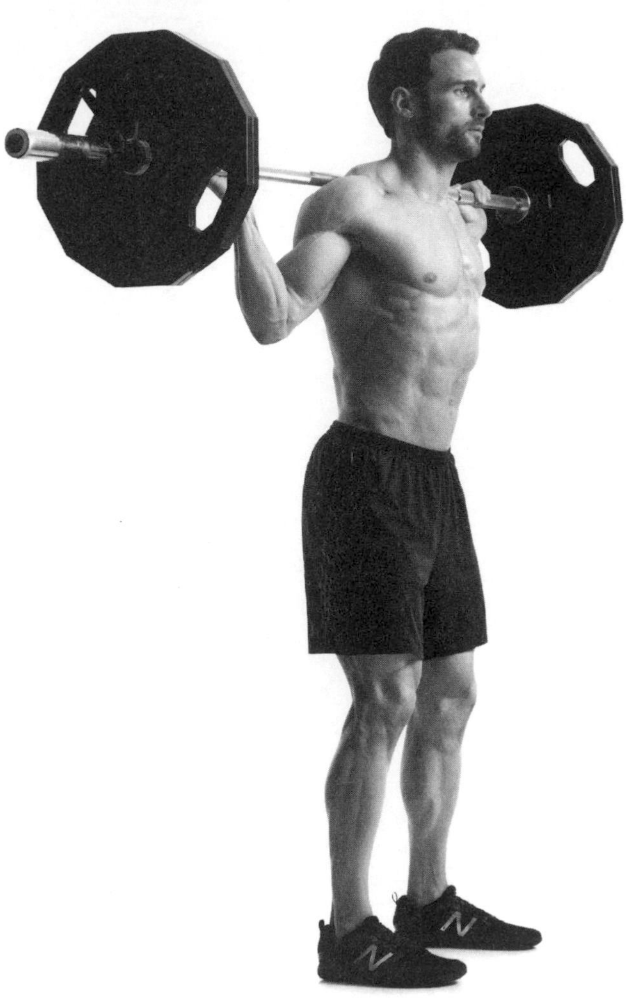

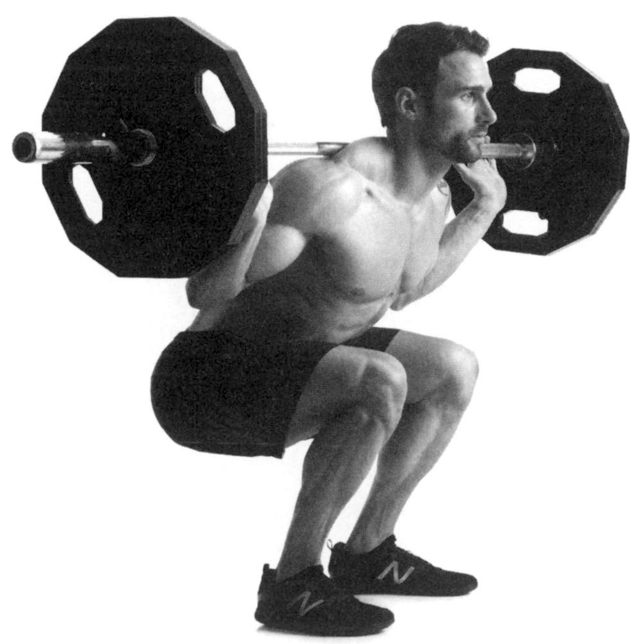

SQUAT

PURPOSE
To create overall leg development through the quadriceps, hamstrings, glutes, and calves.

START
Hold the barbell across your upper back with an overhand grip. Pull your shoulder blades back to create a shelf for the bar to rest. Brace your core. Set your feet shoulder width apart.

MOVEMENT
Maintaining a natural arch in your lower back, lower your body by pushing your hips back while bending at your knees.

FINISH
Pause as deep as you can, then drive your heels into the ground and return to the starting position.

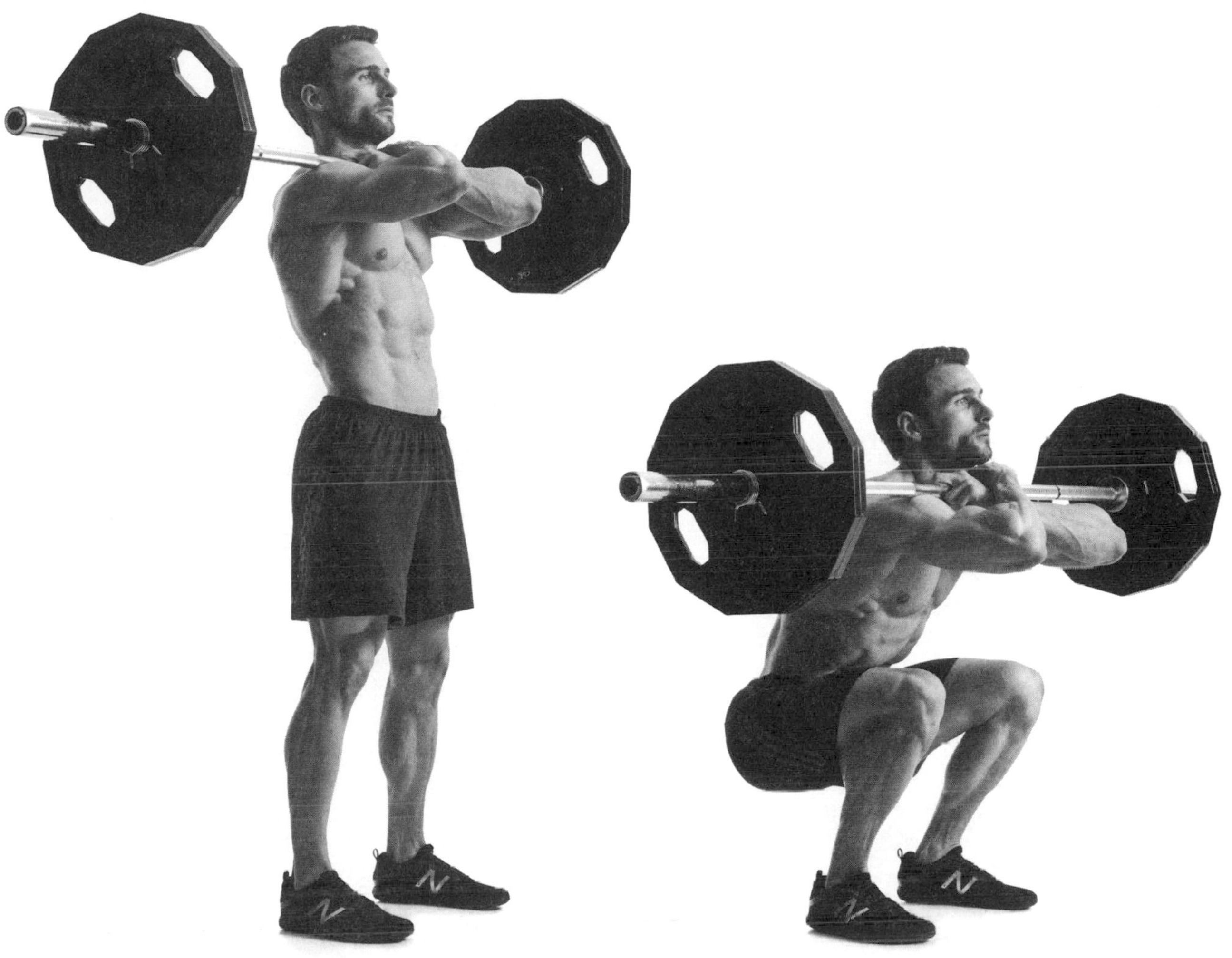

FRONT SQUAT WITH CROSSED ARMS

PURPOSE

A front squat variation made popular by bodybuilders past and a good variation for those who lack shoulder mobility.

START

Step under a barbell on the squat rack then cross your arms in front of you allowing your hands to come over the top of the bar and your thumbs under the bar. Allow the bar to rest on the top of your shoulders.

MOVEMENT

Raise your arms up slightly above your shoulders. Step back away with the barbell resting on your shoulders. Pushing through your heels, core braced, slowly lower your body keeping your arms and thighs parallel to the floor throughout the movement.

FINISH

Pause at the bottom, parallel or deeper. Push through your heels and return to the top position.

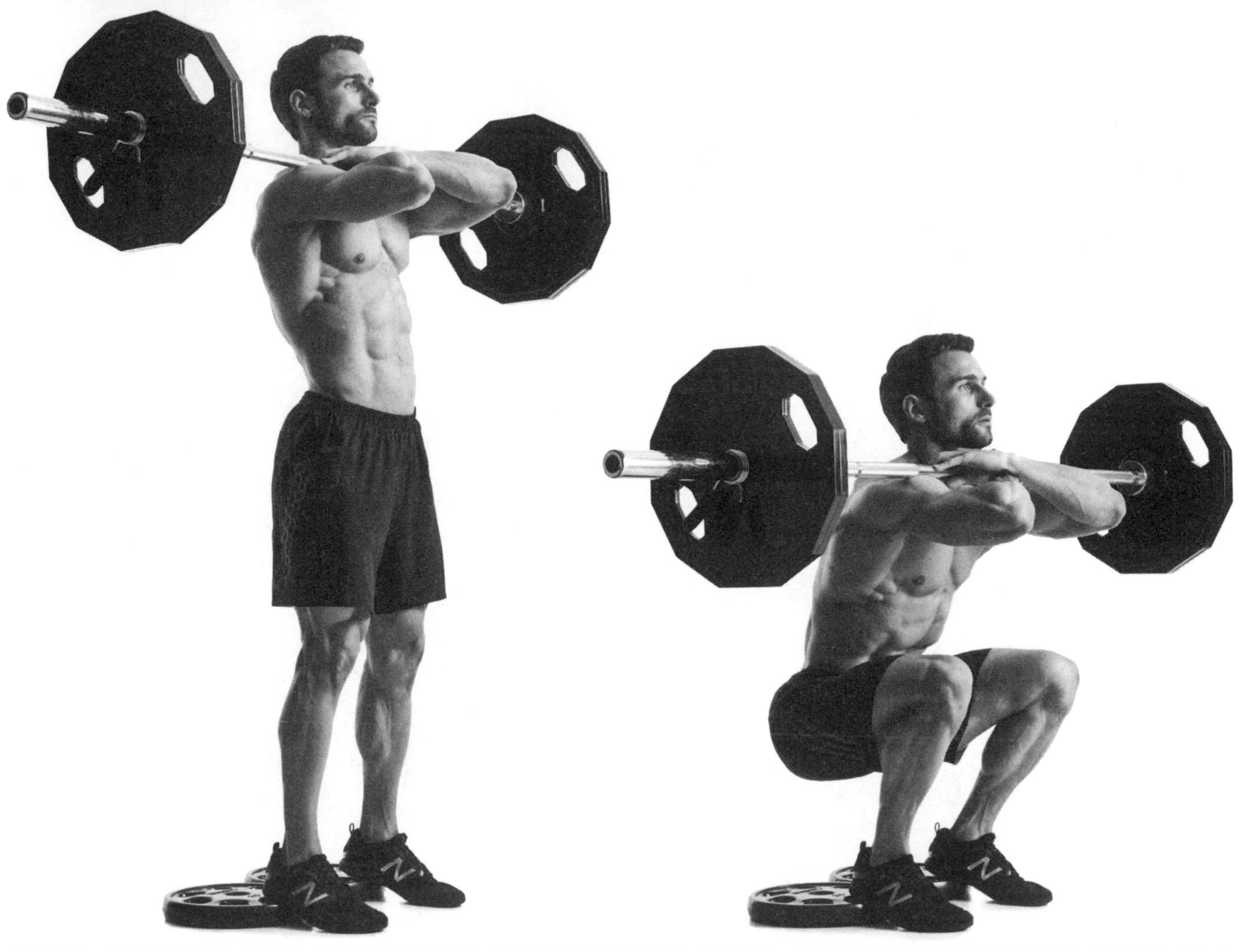

FRONT SQUAT WITH HEELS ELEVATED

PURPOSE

To put greater emphasis on the quadriceps during the squat.

START

Position a pair of 25-pound weight plates behind your heels. Using either the hands shoulder width or crossed-arms position, set the bar in the front squat position on top of your shoulders. Allow the bar to rest on top of the shoulders.

MOVEMENT

Raising your arms to your shoulder height, step away and place your heels on top of the 25-pound weight plates. Push your hips back, bending your knees and pushing through your heels (on top of the weight plates). Lower your body as far as you can.

FINISH

Pause at the bottom, push through the heels and return to the starting position.

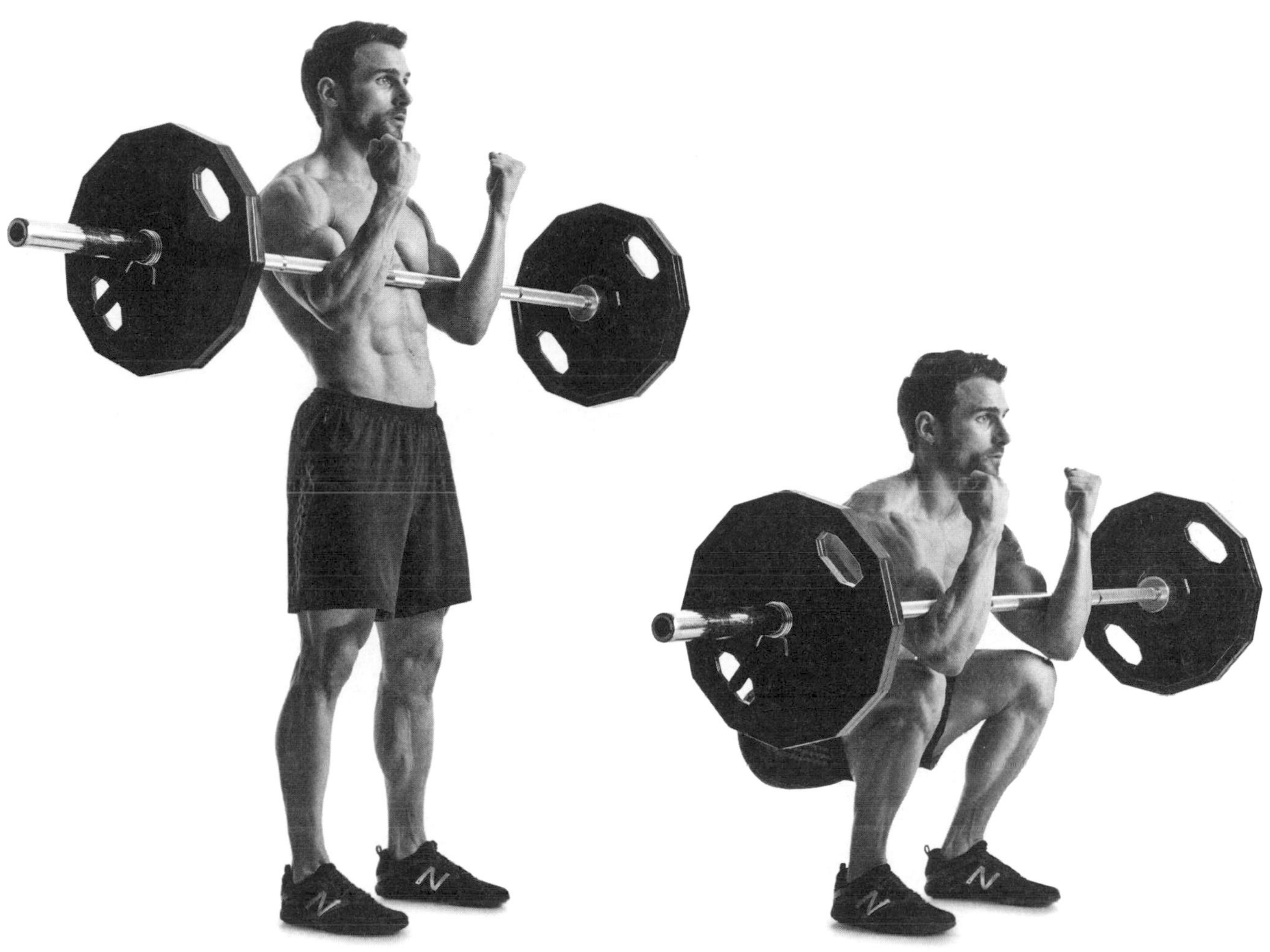

ZERCHER SQUAT

PURPOSE

Target posterior muscle chain as well as the quads and simultaneously activate the shoulders and biceps to control the bar. Invented by 1930s strongman, Ed Zercher, the squat variation allows for a safe deep squat, due to the fact it is front loaded and minimizes spinal load.

START

With the bar placed on a squat rack at mid abdominal height, hold the bar tightly in the crook of your arms—tightly across your chest. Step back away from the rack.

MOVEMENT

Keep your torso tight and hold the bar tightly against your chest with your arms. Lower yourself toward the ground pushing through your heels.

FINISH

Pause, then push yourself back to your starting position.

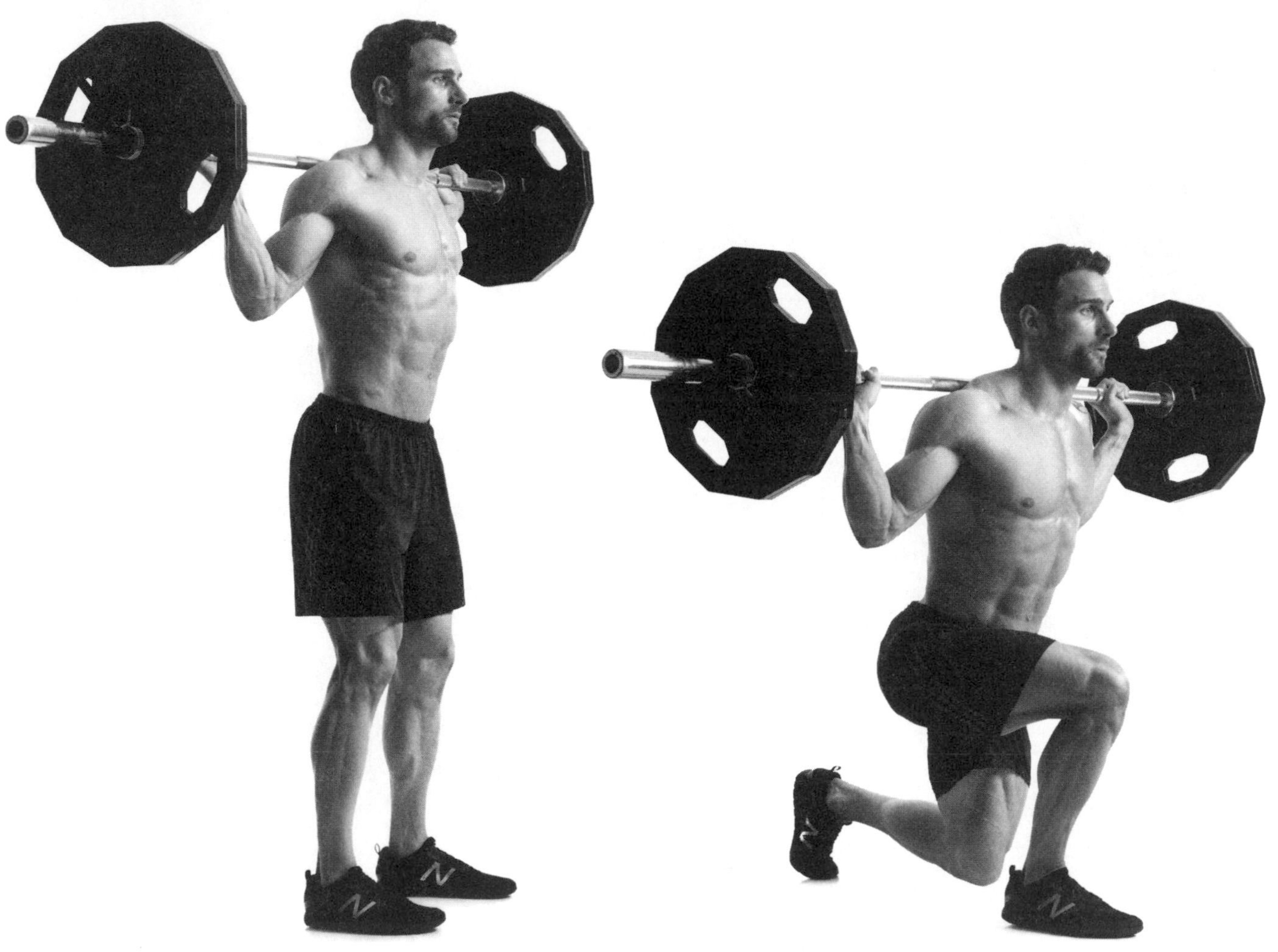

REVERSE LUNGE

PURPOSE
To isolate the quadriceps through unilateral training.

START
Hold the barbell across your upper back with an overhand grip. Pull your shoulder blades back to create a shelf for the bar to rest. Brace your core. Set your feet shoulder width apart.

MOVEMENT
Maintain one leg stationary and take a large backward stride in a lunging fashion, placing your weight on the ball of your foot. Simultaneously sit back into your lunge until your back leg finishes 1 to 2 inches off the floor. The front leg will be bent at 90 degrees with your thigh parallel and shin perpendicular to the floor.

FINISH
Push off your front leg to return to the starting position.

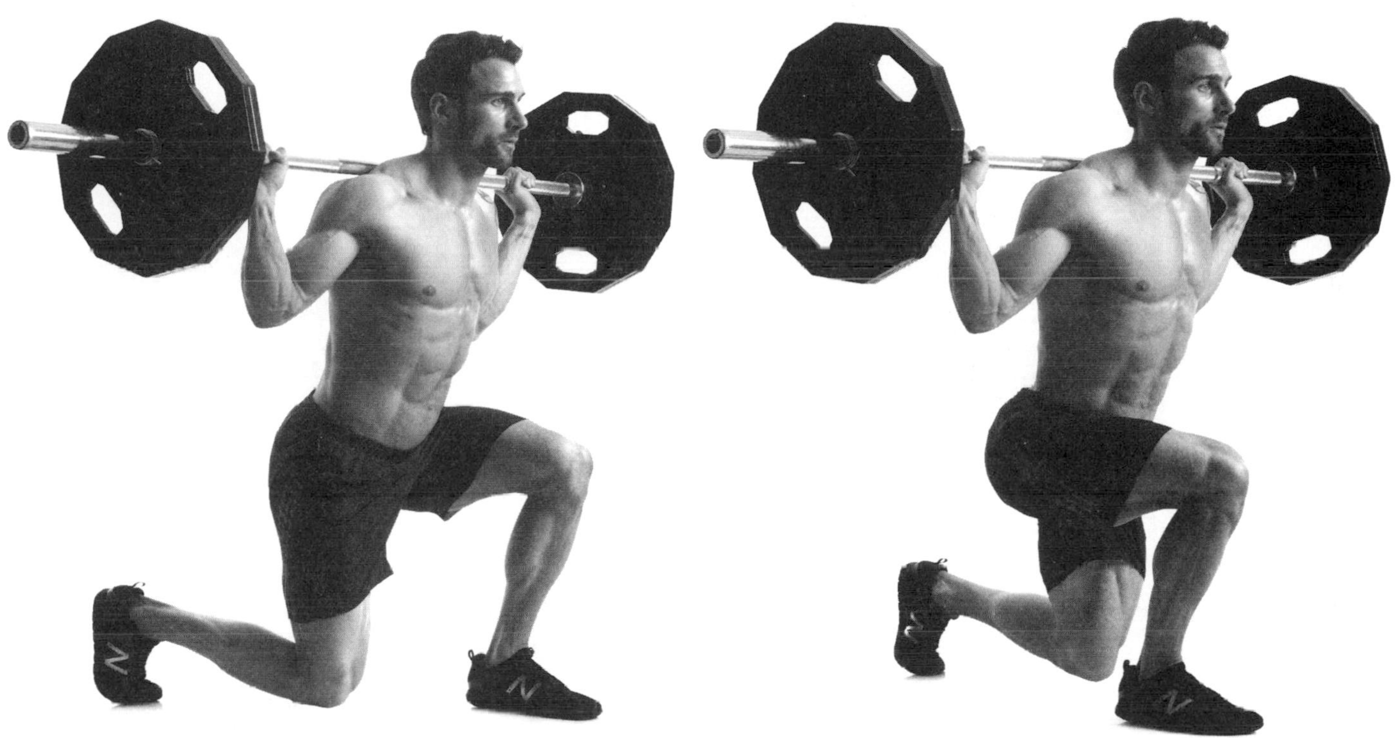

WALKING LUNGE

PURPOSE

Target the quadriceps, glutes, and hamstrings while adding a degree of difficulty by traveling.

START

Hold the barbell across your upper back with an overhand grip. Pull your shoulder blades back to create a shelf for the bar to rest. Brace your core. Set your feet shoulder width apart.

MOVEMENT

Take a large stride forward placing your weight on the heel of your front foot. Simultaneously bend your back knee until it finishes 1 to 2 inches off the ground and your weight is transferred to the ball of your back foot. Pushing through your front heel, return to the starting position while transferring your nondominant (back) leg to the front position in a walking manner. Continue to alternate sides.

FINISH

Return to the shoulder-width apart standing position to rack the barbell.

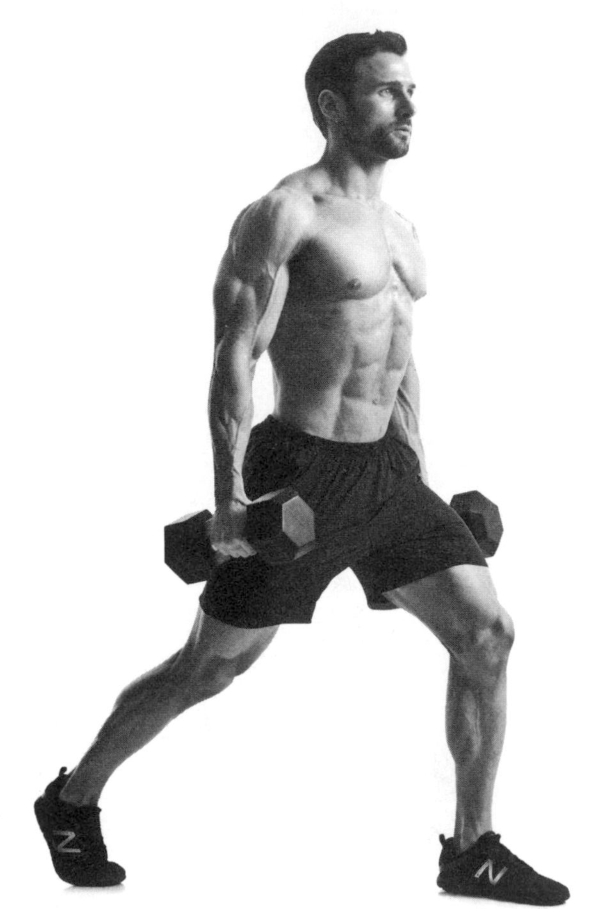

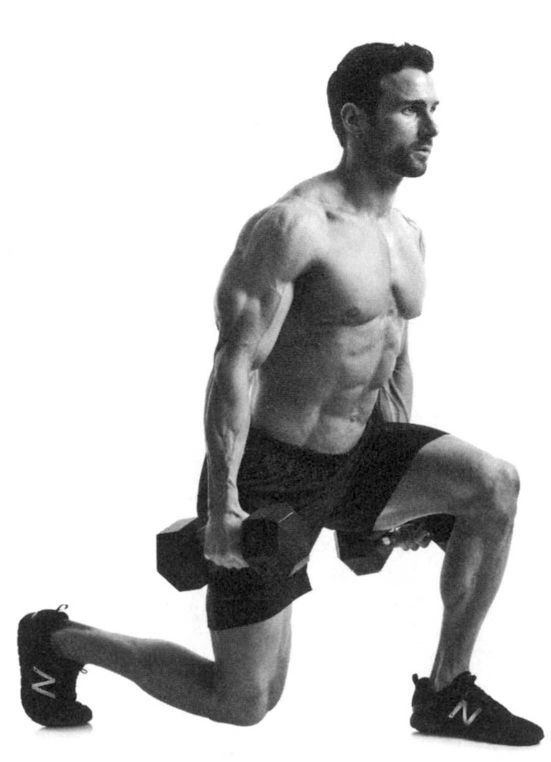

SPLIT SQUAT

PURPOSE

Target the quads, glutes, and calves.

START

Hold two dumbbells and allow them to hang at your sides just outside your hips. Place one foot about 3 feet (depending on your height) in front of the other, maintaining a hip-width placement of your feet.

MOVEMENT

Keeping your front foot flat, push through your heel while your back foot maintains the weight on the ball of your foot. Bending both knees, lower your body until your front quadriceps is parallel to the ground and your back knee finishes just off the floor. Maintain your weight on your front heel and make sure your knee does not come over your front toes.

FINISH

Push through your front heel and return to the top position.

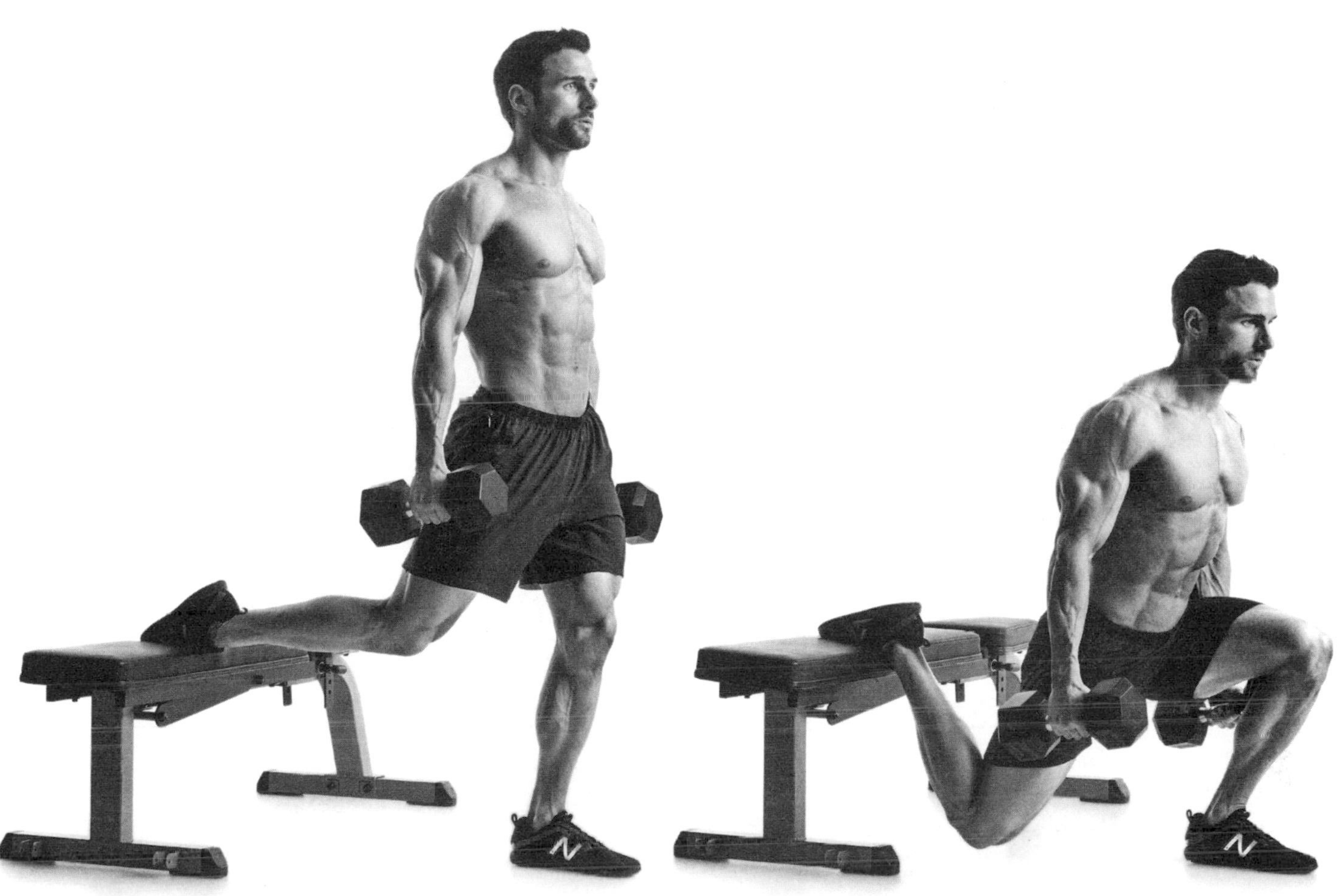

BULGARIAN SPLIT SQUAT

PURPOSE

To put even greater isolation on your quadriceps through unilateral training. Unlike most exercises, this exercise will cause microtrauma to the muscle fibers of the quadriceps.

START

Hold two dumbbells and allow them to hang at your sides just outside your hips. Place one foot about 3 feet (depending on your height) in front of the other, maintaining a hip-width placement of your feet. Place your back toes on a bench.

MOVEMENT

Lower yourself as far as your range of motion will allow (this range can be limited by a lack of hip flexor and quadriceps flexibility). Your front quadriceps may end up lower than parallel, and your weight should stay on your front heel.

FINISH

Pushing through your front heel and flexing your glutes, return to the top.

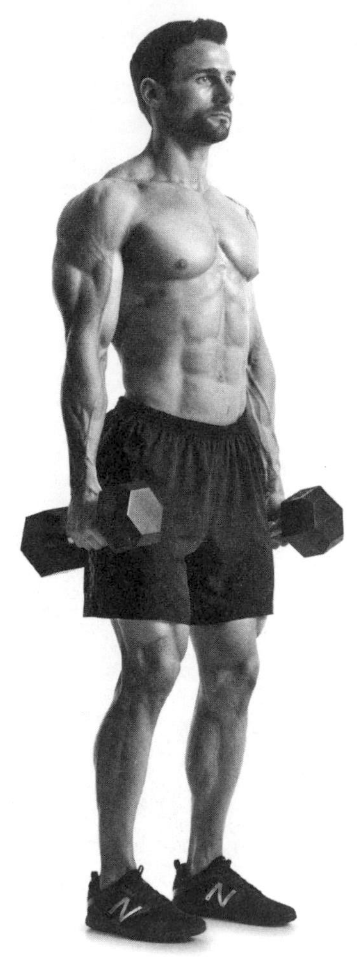

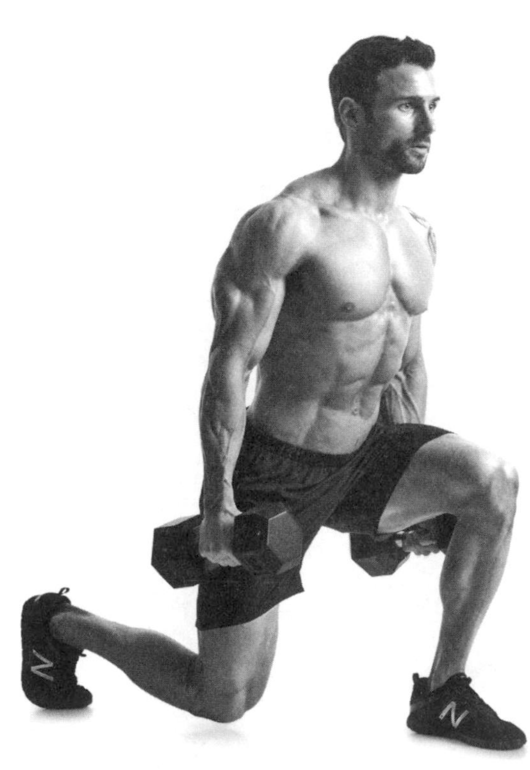

FRONT LUNGE

PURPOSE

Target the quads, glutes, and calves.

START

Stand with feet hip width apart and dumbbells at your sides.

MOVEMENT

Maintaining a hip-width-apart position, step forward into a lunging pattern with your weight on your front heel. Allow your back foot to transfer its weight to the ball of your foot and slowly lower your back knee to 1 to 2 inches off the floor.

FINISH

Using the opposite pattern, push off your front heel and return to your hip-width standing position.

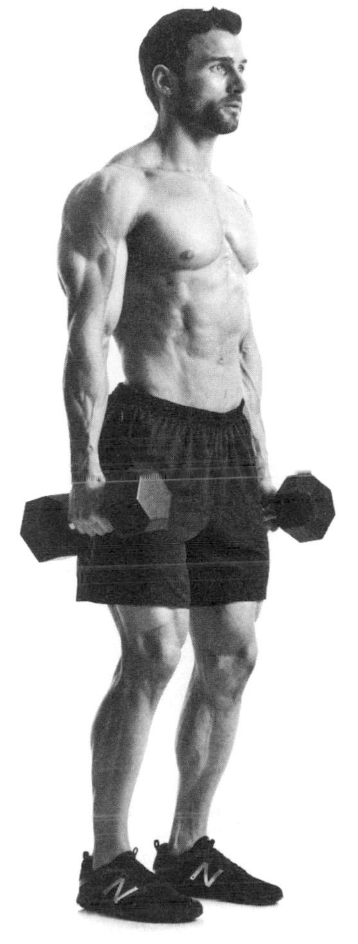

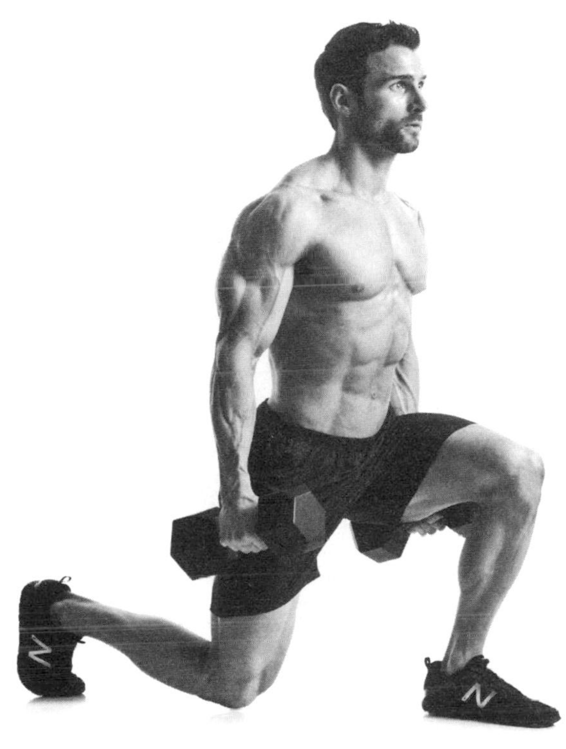

REVERSE LUNGE

PURPOSE

Isolate the quadriceps through unilateral training.

START

Hold two dumbbells at your sides. Brace your core and set your feet shoulder width apart.

MOVEMENT

Keeping one leg stationary, take a large backward stride in a lunging fashion, placing your weight on the ball of your foot. Simultaneously sit back into your lunge until your back leg finishes 1 to 2 inches off the floor. The front leg will be bent at 90 degrees with your thigh parallel and shin perpendicular to the floor.

FINISH

Push off your front leg to return to the starting position.

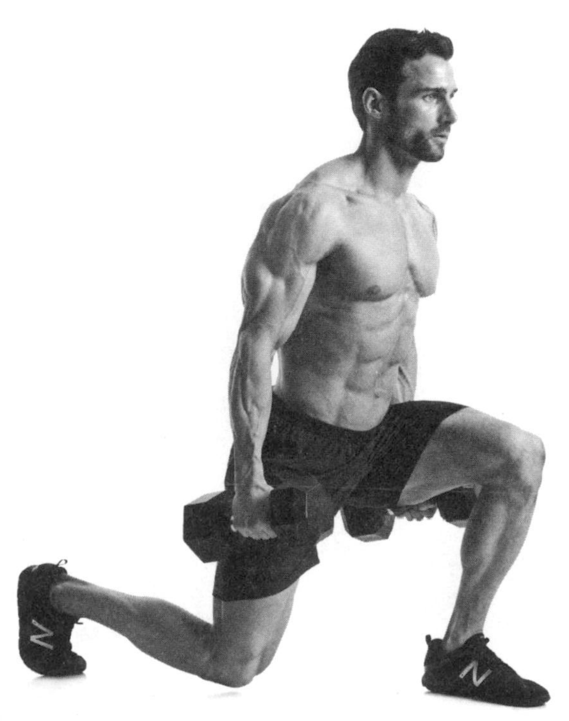

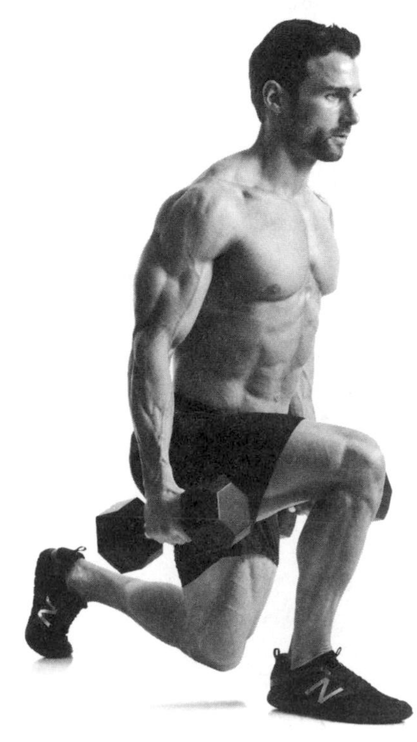

WALKING LUNGE

PURPOSE

Target the quadriceps, glutes, and hamstrings while adding a degree of difficulty by traveling but with less spinal stress than when using a barbell.

START

Hold dumbbells at your sides. Brace your core. Set your feet shoulder width apart.

MOVEMENT

Take a large stride forward placing your weight on your front heel of your foot. Simultaneously bend your back knee until it finishes 1 to 2 inches off the ground and your weight is transferred to the ball of your back foot. Pushing through your front heel, return to the starting position while transferring your non-dominant (back) leg to the front position in a walking manner. Continue to alternate sides.

FINISH

Return to the shoulder-width-apart standing position.

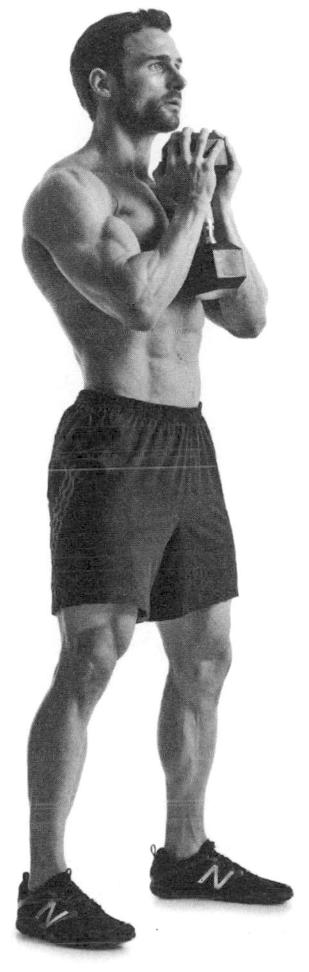

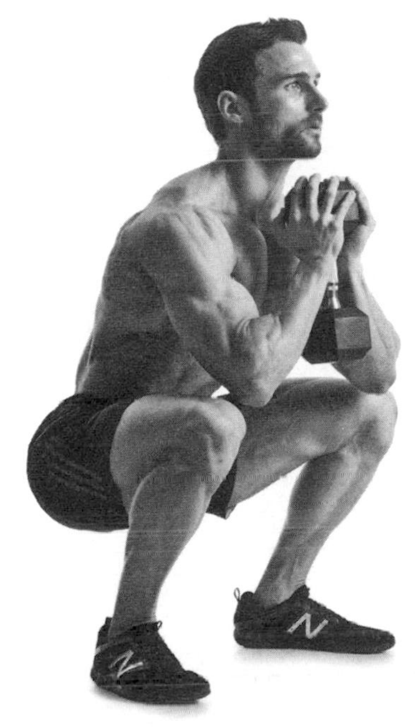

GOBLET SQUAT

PURPOSE

To front load the squatting pattern and place greater emphasis on the quadriceps.

START

Grab a single dumbbell in a bottoms-up position with your palms under the sides of the dumbbell. Set your feet shoulder width apart.

MOVEMENT

Maintain your posture by keeping your chest up and slightly arching your lower back. Push your hips back and push through your heels and lower your body to the floor until your quadriceps finish at parallel or lower. Keep the dumbbell head above your mid chest, elbows down, and shoulder blades flexed.

FINISH

Push through your heels and return to the standing position.

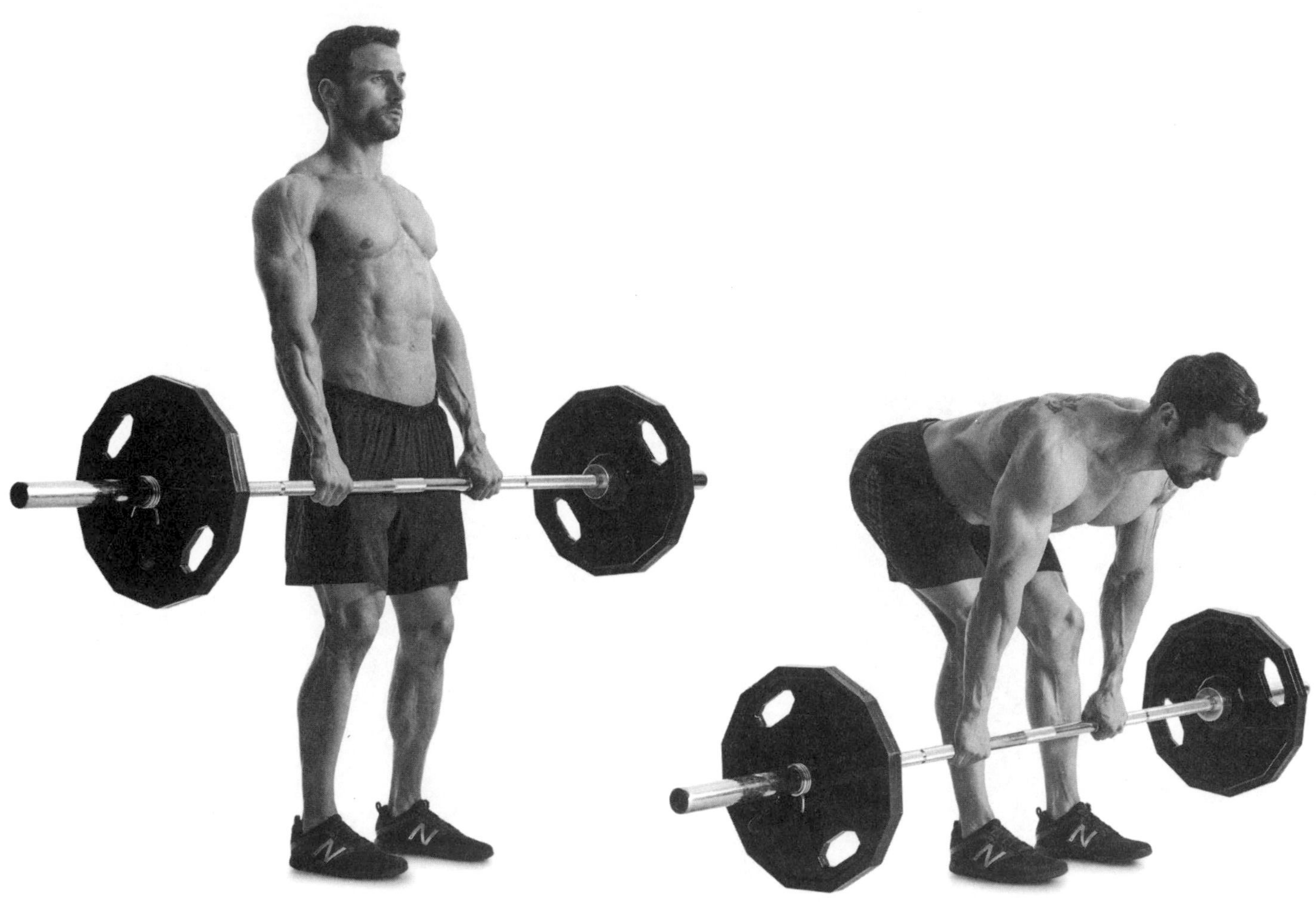

ROMANIAN DEADLIFT

PURPOSE

Target the glutes and hamstrings.

START

Grab a barbell with an overhand grip just wider than shoulder width and hold the bar in front of your hips. Keep your feet hip width apart.

MOVEMENT

Push your chest out and maintain a slight bend in your knees. Keep your back flat but with a natural arch and do not change the slight bend in your knees as you lower your torso to parallel with the floor. Be sure to brace your core through the entire movement.

FINISH

Pause, squeeze your glutes, and push your hips forward, returning to the starting position.

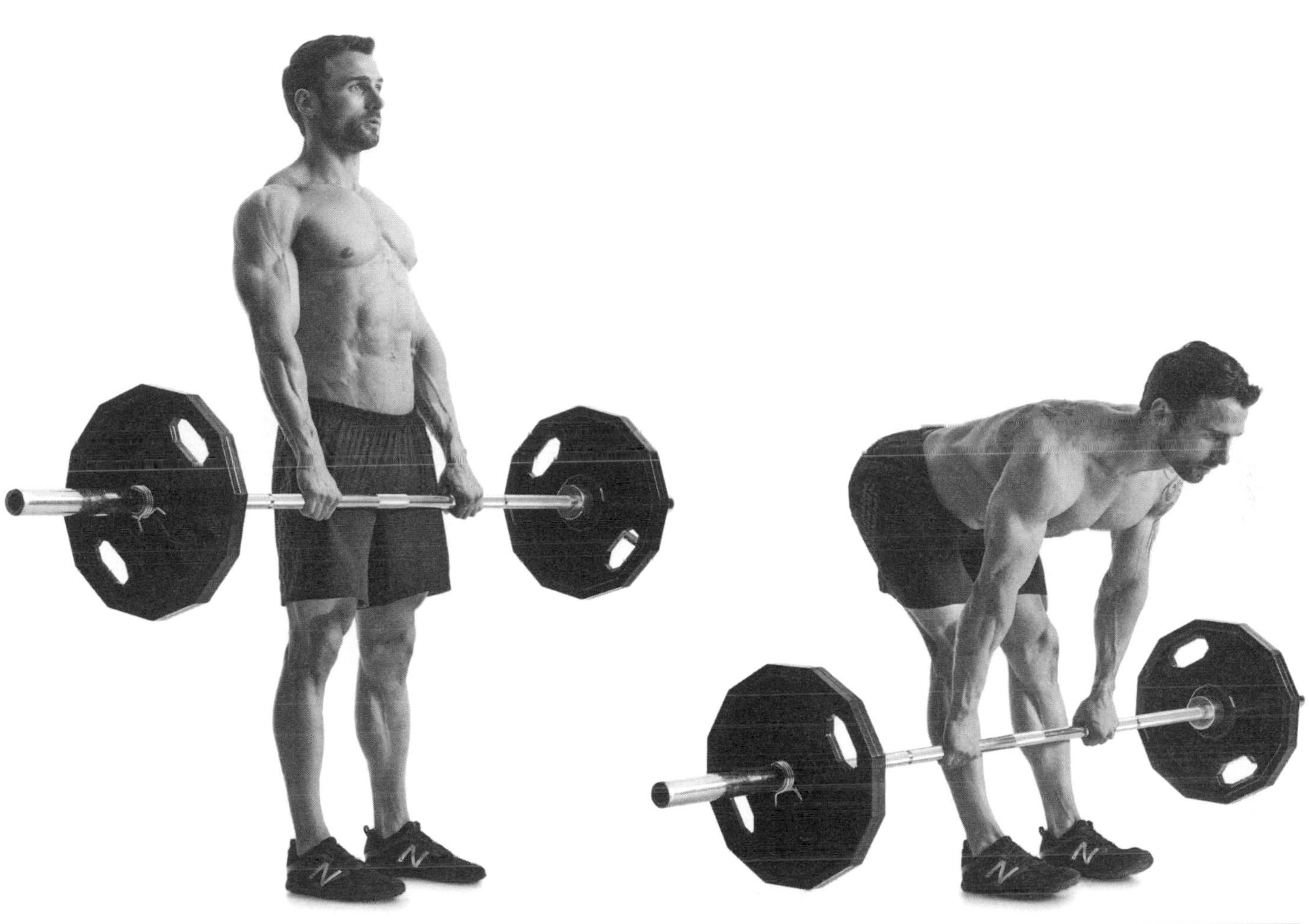

STIFF-LEGGED DEADLIFT

PURPOSE
Target the lower back and hamstrings.

START
Grab a barbell with an overhand grip just wider than shoulder width and hold the bar in front of your hips. Keep your feet hip width apart.

MOVEMENT
Push your chest out and lock out your knees. Keep your back flat but with a natural arch and lower your torso to parallel with the floor. Be sure to brace your core through the entire movement.

FINISH
Pause, squeeze your glutes, and push your hips forward, returning to the starting position.

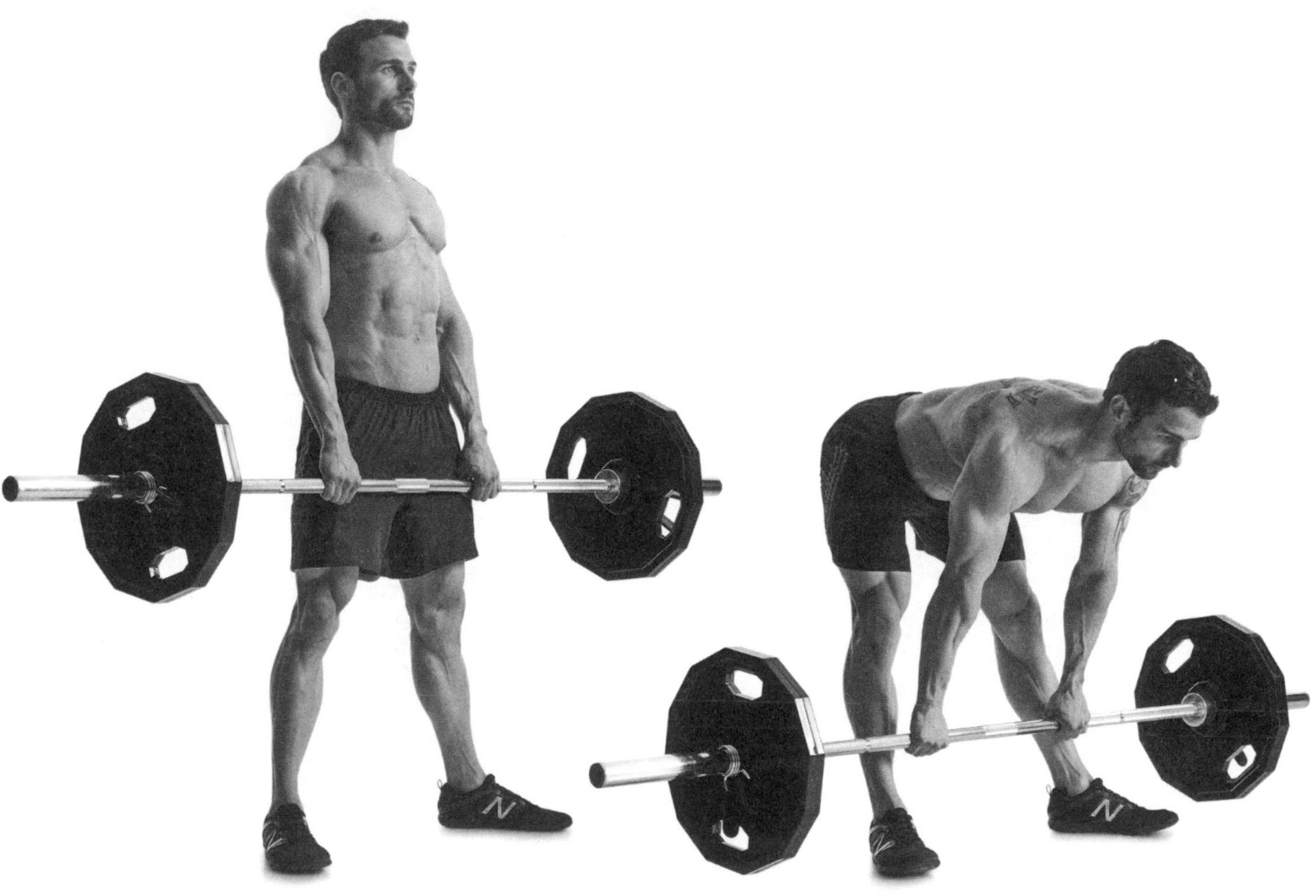

WIDE-STANCE STIFF-LEGGED DEADLIFT

PURPOSE

Target the lower back and hamstrings.

START

Grab a barbell with an overhand grip just wider than shoulder width and hold the bar in front of your hips. Place your feet about twice as wide as shoulder width apart and your toes pointed slightly outward.

MOVEMENT

Push your chest out and lock your knees. Keep your back flat but with a natural arch and lower your torso to parallel with the floor. Be sure to brace your core through the entire movement.

FINISH

Pause, squeeze your glutes, and push your hips forward, returning to the starting position.

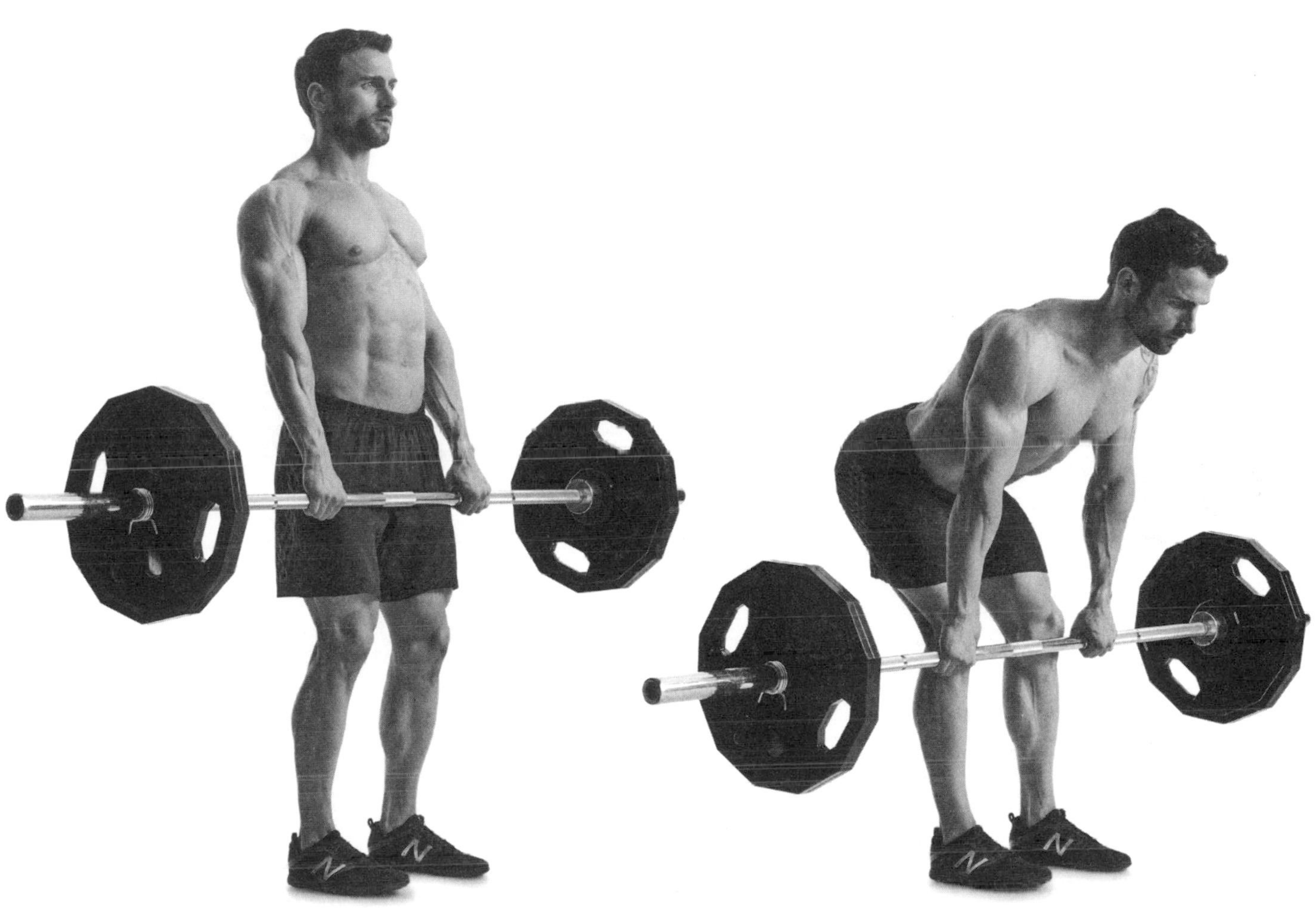

PARTIAL ROMANIAN DEADLIFT

PURPOSE

Target the glutes and hamstrings by creating constant tension on the muscles.

START

Grab a barbell with an overhand grip just wider than shoulder width and hold the bar in front of your hips. Keep your feet hip width apart.

MOVEMENT

Push your chest out and maintain a slight bend in your knees. Keep your back flat but with a natural arch and do not change the slight bend in your knees as you lower your torso to parallel with the floor. Be sure to brace your core through the entire movement.

FINISH

Pause, squeeze your glutes, and push your hips forward, returning halfway to the starting position before lowering and repeating.

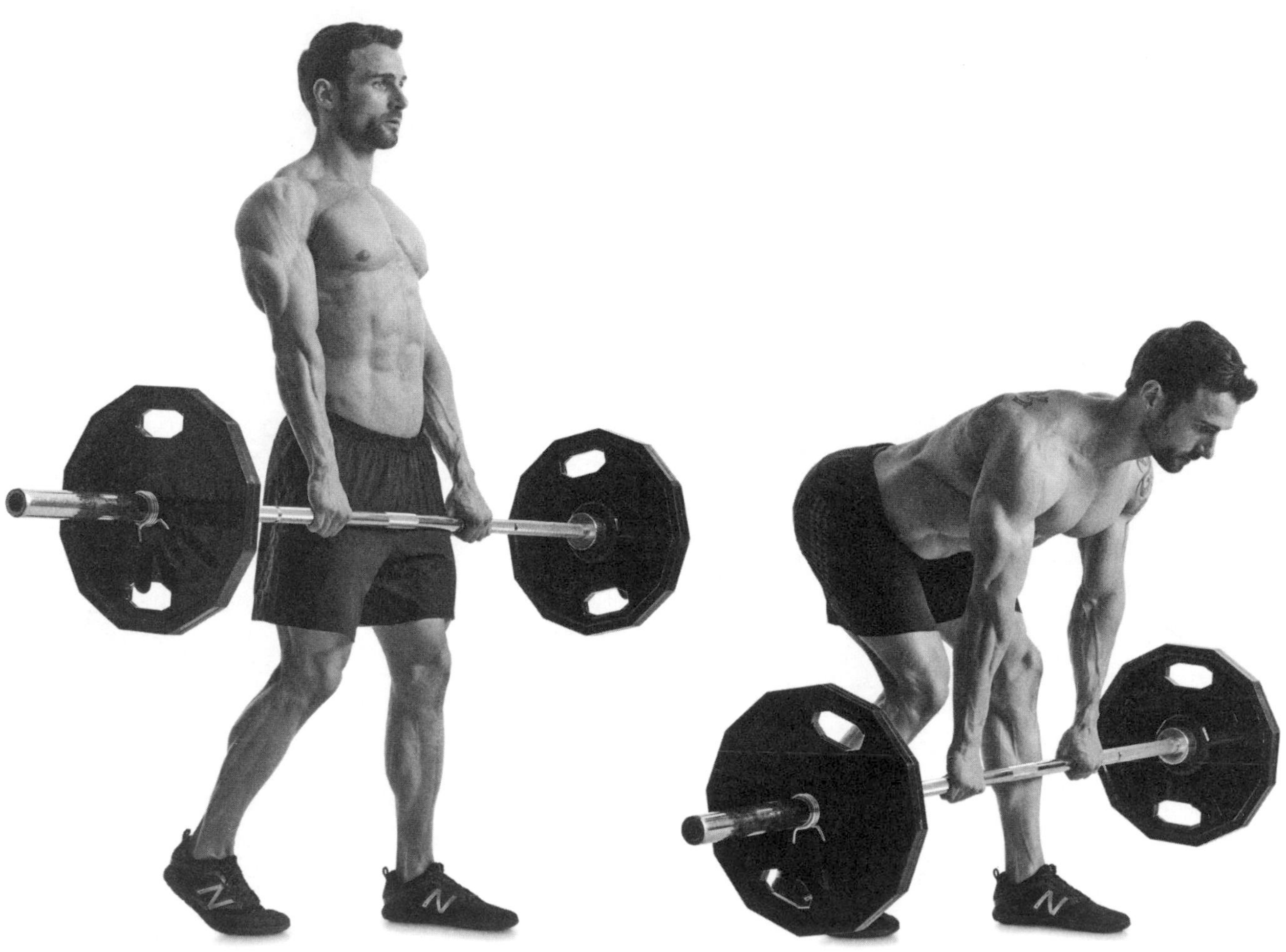

SPLIT-STANCE ROMANIAN DEADLIFT

PURPOSE

Target the glutes and hamstrings through unilateral training.

START

Grab a barbell with an overhand grip just wider than shoulder width and hold the bar in front of your hips. Keep your feet hip width apart and stagger your feet slightly so one foot is only a few inches in front of the other.

MOVEMENT

Push your chest out and maintain a slight bend in your knees. Keep your back flat but with a natural arch and do not change the slight bend in your front knee. Keeping the weight on the heel of your front leg, lower your torso to parallel with the floor and allow your back leg to bend at the knee. Be sure to brace your core through the entire movement.

FINISH

Pause, squeeze your glutes, and push your hips forward, returning to the starting position.

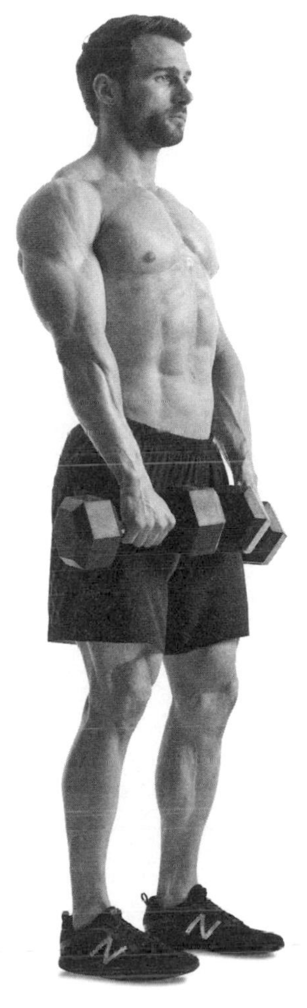

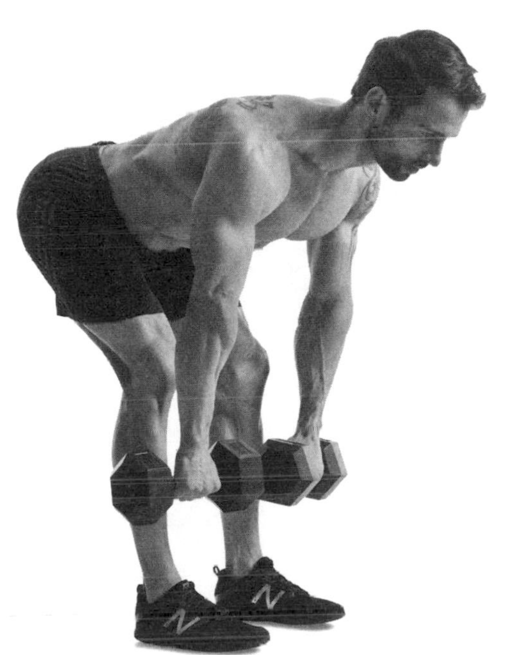

ROMANIAN DEADLIFT

PURPOSE

Target the glutes and hamstrings.

START

Grab a pair of dumbbells with an overhand grip and hold the dumbbells in front of your hips. Keep your feet hip width apart.

MOVEMENT

Push your chest out and maintain a slight bend in your knees. Keep your back flat but with a natural arch and do not change the slight bend in your knees as you lower your torso to parallel with the floor. Be sure to brace your core through the entire movement.

FINISH

Pause, squeeze your glutes, and push your hips forward, returning to the starting position.

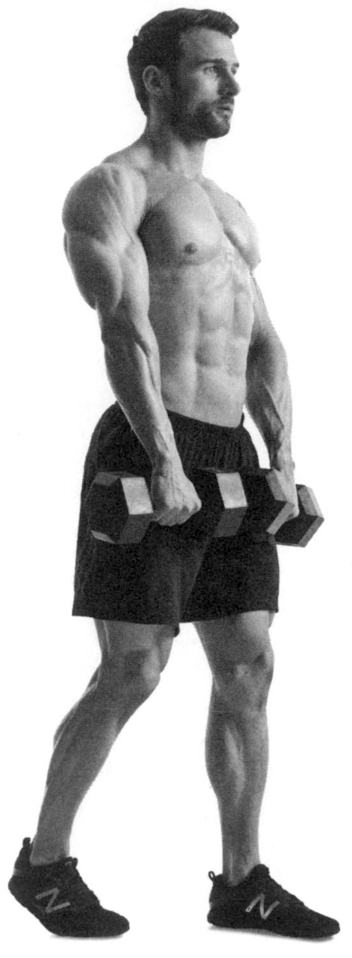

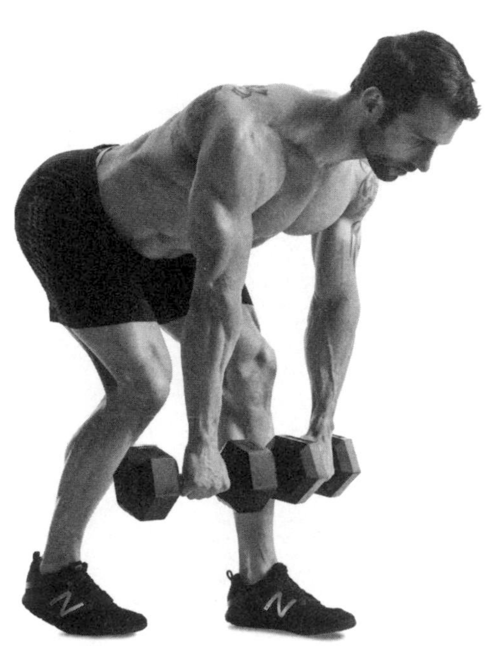

SPLIT-STANCE ROMANIAN DEADLIFT

PURPOSE

Target the glutes and hamstrings through unilateral training.

START

Grab a pair of dumbbells with an overhand grip and hold the dumbbells in front of your hips. Keep your feet hip width apart and stagger your feet slightly so one foot is only a few inches in front of the other.

MOVEMENT

Push your chest out and maintain a slight bend in your knees. Keep your back flat but with a natural arch and do not change the slight bend in your front knee. Keeping the weight on the heel of your front leg, lower your torso to parallel with the floor and allow your back leg to bend at the knee. Be sure to brace your core through the entire movement.

FINISH

Pause, squeeze your glutes, and push your hips forward, returning to the starting position.

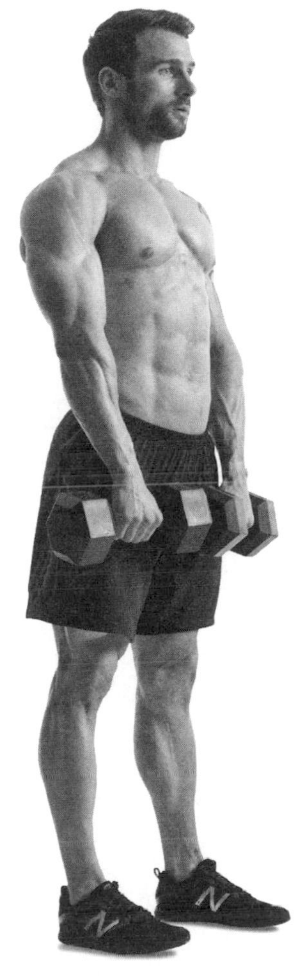

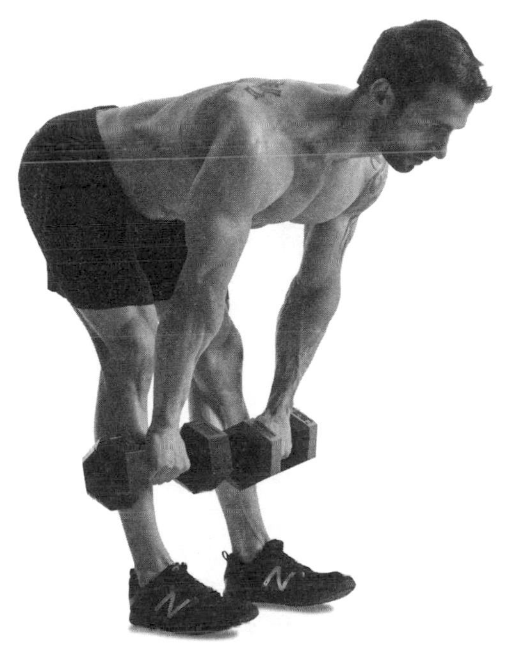

STIFF-LEGGED ROMANIAN DEADLIFT

PURPOSE

Target the lower back and hamstrings.

START

Grab a pair of dumbbells with an overhand grip and hold the dumbbells in front of your hips. Keep your feet hip width apart.

MOVEMENT

Push your chest out and lock out your knees. Keep your back flat but with a natural arch and lower your torso to parallel with the floor. Be sure to brace your core through the entire movement.

FINISH

Pause, squeeze your glutes, and push your hips forward, returning to the starting position.

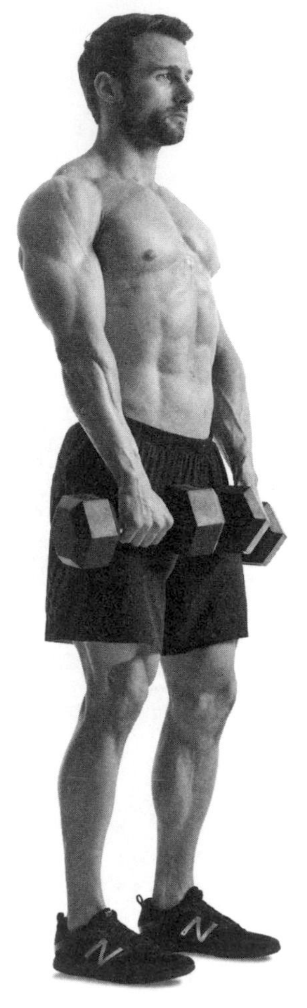

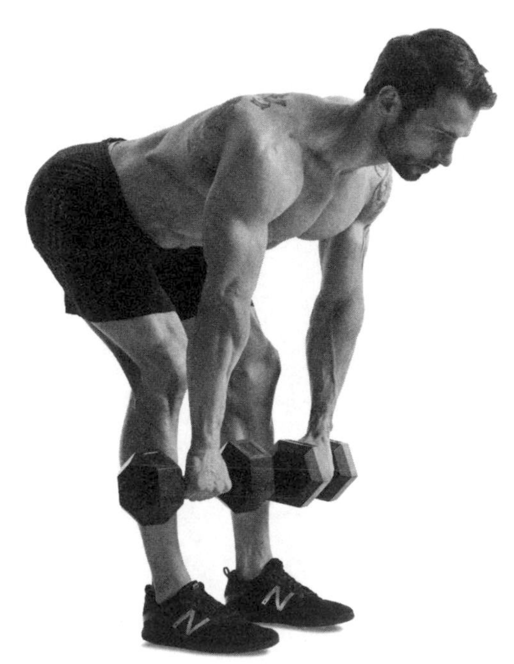

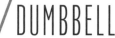

PARTIAL ROMANIAN DEADLIFT

PURPOSE

Target the glutes and hamstrings by creating constant tension on the muscles.

START

Grab a pair of dumbbells with an overhand grip and hold the dumbbells in front of your hips. Keep your feet hip width apart.

MOVEMENT

Push your chest out and maintain a slight bend in your knees. Keep your back flat but with a natural arch and do not change the slight bend in your knees as you lower your torso to parallel with the floor. Be sure to brace your core through the entire movement.

FINISH

Pause, squeeze your glutes, and push your hips forward, returning halfway to the starting position before lowering and repeating.

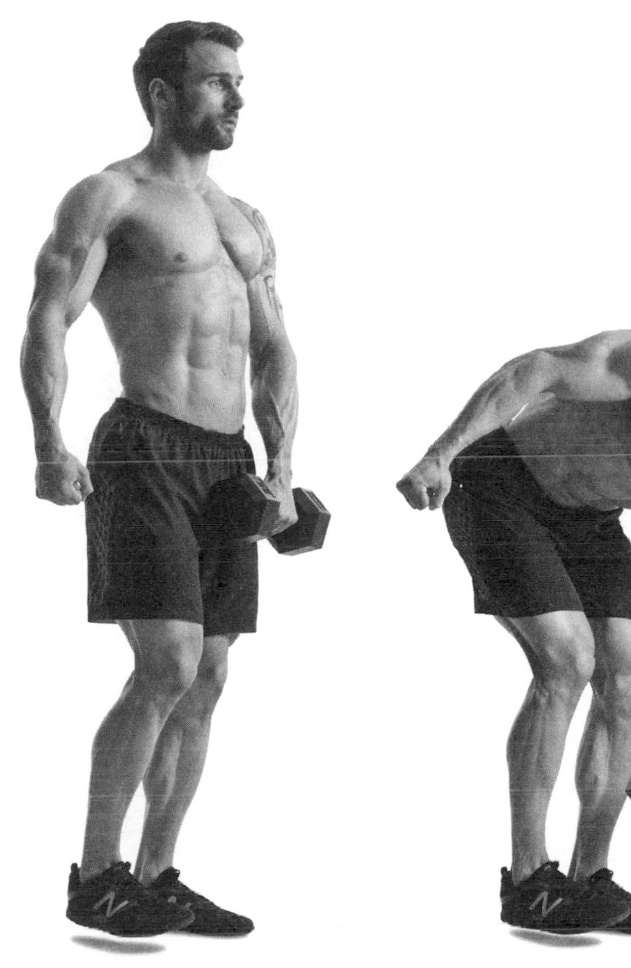

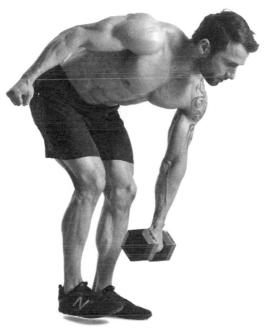

SINGLE-LEG ROMANIAN DEADLIFT

PURPOSE

Target the glutes and hamstrings by creating constant tension on the muscles.

START

Grab a single dumbbell with an overhand grip and hold the dumbbell just over the hip of the grounded leg. Elevate one foot just slightly off the ground. Keep your feet hip width apart.

MOVEMENT

Push your chest out and maintain a slight bend in your knee on your grounded foot. Keep your back flat but with a natural arch and do not change the slight bend in your knee on the grounded leg, as you lower your torso to parallel with the floor. Keep the dumbbell tight to the leg. Be sure to brace your core through the entire movement.

FINISH

Pause, squeeze your glutes, push your hips forward, and return to the starting position with the dumbbell in front of the hip.

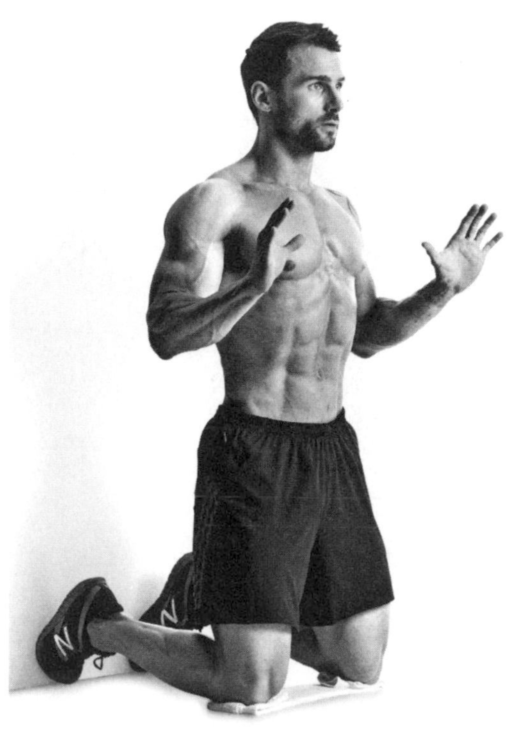

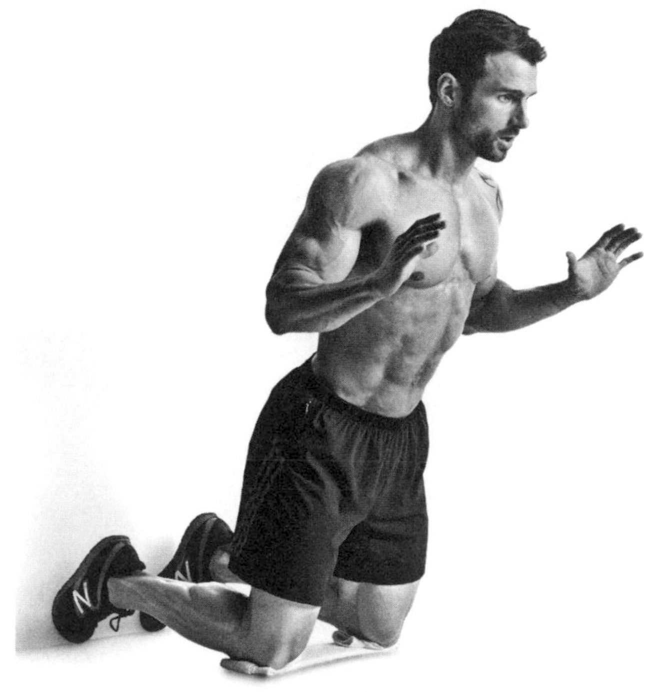

GLUTE-HAM RAISE

PURPOSE

Target the glutes and hamstrings.

START

Place your ankles between the padded supports or wedge your feet against a wall as shown. Create a 90-degree angle with your upper and lower leg. Hold your hands out in front of your chest and squeeze your shoulder blades together.

MOVEMENT

Slowly lower your torso forward while flexing your glutes and maintaining your hips, not allowing your body to bend at the waist.

FINISH

Pull your body upright by flexing at the knees and pulling with your hamstrings and glutes until you return to the starting position.

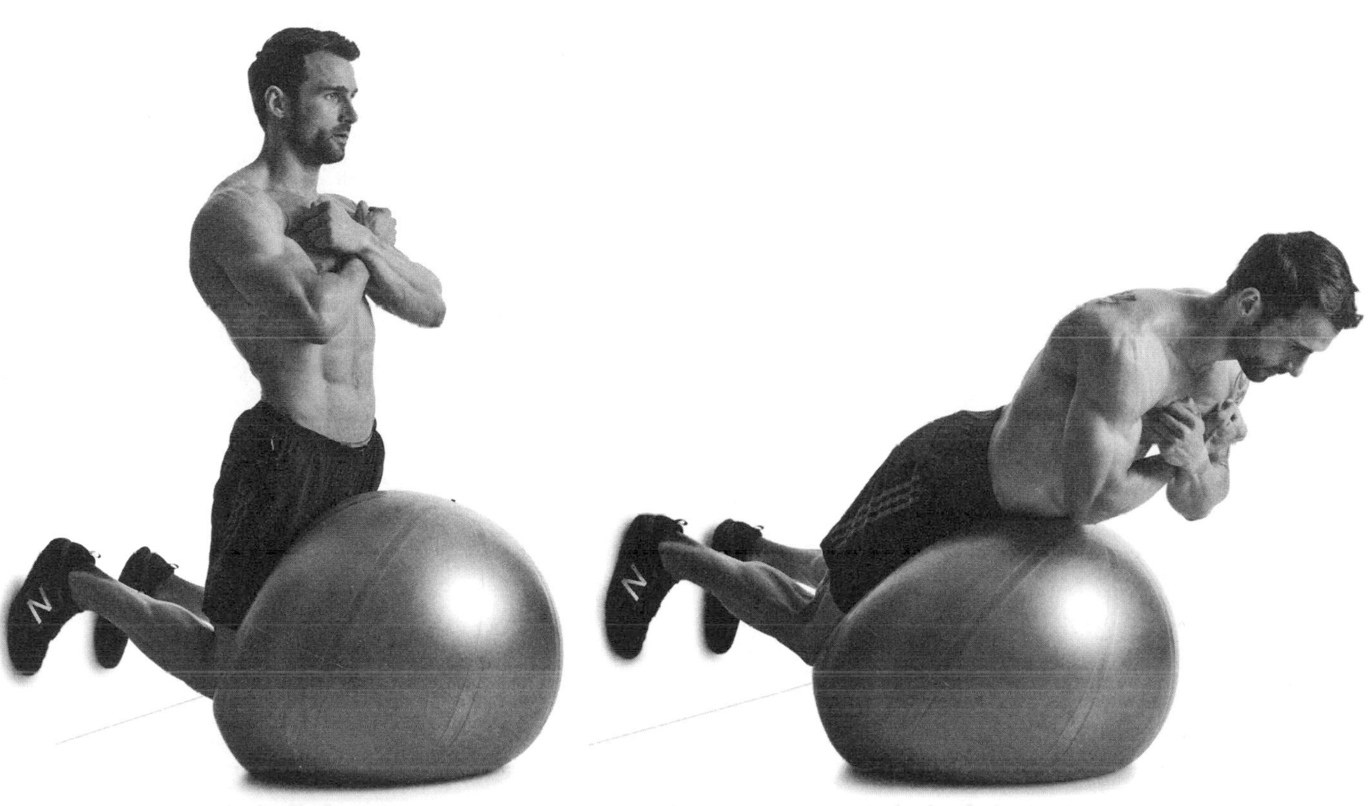

GLUTE-HAM RAISE WITH STABILITY BALL

START

Place your body on top of a stability ball so the stability ball is on your upper quads. Place your feet against a wall and create a 90-degree angle with your upper and lower leg. Cross your arms on your chest and squeeze your shoulder blades together.

MOVEMENT

Slowly lower your torso forward while flexing your glutes and maintaining your hips, not allowing your body to bend at the waist.

FINISH

Pull your body upright by flexing at the knees and pulling with your hamstrings and glutes until you return to the starting position.

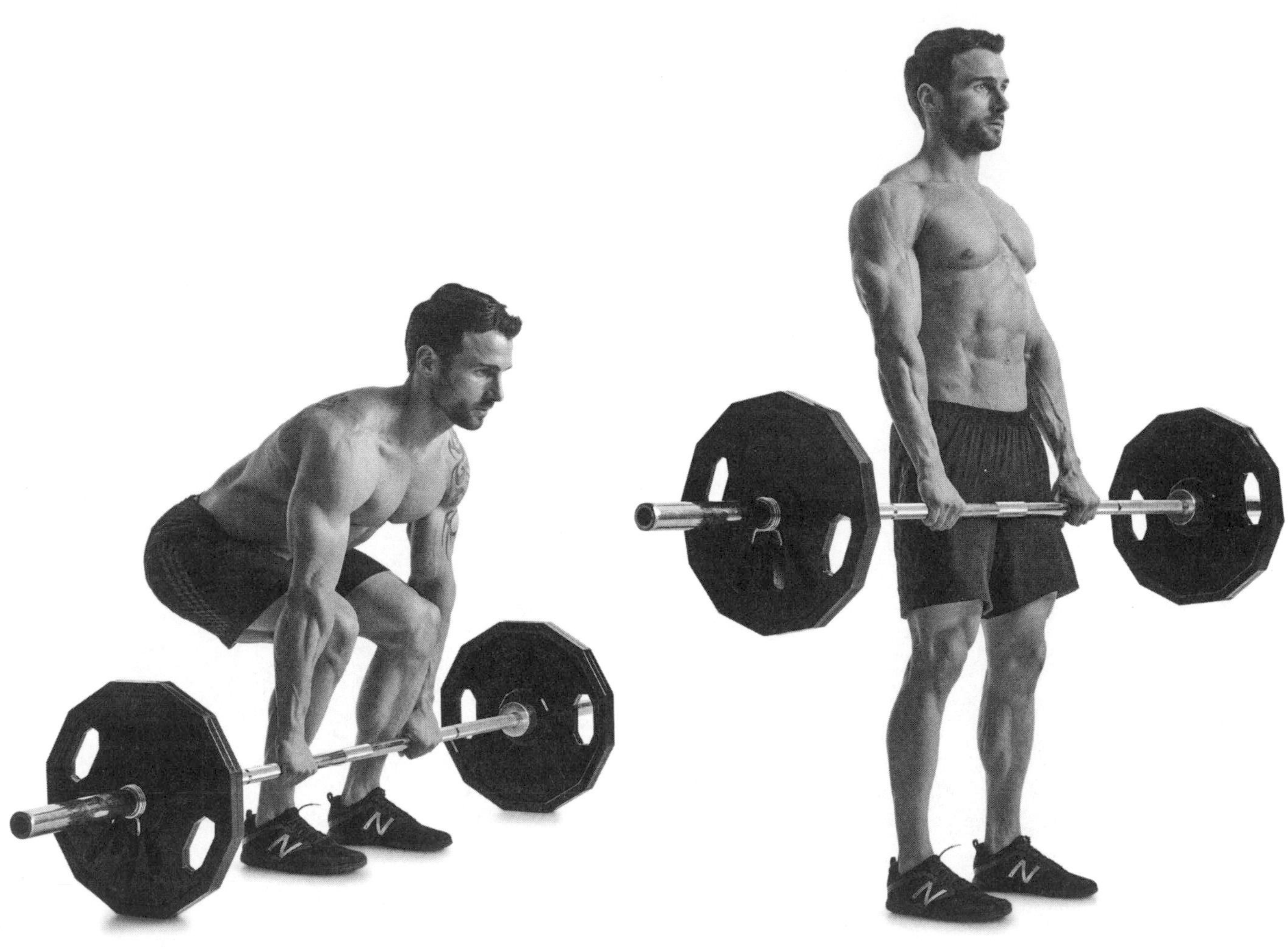

DEADLIFT

PURPOSE
Target the muscles of your back, glutes, and hamstrings.

START
Bend at your hips and knees and grab the bar with an overhand grip, keeping your hands shoulder width apart. Roll the bar to your shins.

MOVEMENT
Do not round your lower back while you pull your torso back and up, thrusting your hips forward and simultaneously standing up with the barbell. (Flex your glutes throughout the movement.)

FINISH
Keep the bar close to the body as you lower the bar to the floor.

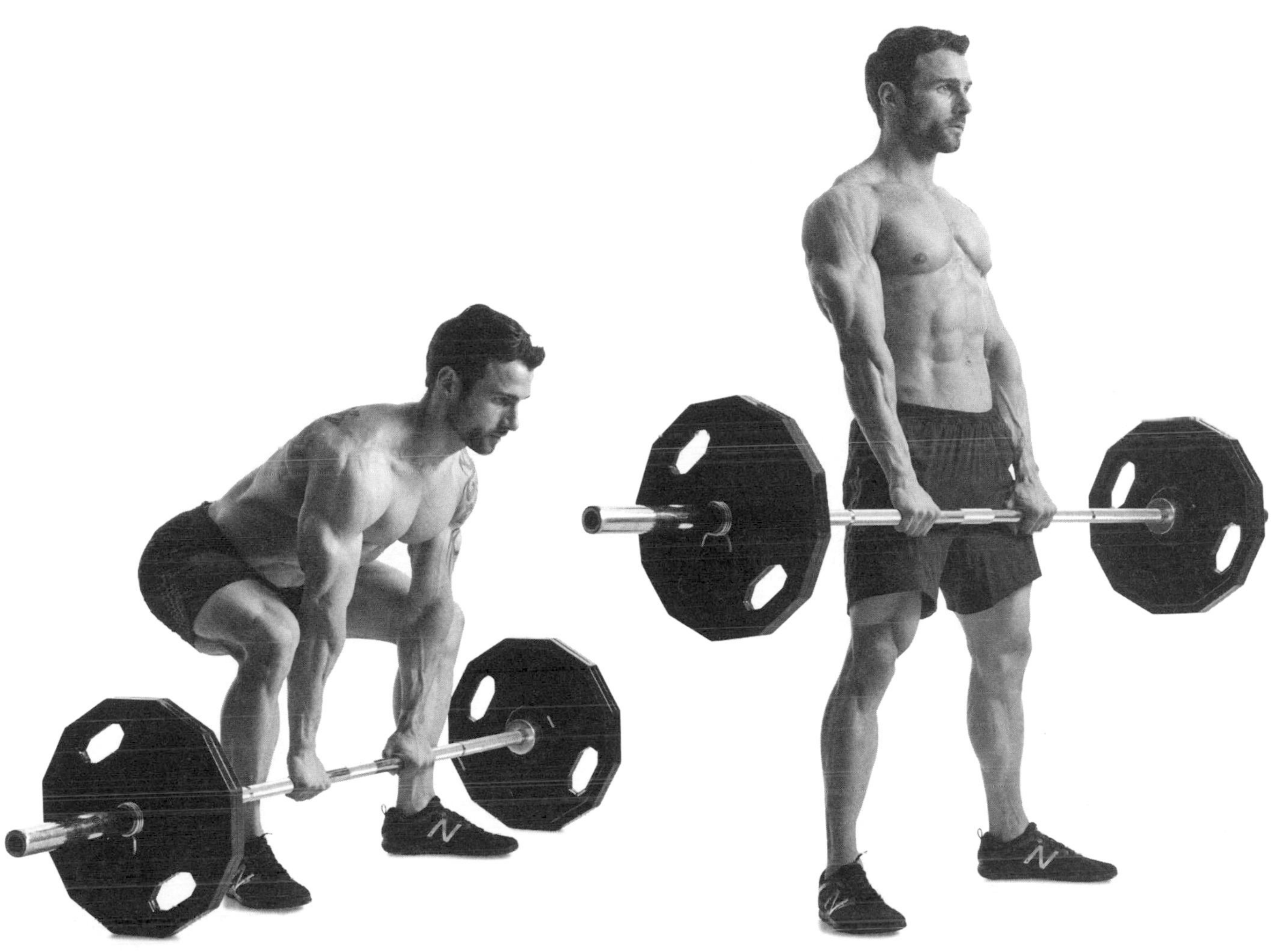

SUMO DEADLIFT

PURPOSE

Target the muscles of your back, glutes, and hamstrings.

START

Stand with your feet twice as wide as shoulder width apart and your toes pointed out at an angle. Grab the center of the bar with your hands about 10 to 12 inches apart and palms facing you.

MOVEMENT

While holding the bar with an overhand grip roll the barbell to your shins and bend at your hips and knees. Do not allow your back to round while you pull your torso back and up, push your hips forward, and stand up with the barbell. (Be sure to squeeze your glutes throughout the movement.)

FINISH

Lower the bar to the floor while keeping the bar as close to your body as possible.

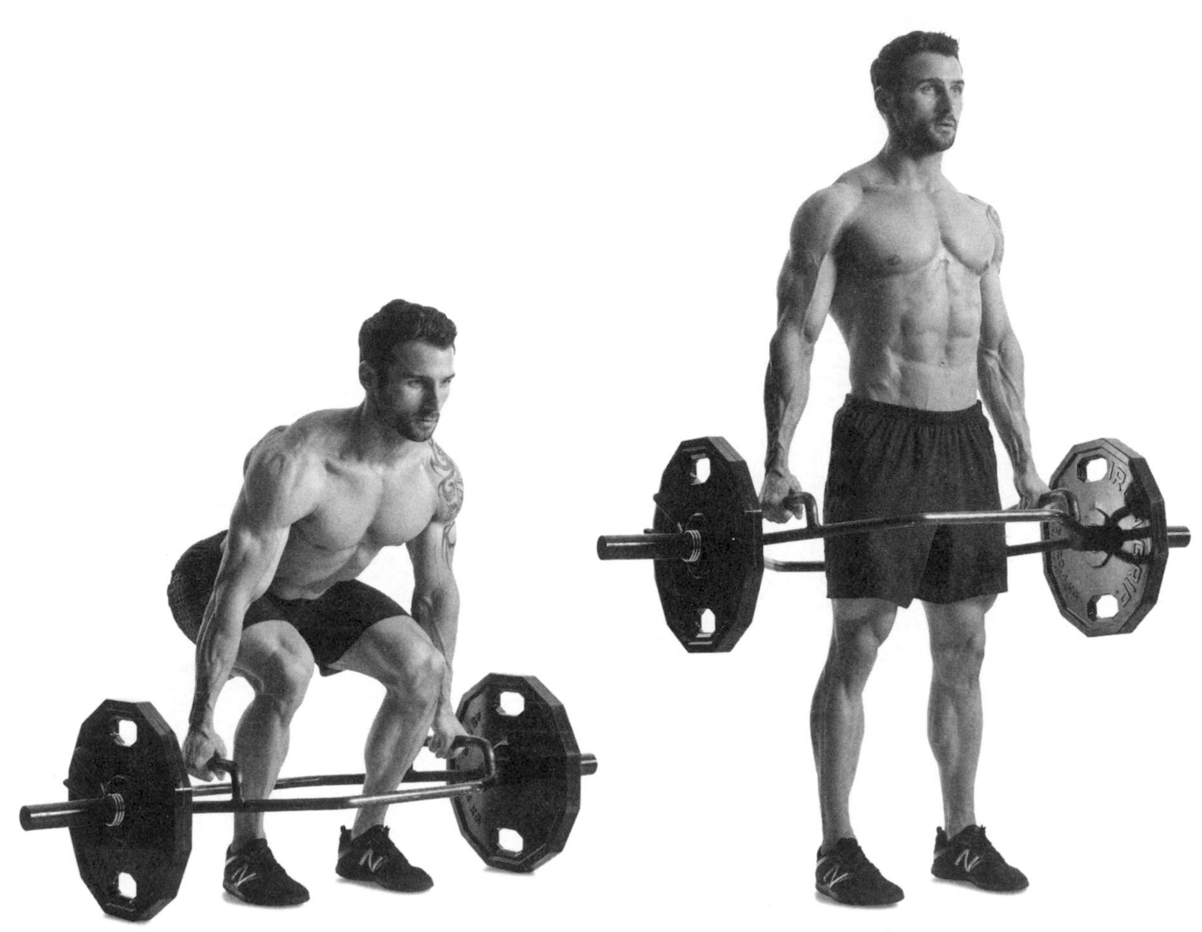

TRAP BAR DEADLIFT

PURPOSE

Target the muscles of the back, glutes, and hamstrings.

START

Step inside the trap bar and grab the bar with a neutral grip. Bend at your hips and knees keeping a slight arch in your back while not allowing your lower back to arch.

MOVEMENT

Pull your torso back and up, push your hips forward, and stand up with the trap bar. (Lead with your chest and flex your glutes on the way up.)

FINISH

Lower the trap bar to the floor.

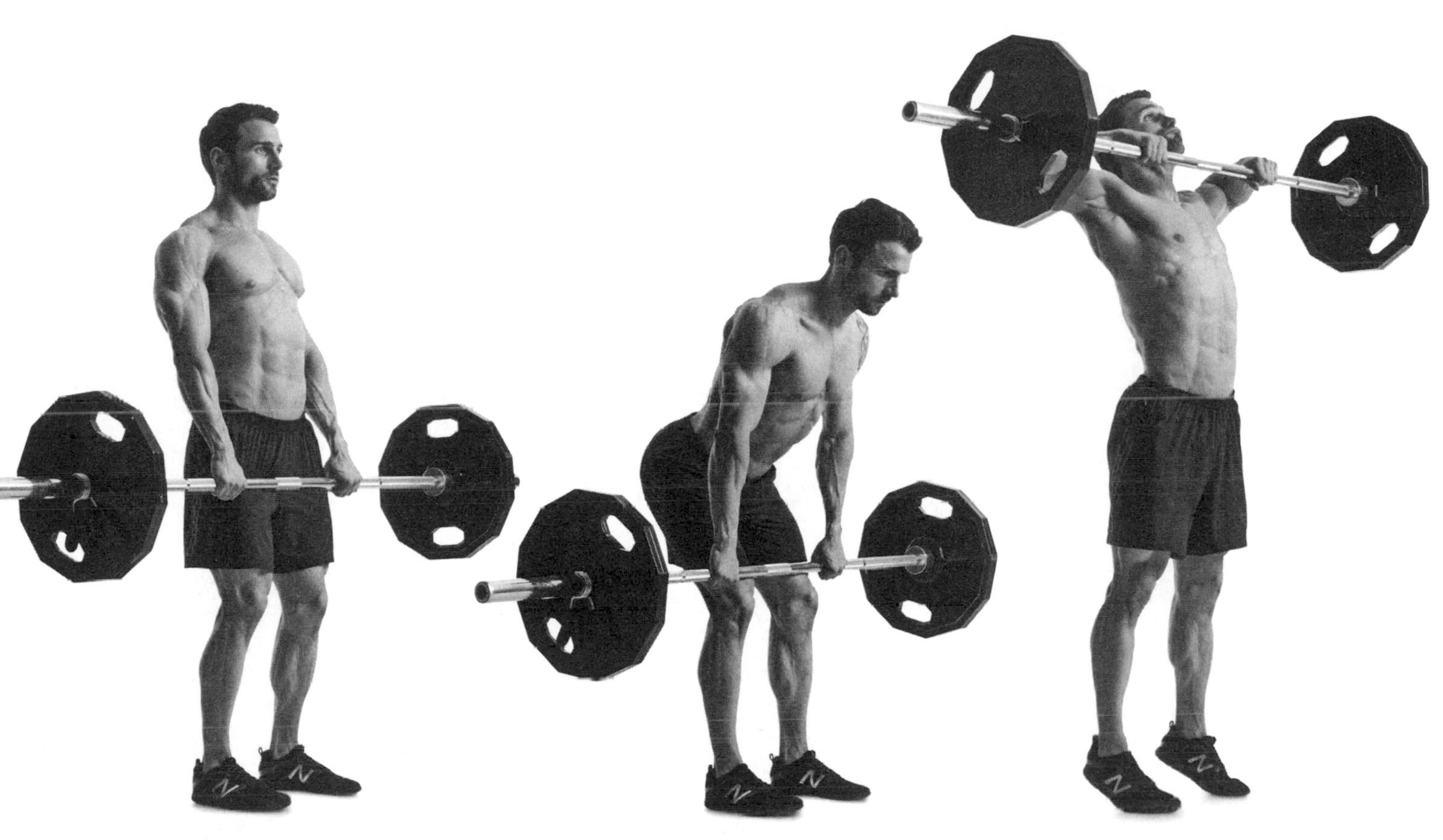

HIGH PULL

PURPOSE

Target the muscles of the upper back.

START

Grab the barbell with an overhand grip that's just beyond shoulder width. Bend at your hips and knees to squat down to the bar. Roll the bar to your shins.

MOVEMENT

Pull the bar as high as you can by explosively standing up as you bend your elbows and raise your upper arms. Pull your torso backward and thrust your hips forward forcefully. (You should explode up on your toes.)

FINISH

Reverse the movement back to the starting position.

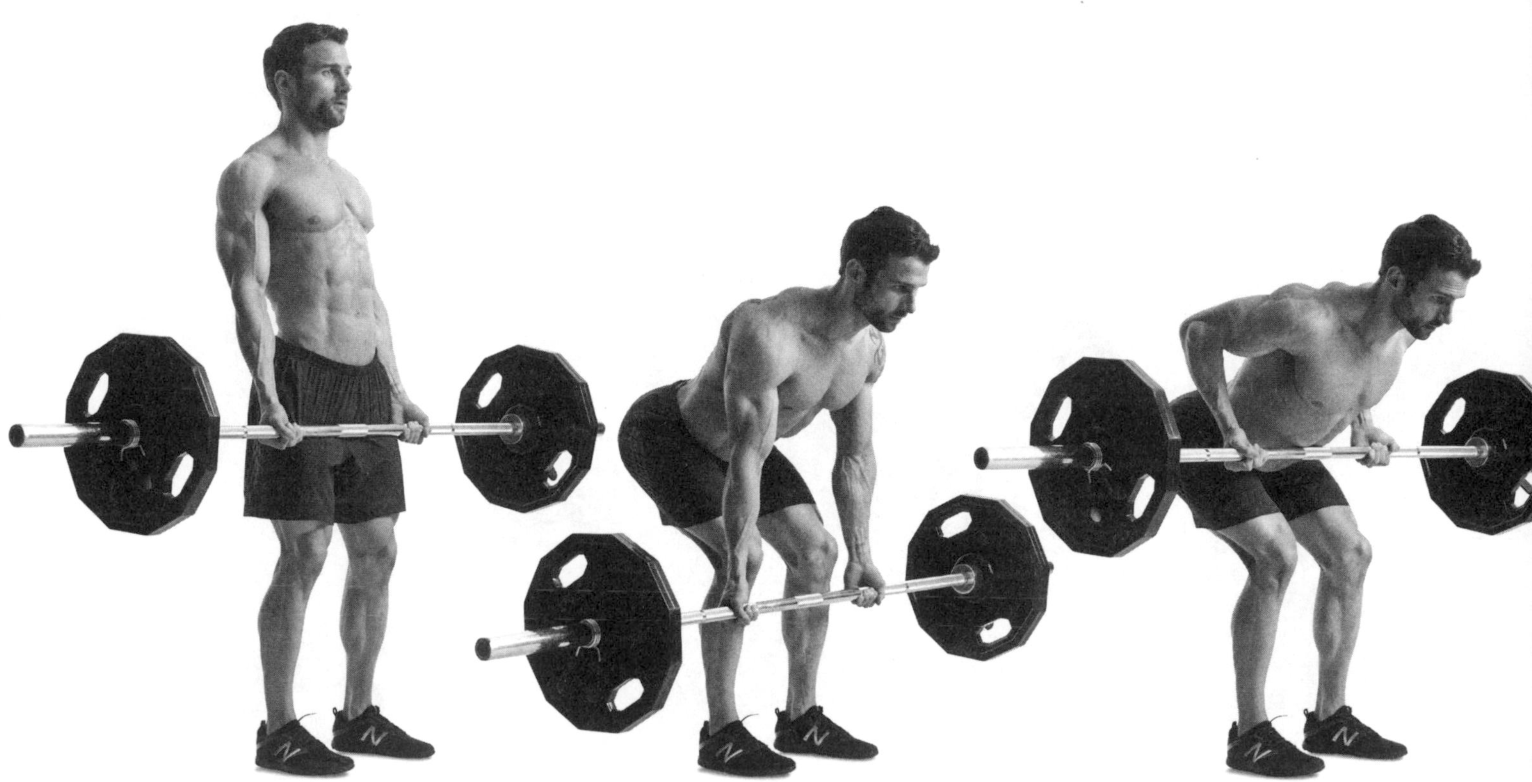

UNDERHAND-GRIP ROW

PURPOSE

Target the muscles of the mid-back, lats, and rhomboids.

START

Grab a barbell with an underhand grip that's just beyond shoulder width and hold the bar at arm's length. Bend at your hips and create a bend in your knees. Lower your torso until it's just above parallel to the floor.

MOVEMENT

Maintain a slight knee bend and a natural arch to your lower back. Pull the bar to your upper abs. Bend your elbows and raise your upper arms while squeezing your shoulder blades toward each other. (Do your best to not lift your torso during the lift.)

FINISH

Lower the bar to hang straight down from your shoulders.

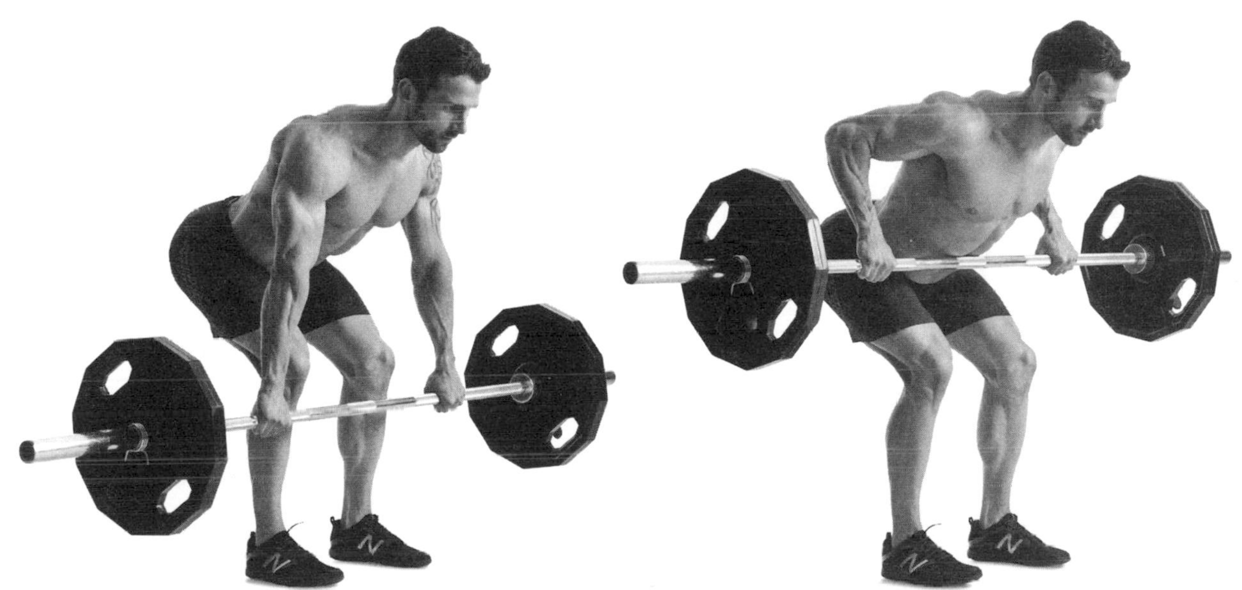

OVERHAND-GRIP ROW

PURPOSE

Target the muscles of the lats and rhomboids.

START

Grab a barbell with an overhand grip that's just beyond shoulder width and hold the bar at arm's length. Bend at your hips and create a bend in your knees. Lower your torso until it's just about parallel to the floor.

MOVEMENT

Maintain a slight knee bend and a natural arch to your lower back. Pull the bar to your upper abs. Bend your elbows and raise your upper arms while squeezing your shoulder blades toward each other. (Do your best to not raise your torso during the lift.)

FINISH

Lower the bar to hang straight down from your shoulders.

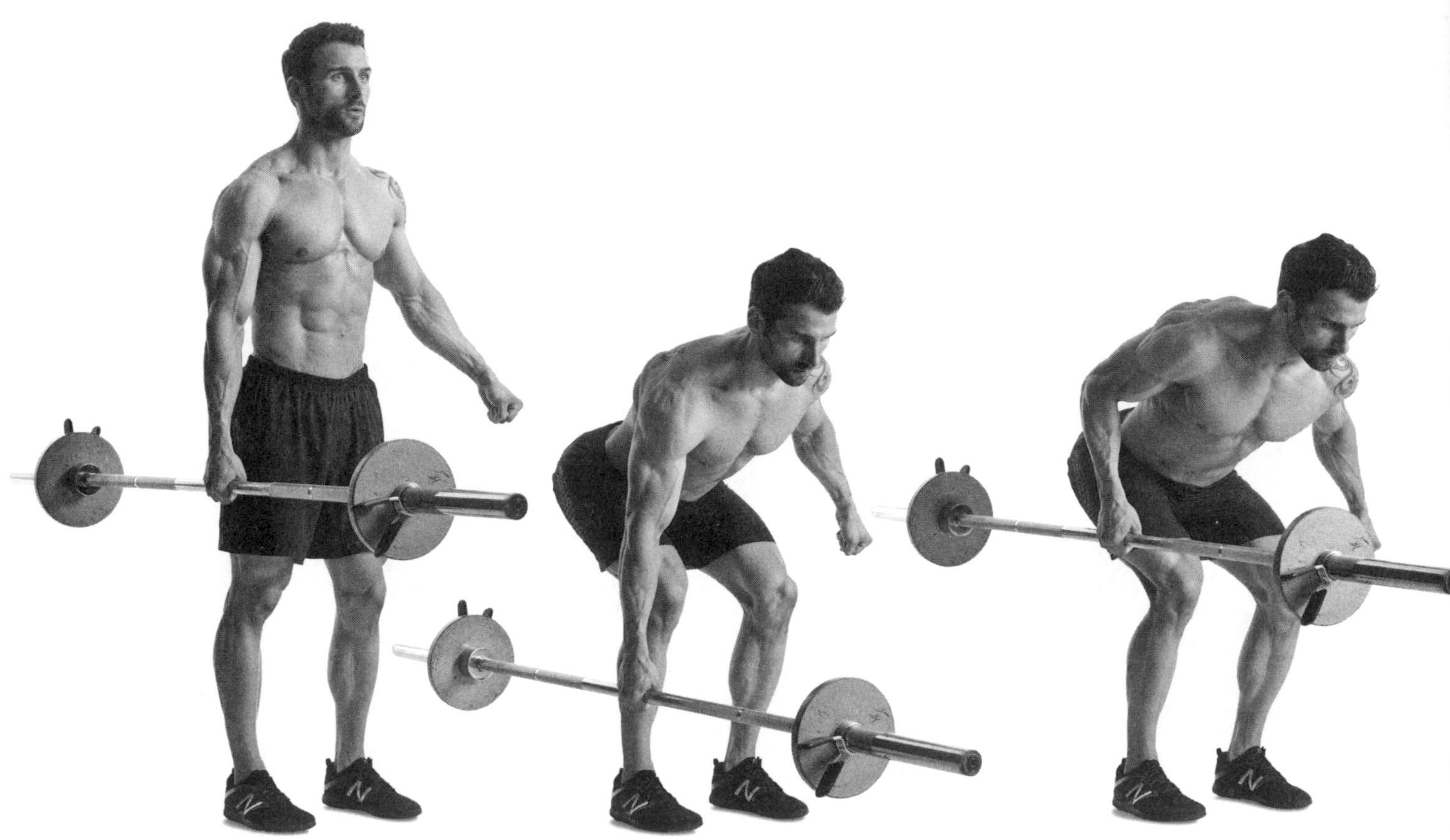

SINGLE-ARM ROW

PURPOSE

Target the muscles of the lats.

START

Place a barbell on one side of the body. Grab the barbell in the center with one hand. Hold the bar at arm's length and let it hang at your side. Bend at your hips and create a bend in your knees. Lower your torso until it's just about parallel to the floor.

MOVEMENT

Maintain a slight knee bend and a natural arch to your lower back. Pull the bar back, bending your elbow, keeping your palm facing in. (The bar will require your forearms to work overtime to maintain a controlled balance.)

FINISH

Lower the bar back to arm's length at your side.

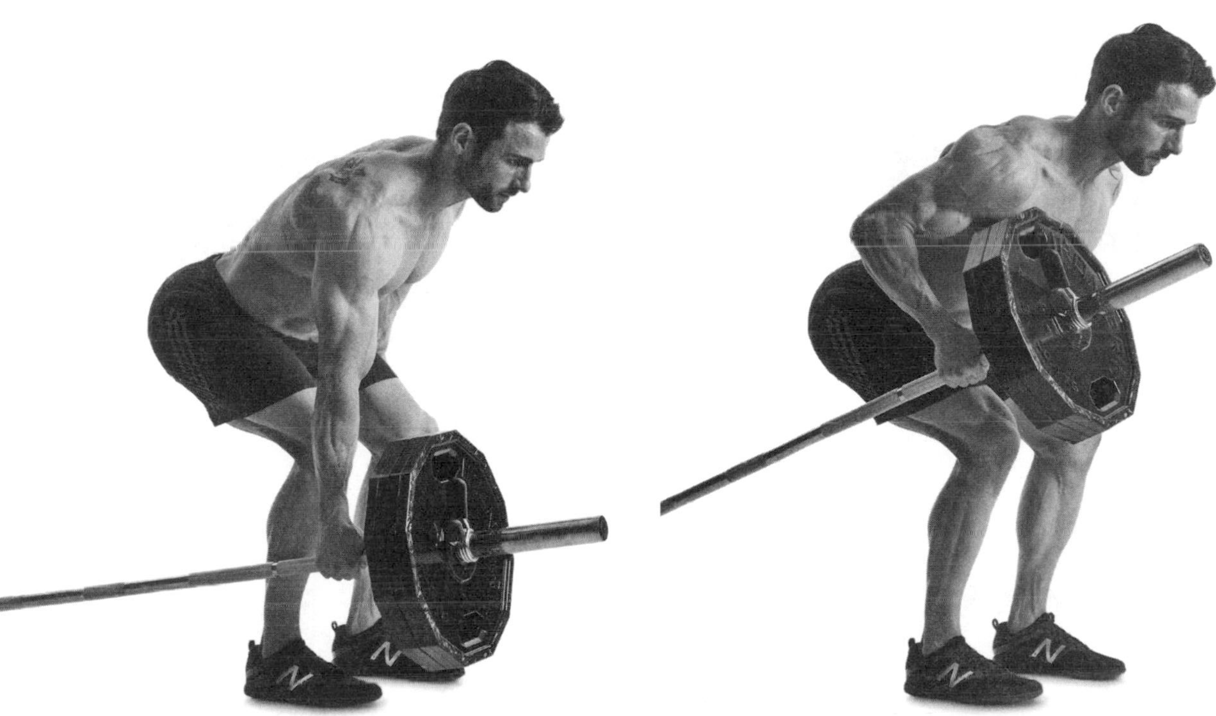

LANDMINE ROW

PURPOSE

Target the muscles of the rhomboids and lats.

START

Place a barbell in a corner of a squat rack to prevent it from sliding. Stand on one side of the barbell and grab the bar in front or in back of the loaded weight. Hold the bar at arm's length. Bend at your hips and create a bend in your knees. Lower your torso until it's about 45 degrees to the floor.

MOVEMENT

Maintain a slight knee bend and a natural arch to your lower back. Pull the bar back bending your elbow, keeping your palm facing in. (Avoid using momentum from your torso.)

FINISH

Slowly lower the bar back to arm's length at your side.

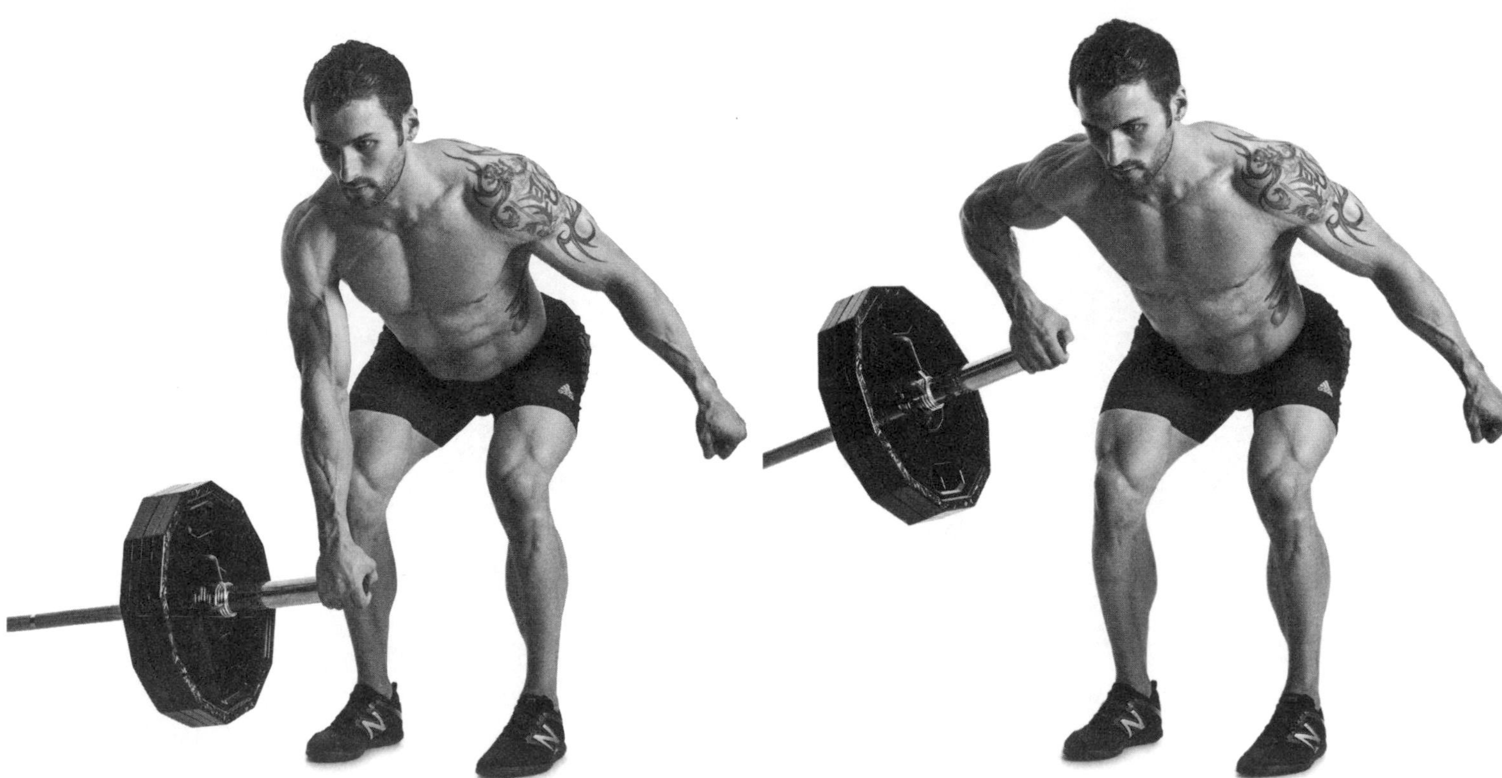

ELBOWS-OUT LANDMINE ROW

PURPOSE

Target the muscles of the rhomboids and lats.

START

Place a barbell in a corner of a squat rack to prevent it from sliding. Stand perpendicular to the barbell and grab the bar with one hand in front of the loaded weight (around the thick portion of the bar). Hold out the bar at arm's length in front of your shoulder. Bend at your hips and create a bend in your knees. Lower your torso until it's just about parallel to the floor.

MOVEMENT

Maintain a slight knee bend and a natural arch to your lower back. Pull the bar back while bending your elbow, keeping it flared out and keeping your palm facing your back. (Avoid using momentum from your torso.)

FINISH

Slowly lower the bar back to arm's length at your side.

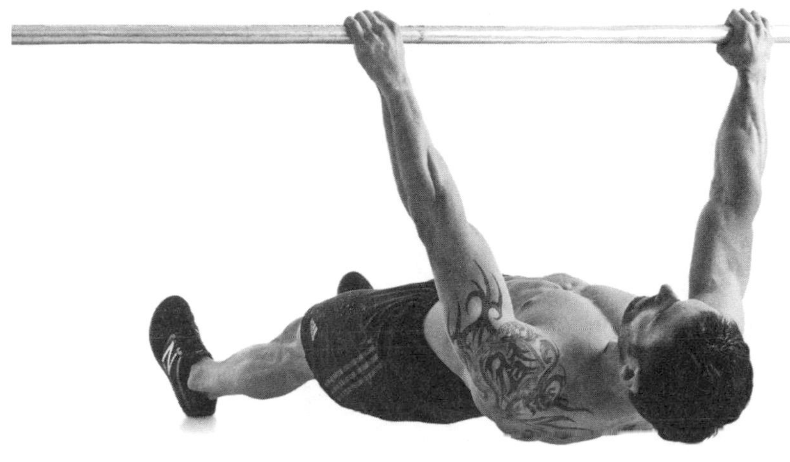

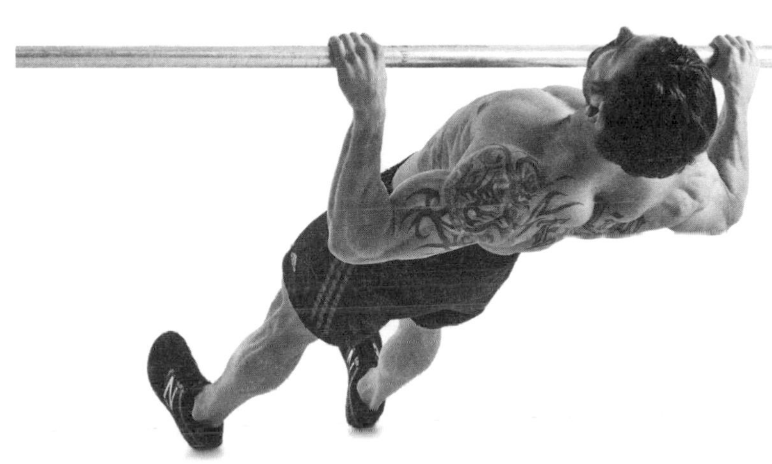

INVERTED ROW

PURPOSE

Target the lower traps, rhomboids, rear delts, and latissimus dorsi.

START

Place a barbell in a locked position on a squat rack or use a Smith machine bar. Position your body under the bar and grab the barbell with an overhand grip. Start with your hands on the bar wider than shoulder width apart. Your legs should be straight and your body should be at a 45-degree angle from your heels to your shoulders when you raise your upper body to the bar. Start with your arms extended (slight elbow bend). Keep your feet shoulder width apart and your weight on your heels.

MOVEMENT

Squeezing your shoulder blades together and bracing your core, pull your body up toward the ceiling until your chest touches the barbell.

FINISH

Pause, then return to the starting position.

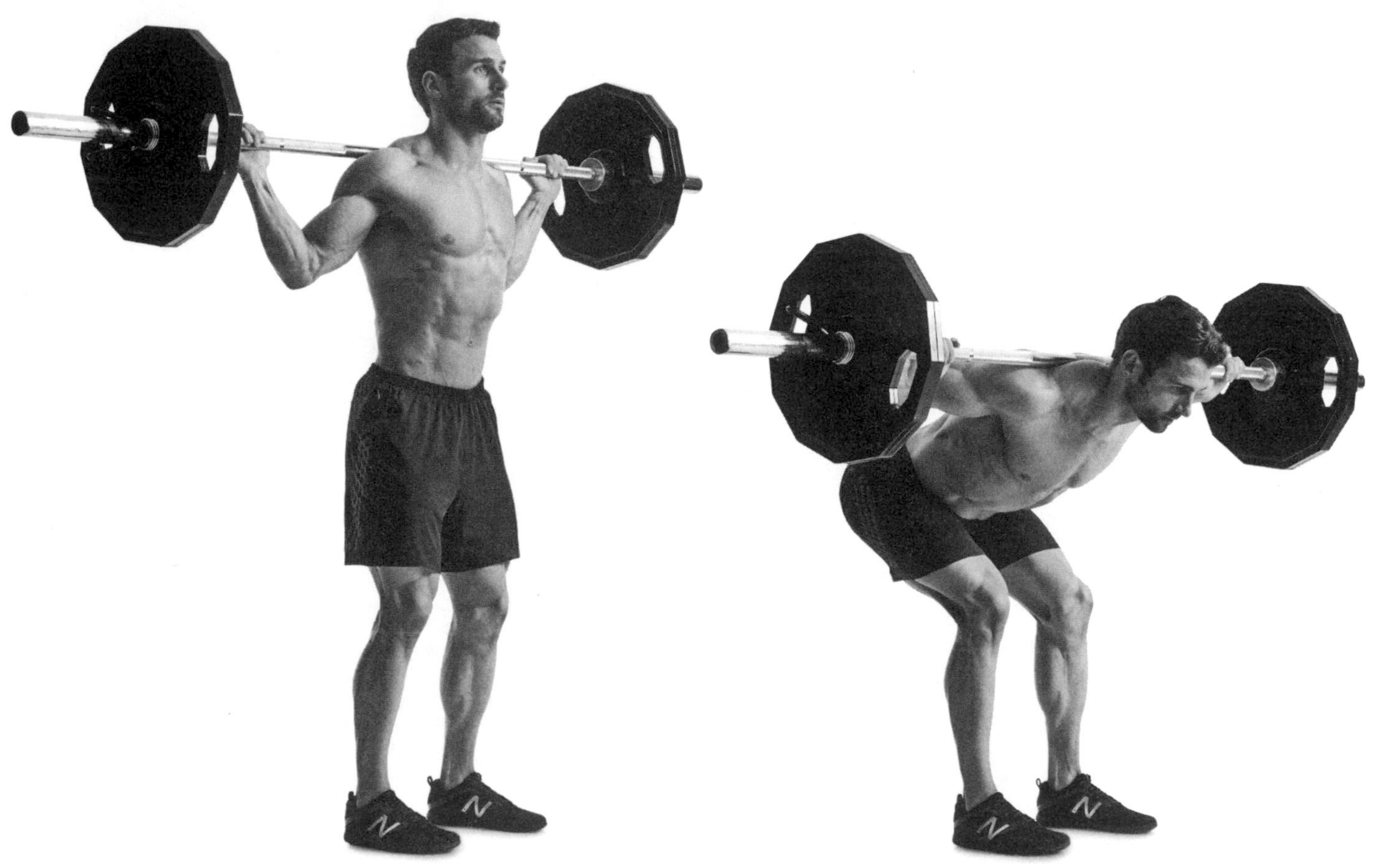

GOOD MORNING

PURPOSE
Target the lower back and hamstrings.

START
Place the barbell on your upper back and pinch your shoulder blades together. Create a slight bend to your knees.

MOVEMENT
Keep your shoulders pinched and your elbows down and back. Hinge (bend) at your hips keeping your chest up and maintain the slight bend in your knees.

FINISH
Pause, flex your glutes, and push your hips forward to return to the starting position.

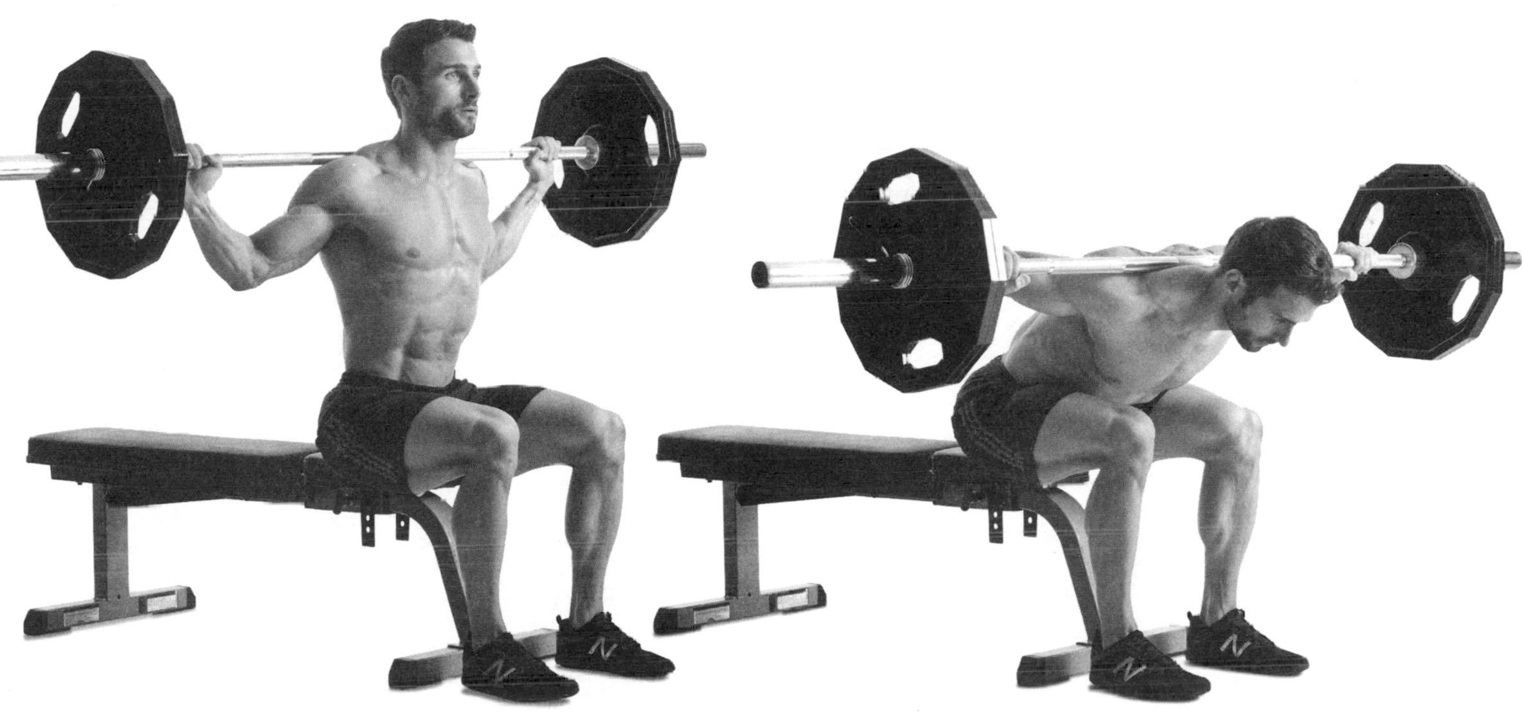

SEATED GOOD MORNING

PURPOSE

Target lower back and hamstrings.

START

Sit upright on a bench with a barbell across your upper back.

MOVEMENT

Maintaining a natural arch to your lower back, bend forward at your hips and lower your torso as far as you can while keeping a tight core and without rounding your back.

FINISH

Pause, then raise your torso back to the upright position.

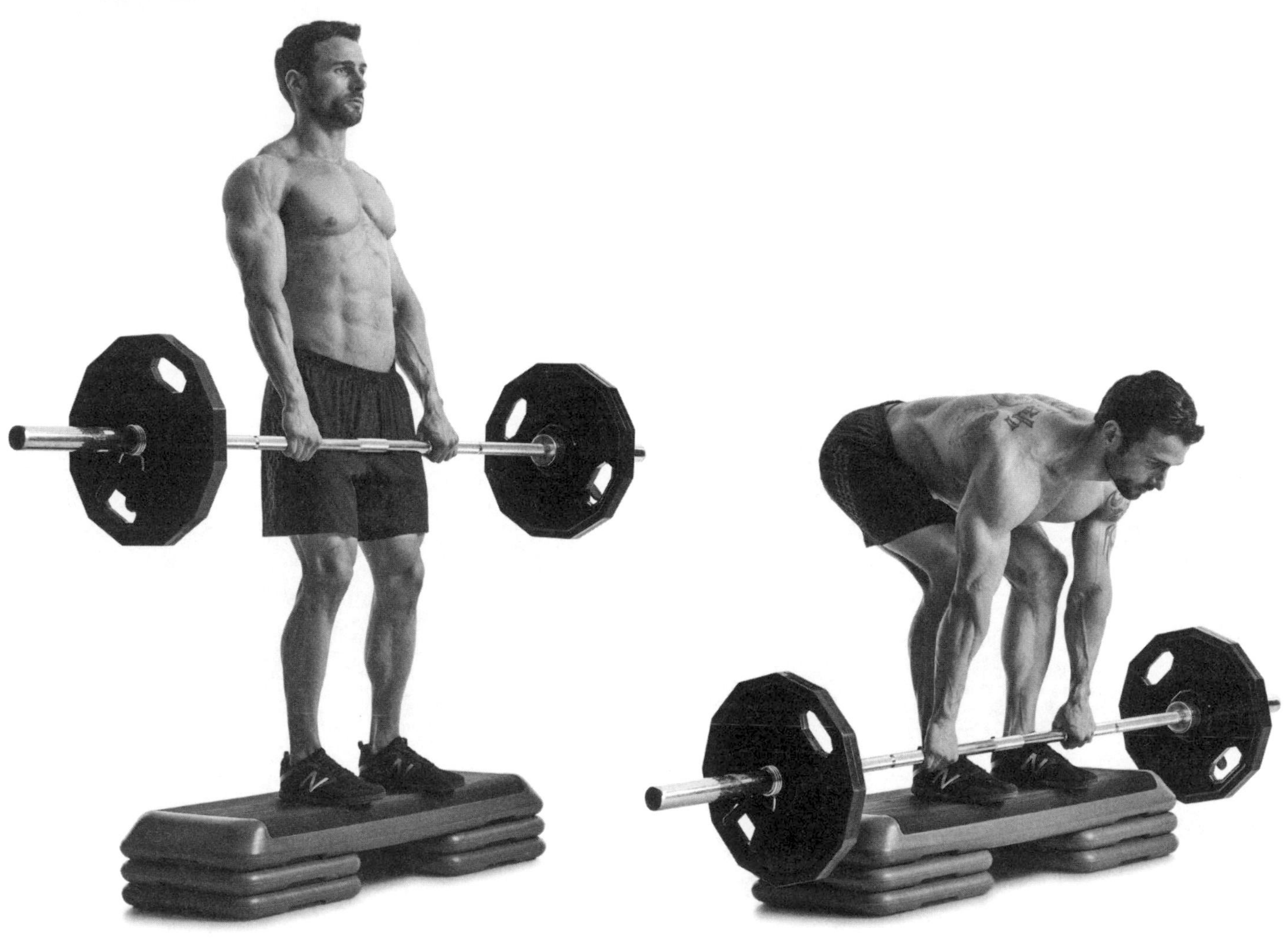

DEFICIT DEADLIFT

PURPOSE
Target the lower back muscles.

START
Stand on a step and grab a barbell with an overhand grip just wider than shoulder width and hold the bar in front of your hips. Keep your feet hip width apart.

MOVEMENT
Push your chest out and maintain a slight bend to your knees. Keep your back flat with a natural arch and do not change the slight bend in your knees as you lower your torso to just below parallel with the floor. Be sure to brace your core through the entire movement.

FINISH
Pause, squeeze your glutes, and push your hips forward, returning to the starting position.

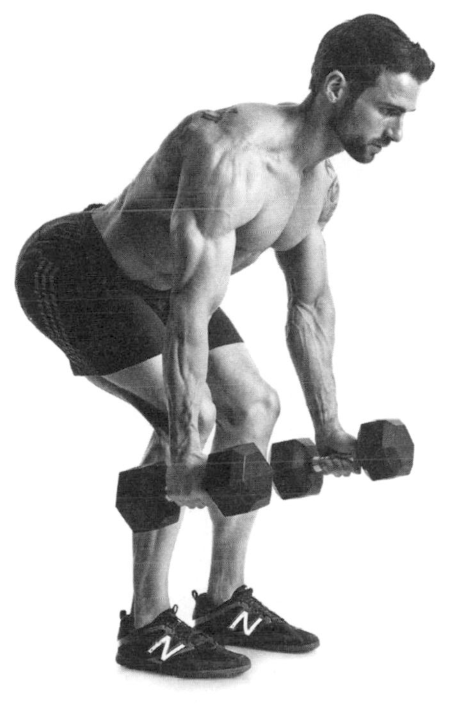

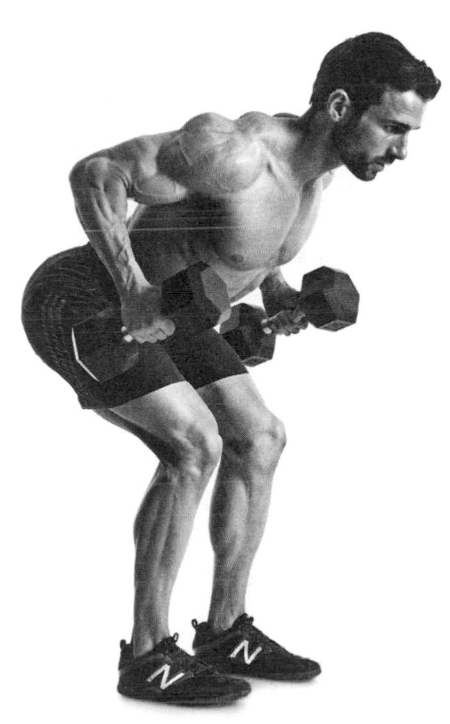

DUAL ROW

PURPOSE

Target the lats and rhomboids.

START

Grab a pair of dumbbells and bend at your hips. Keep a slight bend to your knees and place the dumbbells out in front of your torso.

MOVEMENT

Keep the natural arch to your lower back and from an extended position of your arms, pull the dumbbells back flexing your back. Allow the dumbbells to finish just in front of the side of your body or when your elbows pass behind your back.

FINISH

Pause, then return the dumbbells to the front of the body.

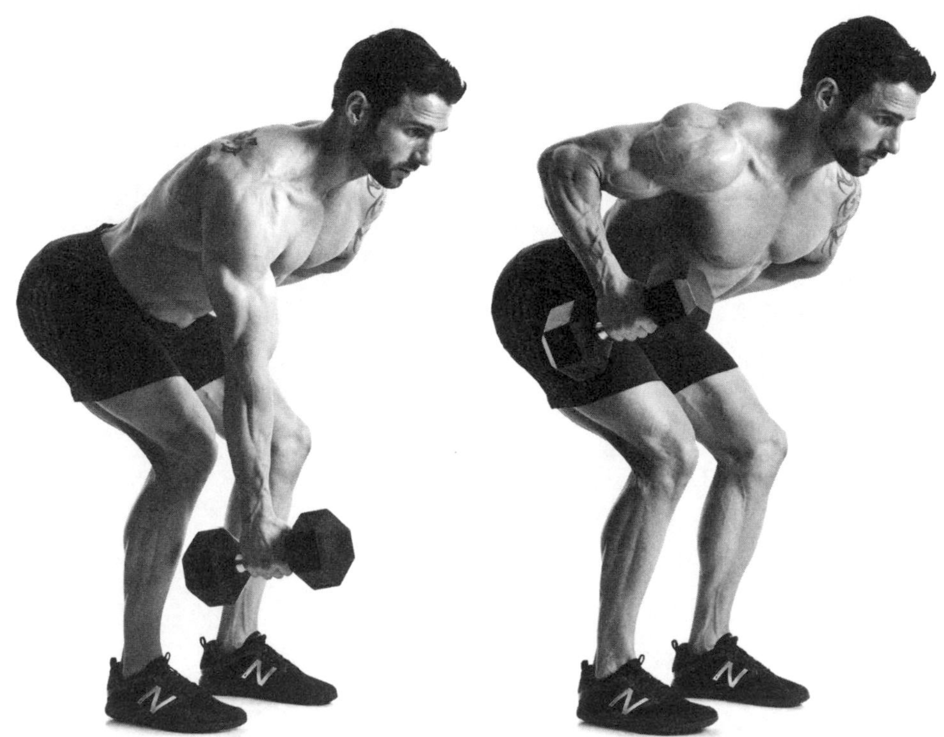

SINGLE-ARM ROW

PURPOSE

Target the muscles of the middle and upper back.

START

Grab a dumbbell in one hand using a neutral grip. Bend at the hips while lowering your torso. Let the dumbbell hang at arm's length from your shoulders.

MOVEMENT

Brace your core and pull the dumbbell to the side of your torso, keeping your elbow tucked close to your side. (Do not rotate or elevate your torso during the lift.)

FINISH

Return the dumbbell to arm's length from your shoulder.

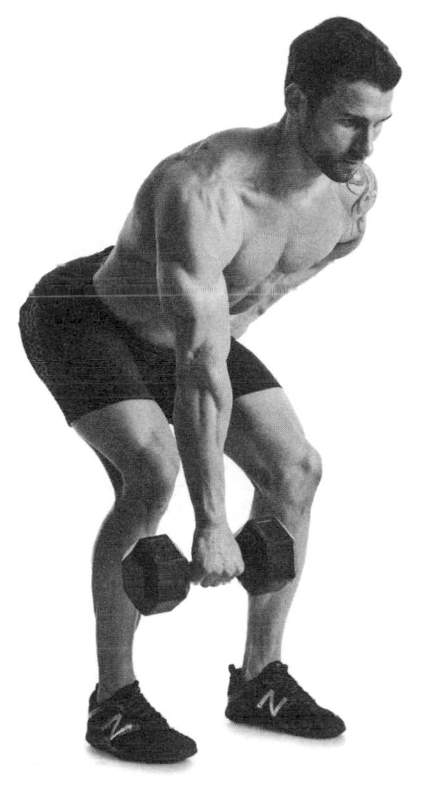

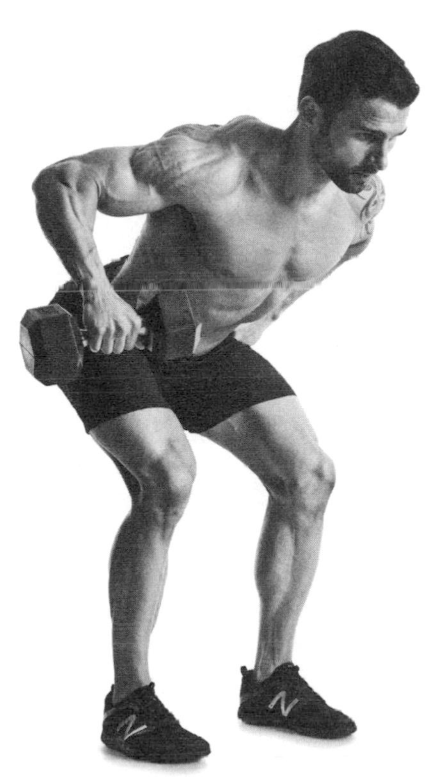

SINGLE-ARM ELBOW-OUT ROW

PURPOSE

Target the muscles of the middle and upper back.

START

Grab a dumbbell in one hand. Bend at the hips while lowering your torso. Let the dumbbell hang at arm's length from your shoulders. Rotate your palm to use an overhand grip.

MOVEMENT

Brace your core and pull the dumbbell back while keeping your elbow outside your torso, allowing your elbow to flare out. (Do not rotate or elevate your torso during the lift.)

FINISH

Return the dumbbell to arm's length from your shoulder.

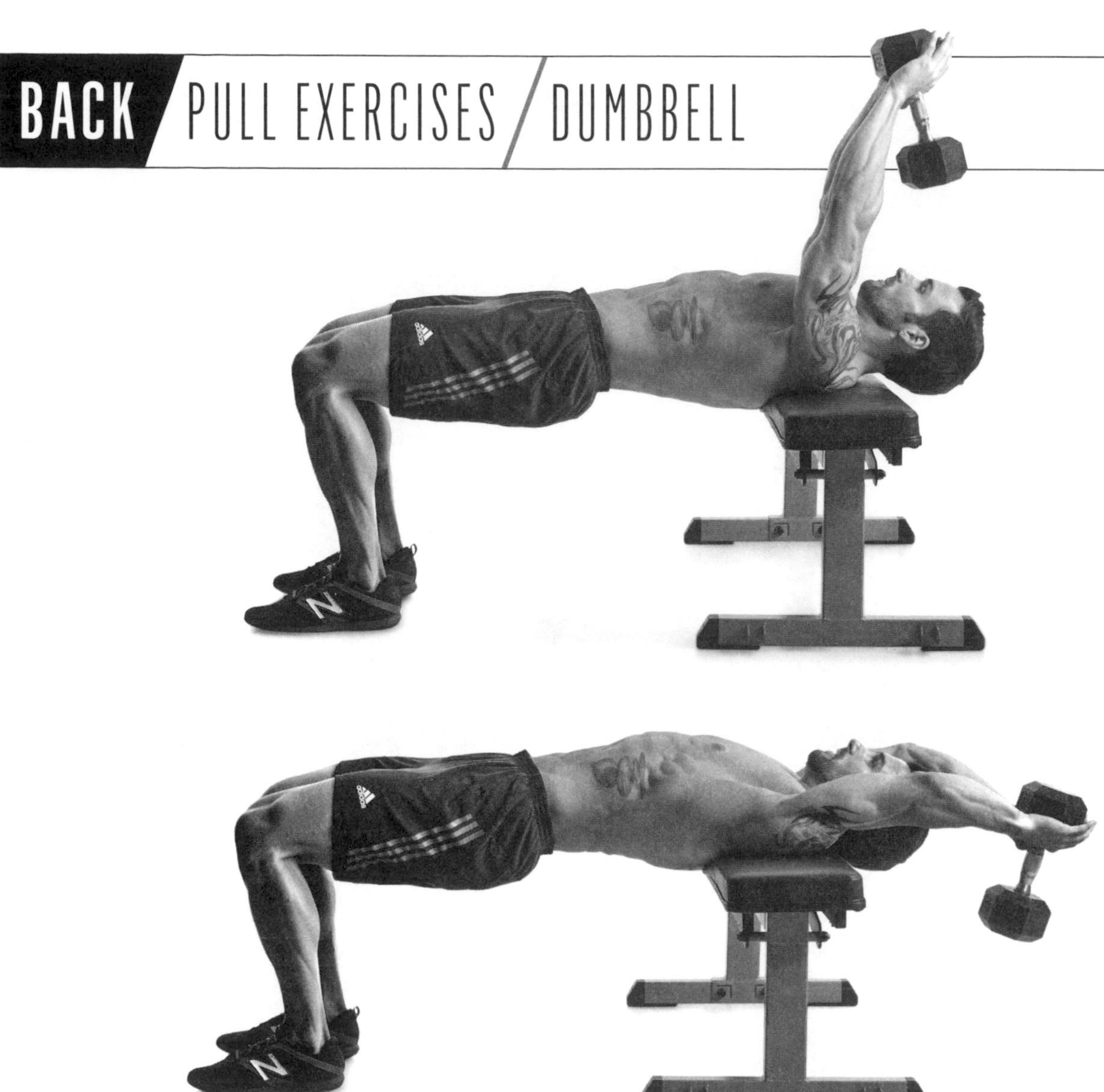

PULLOVER

PURPOSE
Target the lat muscles.

START
Grab a dumbbell, holding it underneath one end, with both hands. Lie on your back on a flat bench and hold the dumbbell straight over your chin.

MOVEMENT
Without changing the angle of your elbow, slowly lower the dumbbell back beyond your head until the upper arms are in line with your body or parallel to the floor. (Keep your feet flat on the ground.)

FINISH
Pause, then slowly raise the dumbbell back to the starting position.

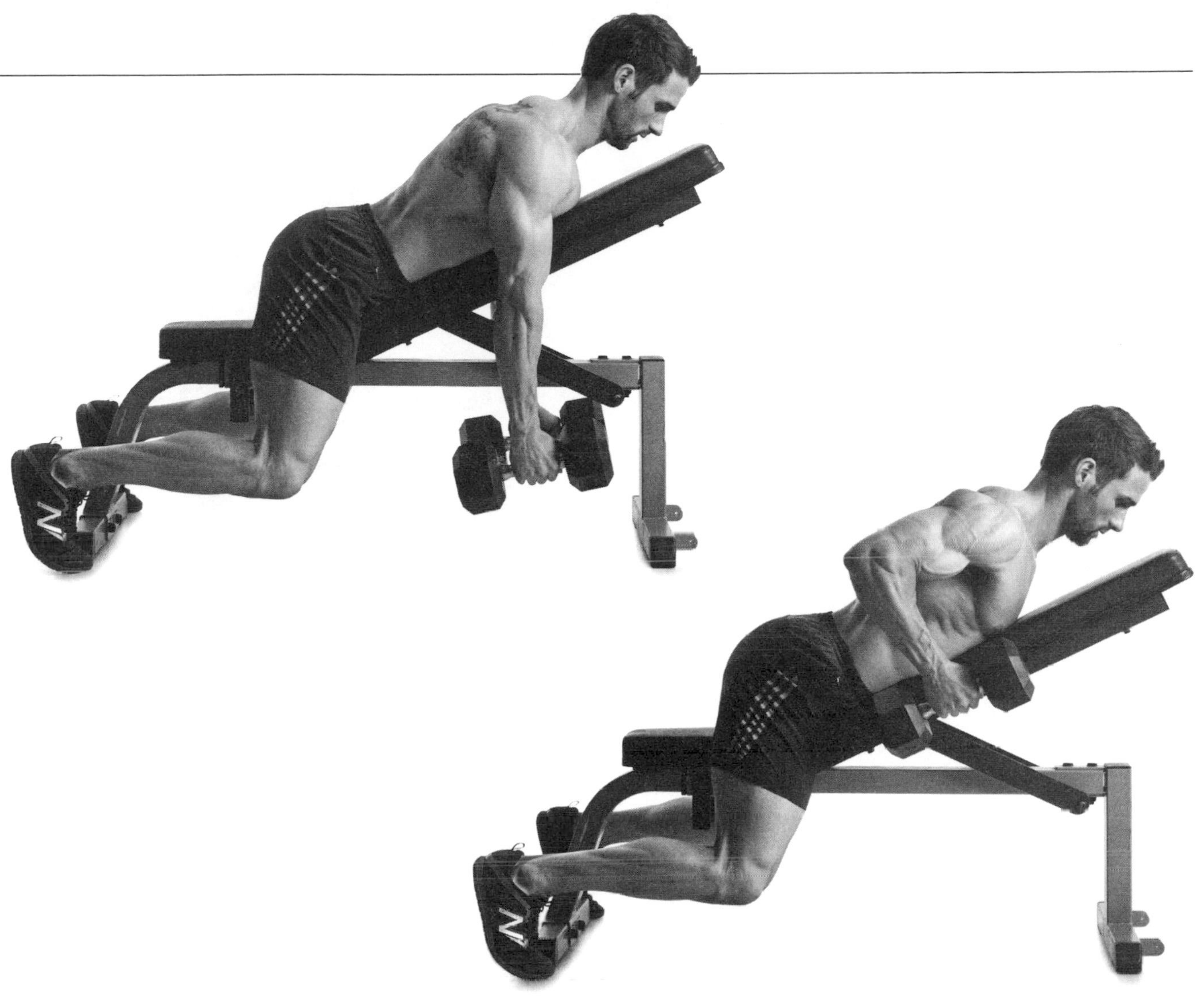

CHEST-SUPPORTED ROW

PURPOSE

Target the middle and upper back muscles.

START

Lie chest down on an incline bench (set to the lowest incline). Let the dumbbells hang at arm's length from your shoulders. Use a neutral grip.

MOVEMENT

Keep your lower back in a natural arch, and keep your elbows in as you pull the dumbbells back and toward the sides of your back.

FINISH

Pause, then lower the dumbbells back to a hanging position arm's length from your shoulders.

 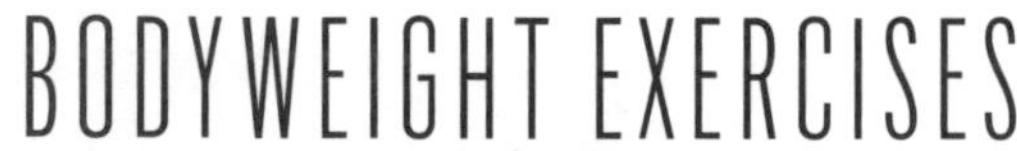

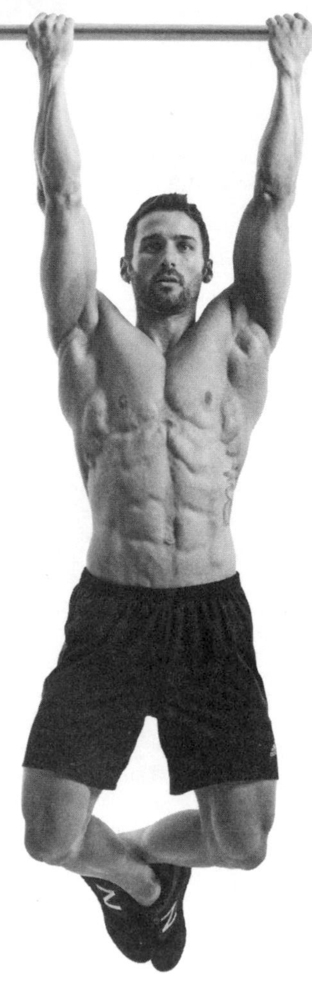

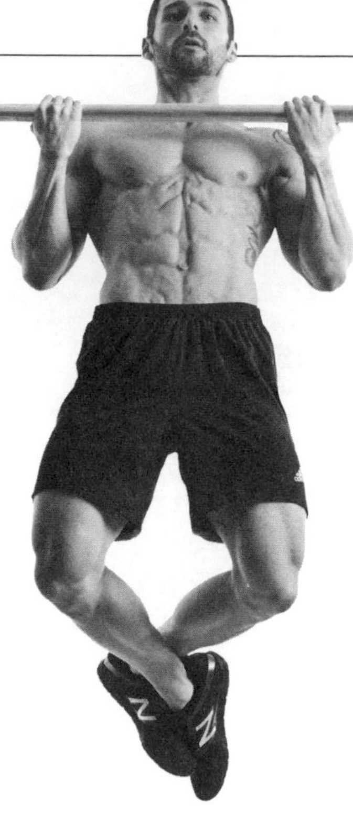

CHINUP

PURPOSE

Target your lats and hit your teres major and biceps.

START

Grab a chinup bar with an underhand grip shoulder width apart.

MOVEMENT

Hang at arm's length. Squeeze your shoulder blades together as you bend your arms and pull your chest to the bar.

FINISH

Pause, then slowly lower your body back to an arm's length hang position, also called a dead hang position.

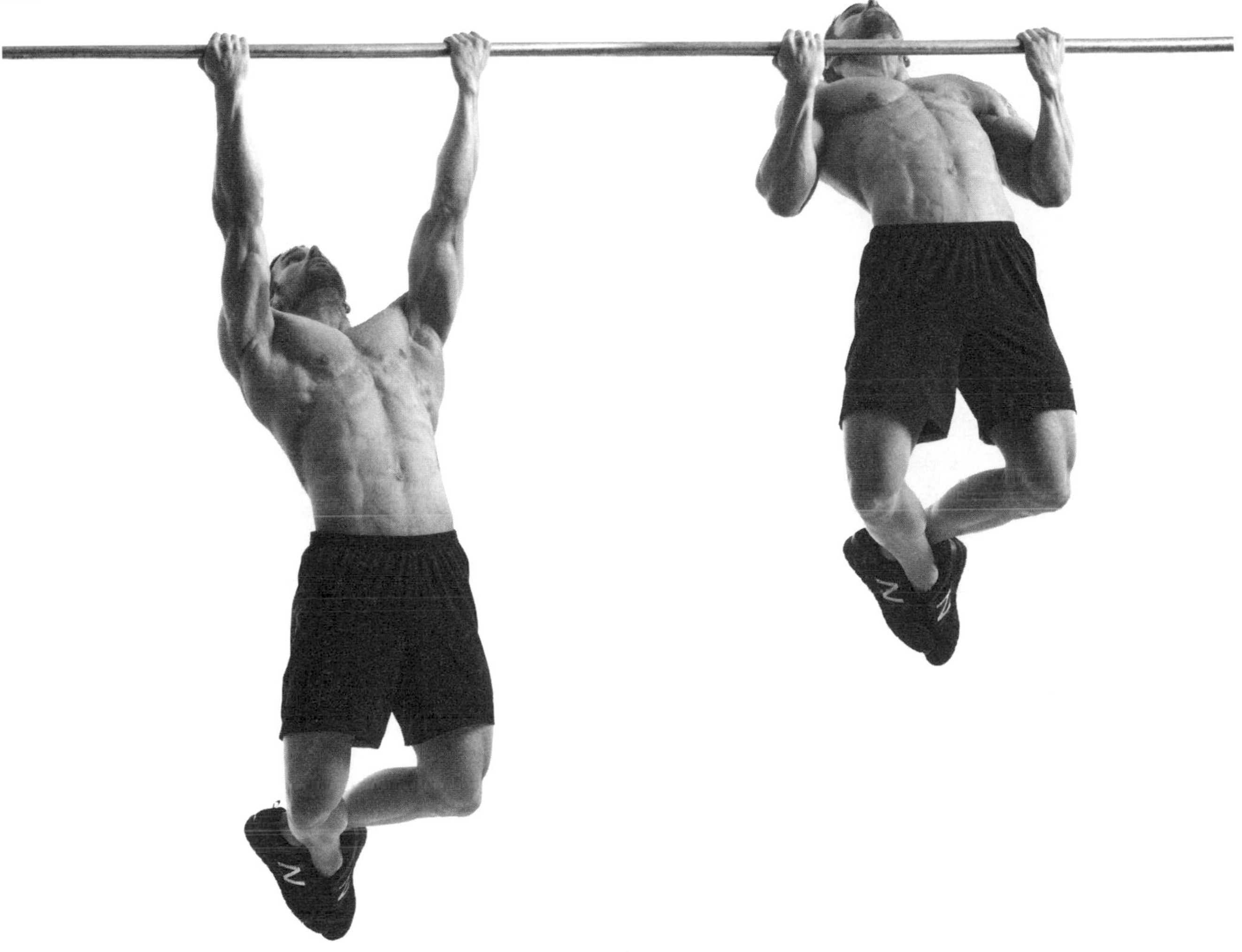

STERNUM CHINUP

PURPOSE
Target your lats.

START
Grab a chinup bar with an underhand grip shoulder width apart. Attempt to create an over-pronounced arch to your back.

MOVEMENT
Hang with the over-pronounced arch to your back, then pull your sternum toward the bar.

FINISH
Pause, then slowly lower your body back to the over-pronounced arched position.

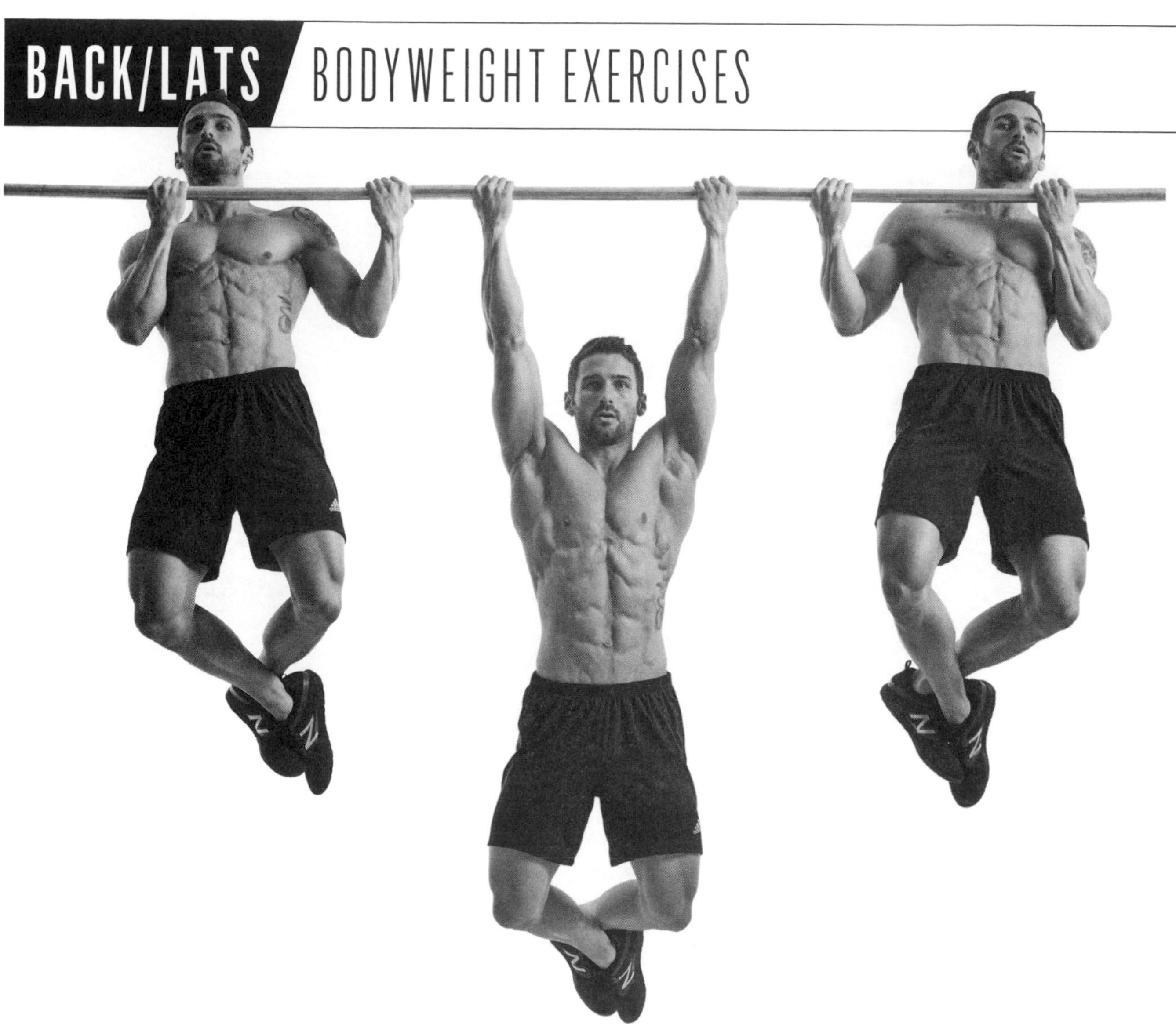

SIDE-TO-SIDE CHINUP

PURPOSE
Target your lats and hit your teres major and biceps.

START
Grab a chinup bar with an underhand grip shoulder width apart.

MOVEMENT
Hang at arm's length. Squeeze your shoulder blades together as you pull your chest to the bar and to the right. Once your chest is at the bar, return to the dead hang position and pull yourself to the left side of your chest.

FINISH
Pause, then slowly lower your body back to an arm's length hang, or dead hang position.

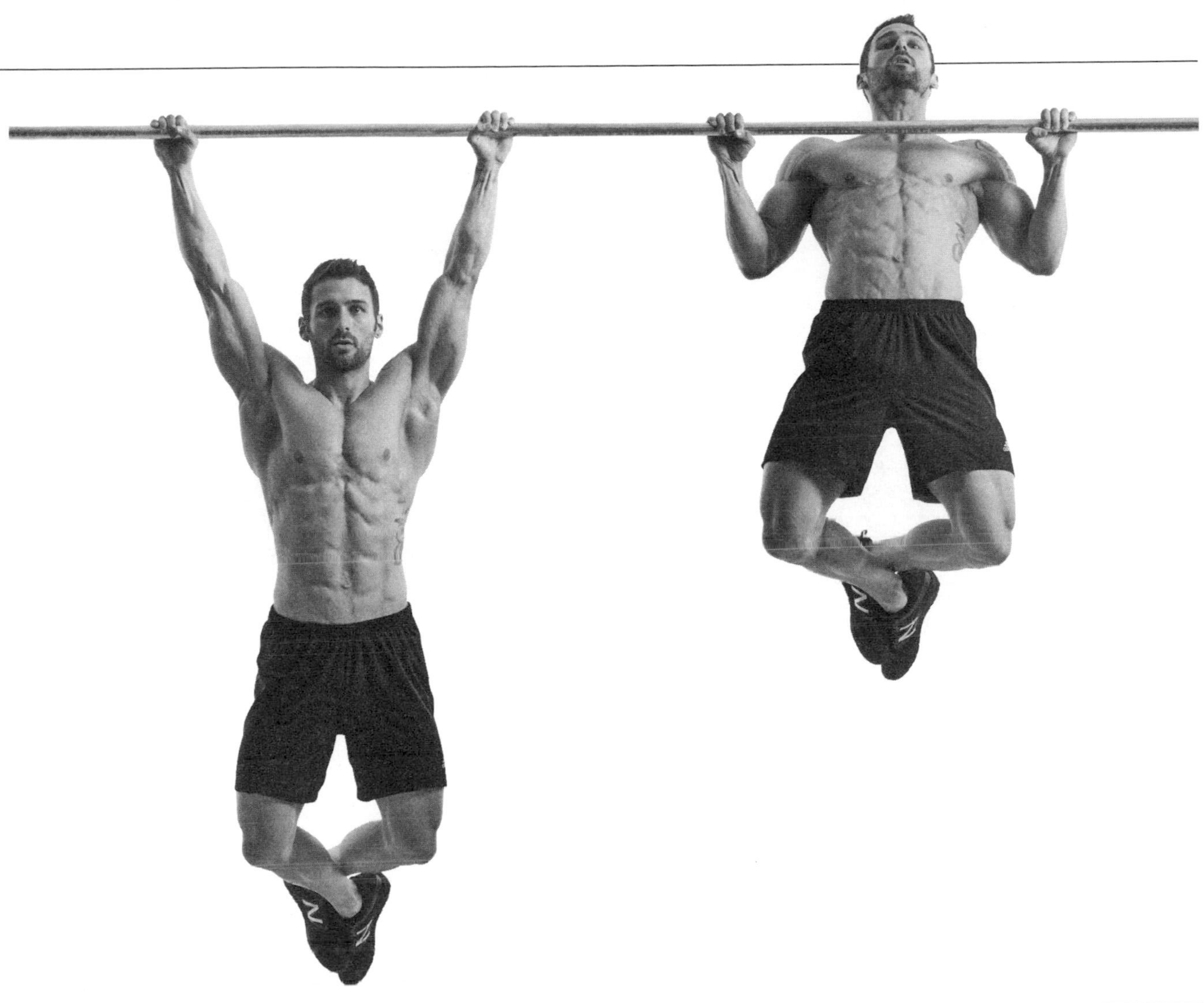

PULLUP

PURPOSE

Target your lats and hit your teres major and biceps.

START

Grab a chinup bar with an overhand grip slightly wider than shoulder width apart.

MOVEMENT

Hang at arm's length. Squeeze your shoulder blades together as you pull your chest to the bar.

FINISH

Pause, then slowly lower your body back to an arm's length hang, or dead hang position. (Note: To do an eccentric or negative pullup, or chinup, on the finish, lower yourself slowly to a three-count.)

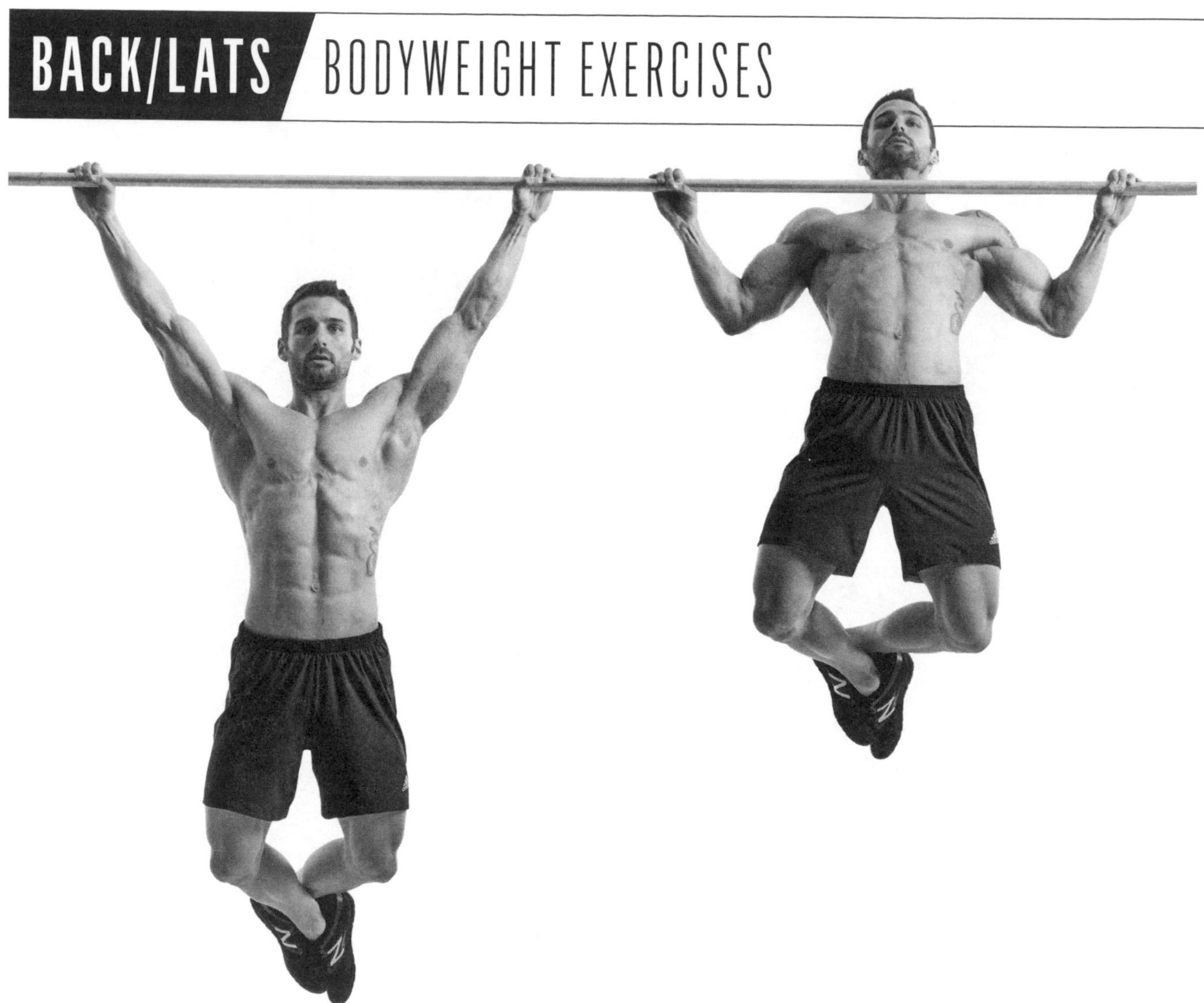

WIDE-GRIP PULLUP

PURPOSE

Target your lats and hit your teres major and biceps.

START

Grab a chinup bar with an overhand grip one and a half times as wide as your shoulders.

MOVEMENT

Hang at arm's length. Squeeze your shoulder blades together and pull your chest to the bar.

FINISH

Pause, then slowly lower your body back to an arm's length hang, or dead hang position.

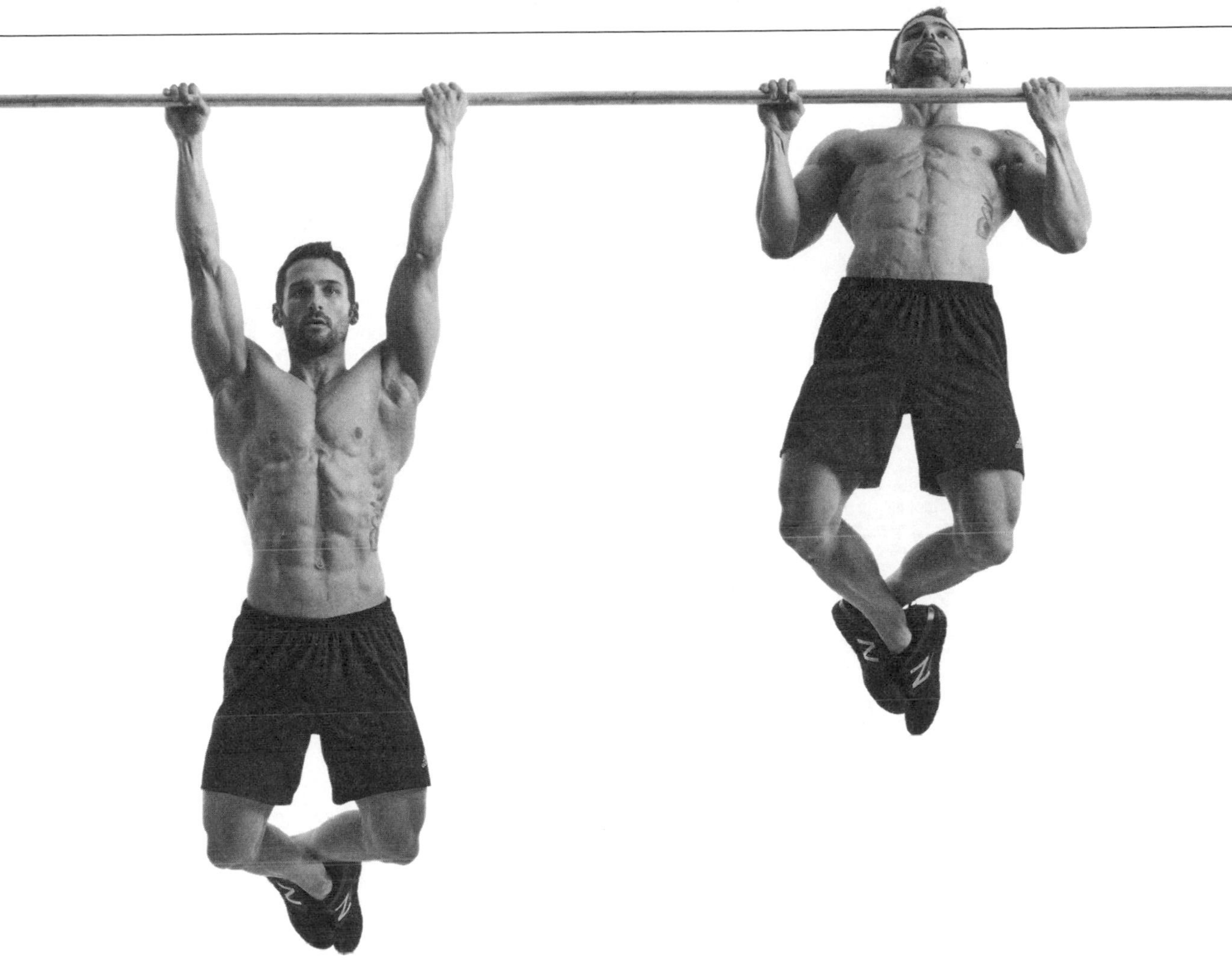

MIXED-GRIP CHINUP

PURPOSE
Target your lats and hit your teres major and biceps.

START
Grab a chinup bar with your hands shoulder width apart and with one hand in an underhand grip and one hand in an overhand grip.

MOVEMENT
Hang at arm's length. Squeeze your shoulder blades together and pull your chest to the bar.

FINISH
Pause, then slowly lower your body back to the dead hang position.

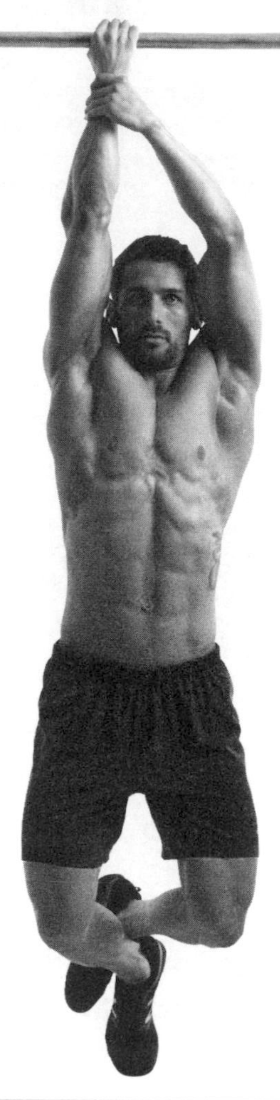

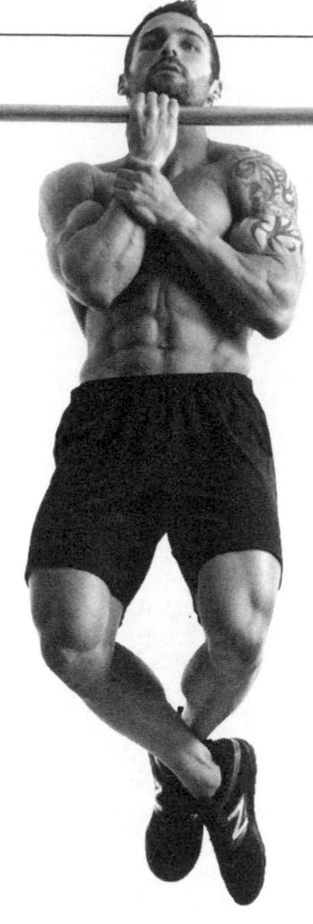

ONE-ARM GRIP CHINUP

PURPOSE

Target your lats and hit your teres major and biceps.

START

Grab a chinup bar with one hand and hold your wrist with the other hand for support.

MOVEMENT

Hang at arm's length. Pull your chin to the bar.

FINISH

Pause, then slowly lower your body back to the dead hang position.

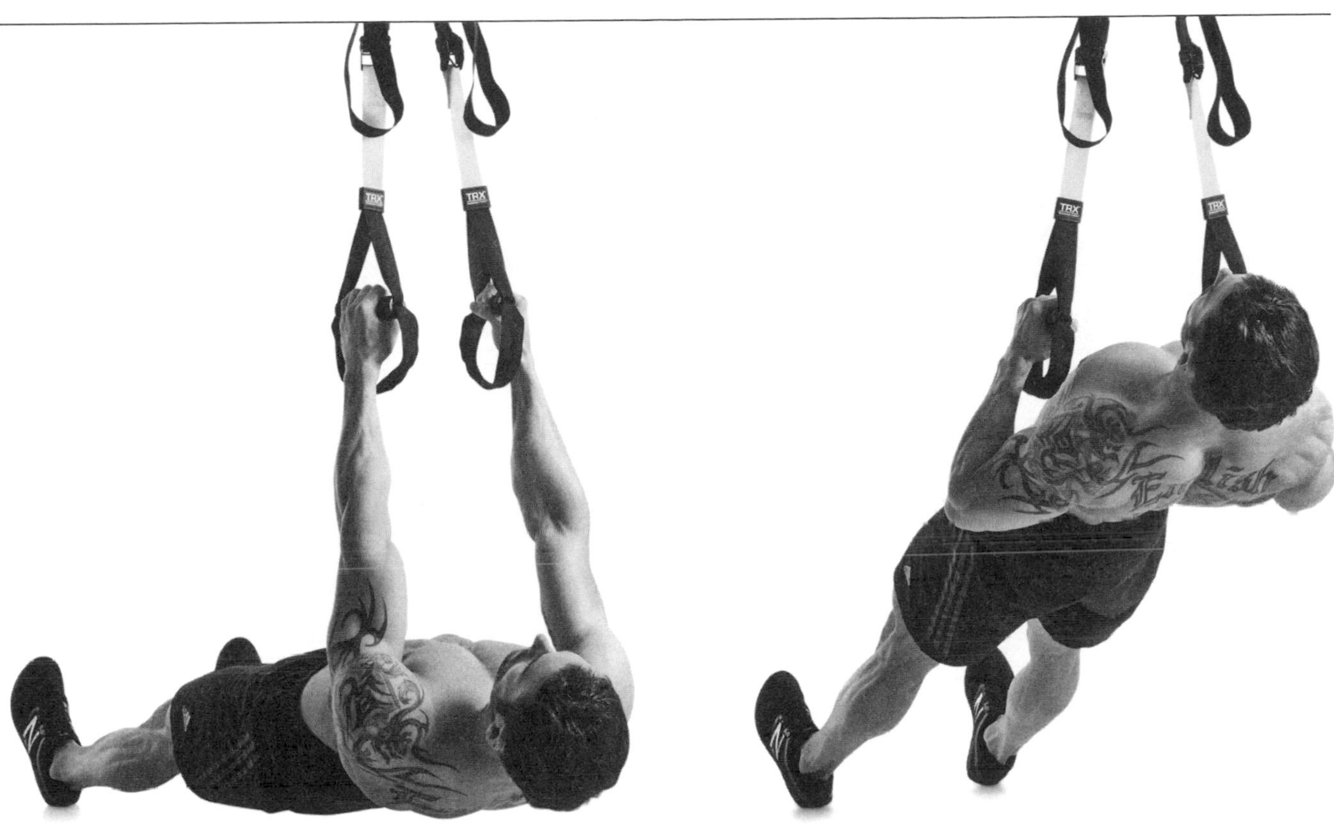

SUSPENDED INVERTED ROW WITH TRX

PURPOSE

Target the rhomboids and latissimus dorsi.

START

Place your body anywhere from parallel to a 45-degree angle while grabbing the handles of TRX straps so your palms are facing each other. Start with the handles just outside your chest with your arms extended (slight elbow bend). Keep your feet shoulder width apart and your weight on the balls of your heels.

MOVEMENT

Squeezing your shoulder blades and bracing your core, pull your body toward the ceiling.

FINISH

Pause, then return to the starting position.

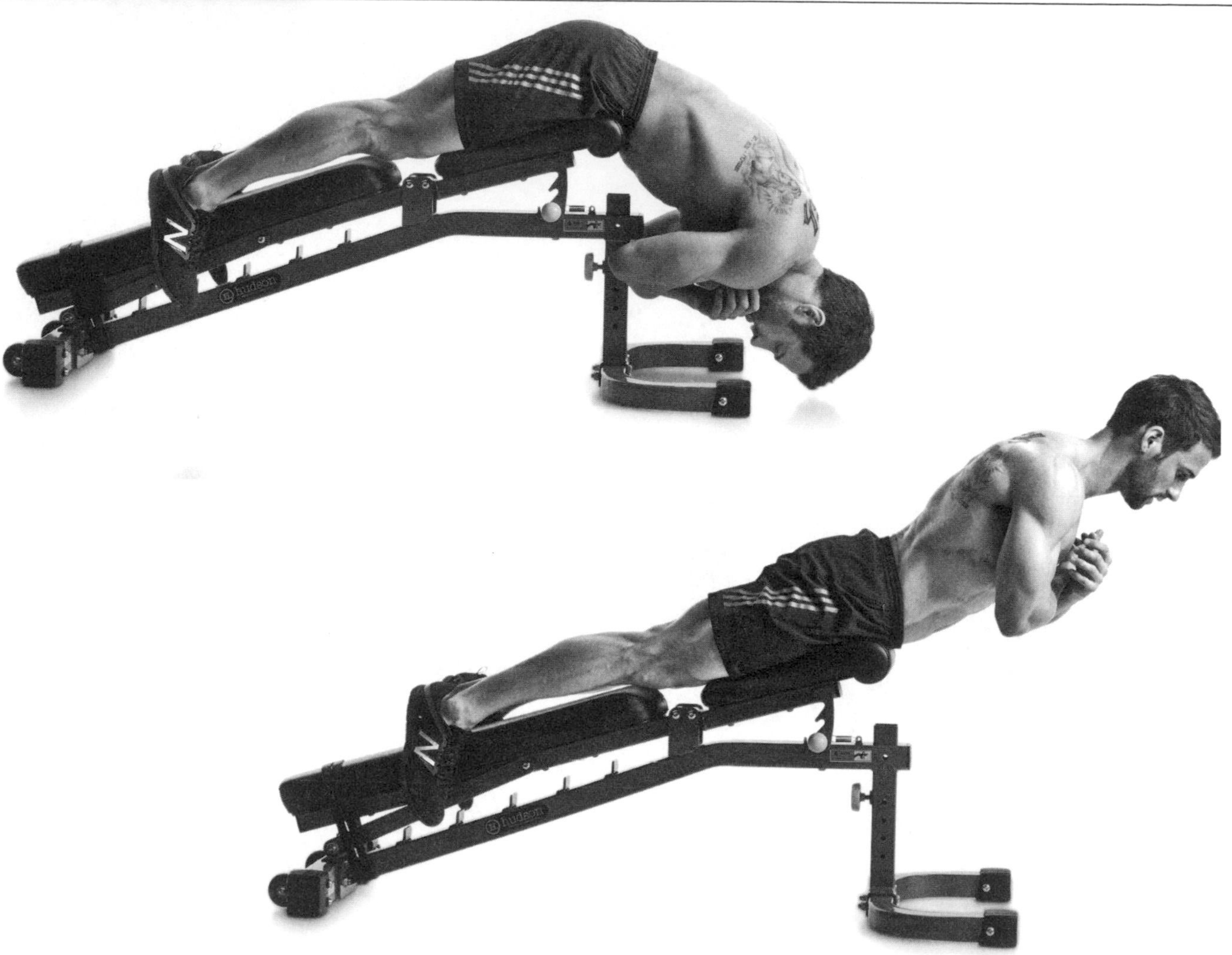

BACK EXTENSION

PURPOSE

Target the lower back muscles and hamstrings.

START

Lie face forward on a Roman chair or bench (as shown) so that your hips are on it but your upper body, starting at your navel, hangs off. Tuck your ankles under foot-pads if available or hold yourself by squeezing your feet against the bench.

MOVEMENT

Cross your arms in front of your chest and slowly bend forward at the waist as far as you can while keeping your back flat. Feel the nice stretch in your hamstrings. Do not round your back.

FINISH

Pause, then slowly raise your torso until your body forms a straight line from heels to head. Avoid the temptation to arch your back past the straight line to avoid injury.

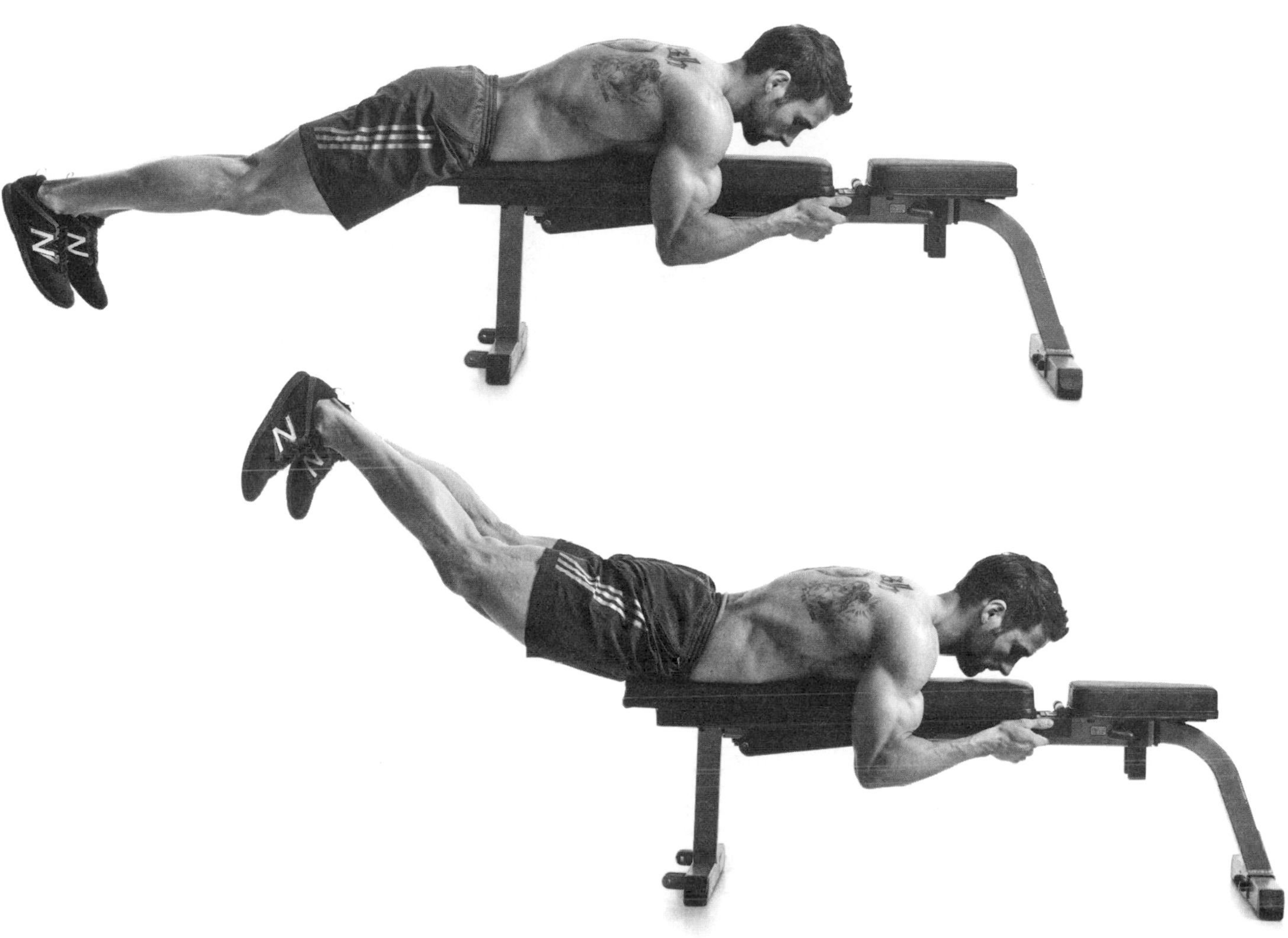

REVERSE HYPER-EXTENSION

PURPOSE

Target the lower back muscles.

START

Lie prone (facedown) with your torso on a flat bench from the navel up and your legs hanging off behind you.

MOVEMENT

Holding on to the bench, lift your legs and feet until they are parallel to slightly above parallel with the floor.

FINISH

Pause, then lower your legs to the starting position.

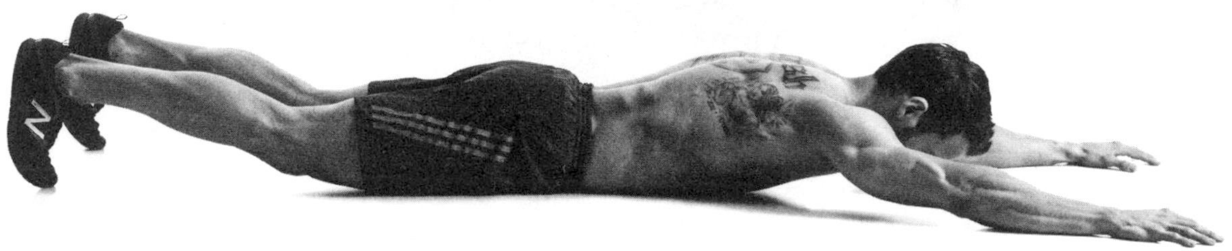

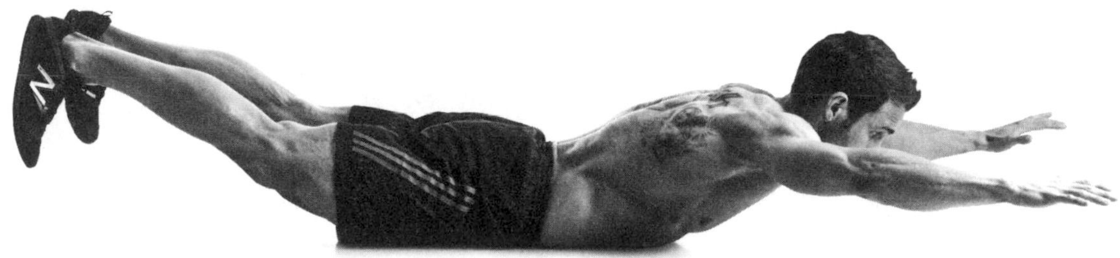

SUPERMAN

PURPOSE
Target the lower back muscles.

START
Lie prone (face-down) on the ground. Place your arms overhead just outside your shoulders. Keep your feet hip width apart.

MOVEMENT
Simultaneously lift your arms, chest, and legs off the ground, flexing your middle and lower back.

FINISH
Pause, then return to the starting position.

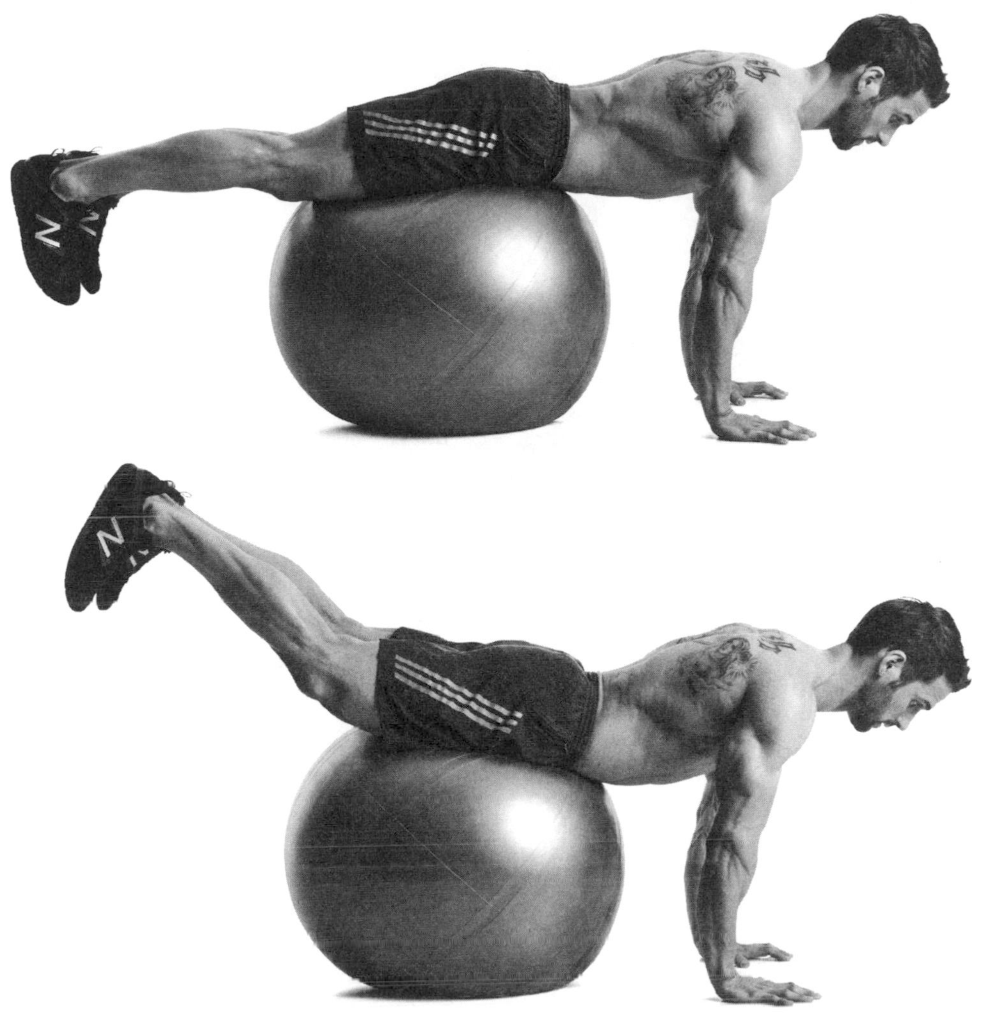

STABILITY BALL HYPER-EXTENSION

PURPOSE
Target the muscles of the lower back.

START
Lie on a stability ball with your upper abdominal region on the ball. Place your hands on the ground.

MOVEMENT
Flexing your glutes and maintaining a natural arch to your lower back, elevate your legs and feet as high as your flexibility will allow.

FINISH
Pause, then lower your legs to the starting position.

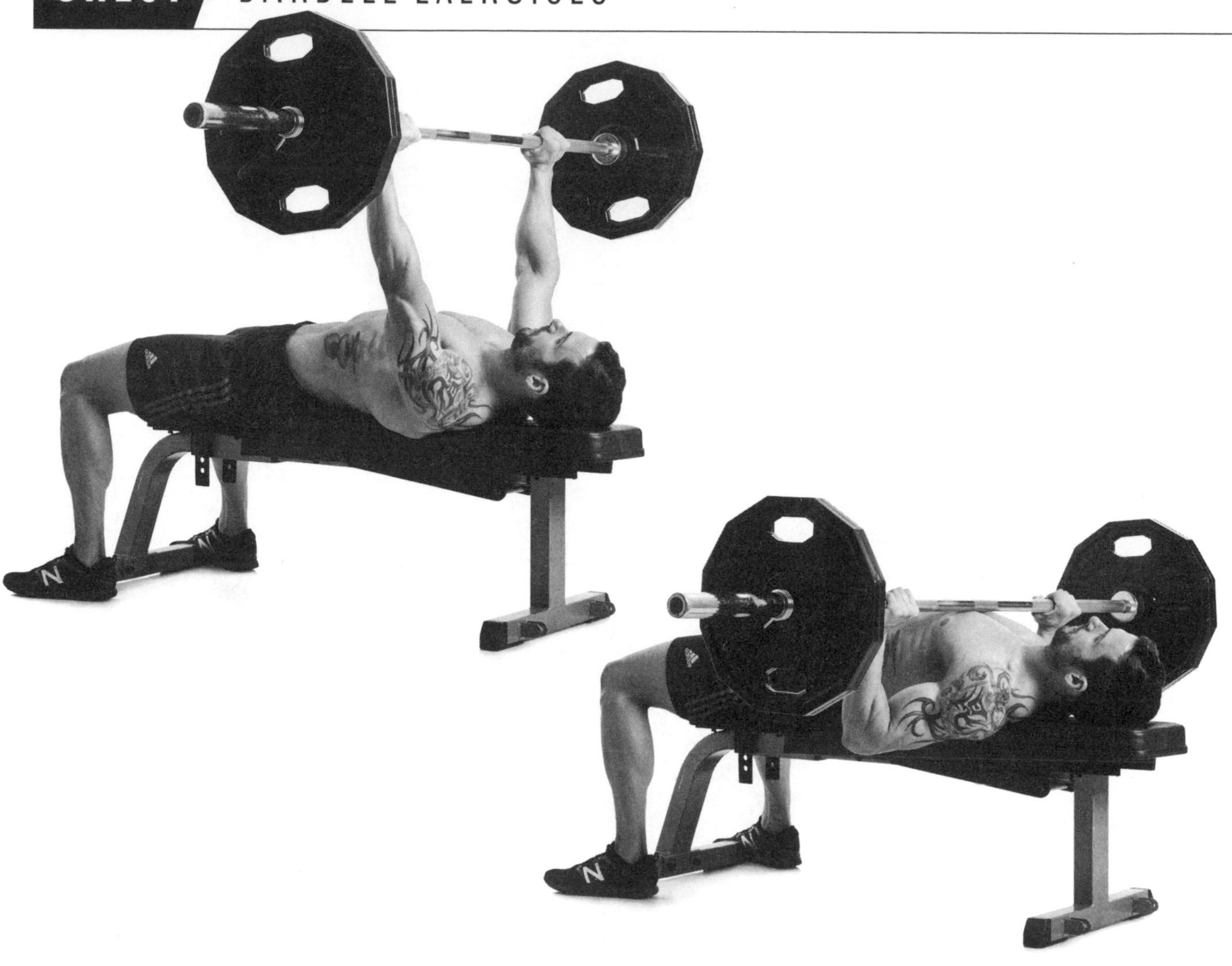

BENCH PRESS

PURPOSE

For overall chest development.

START

Lie on a bench with your head, torso, and hips pressed against the bench and keep your feet flat on the floor. Use an overhand grip (wrapping your thumbs around the barbell) and place your hands just outside your shoulders (slightly wider than shoulder width). Remove the bar from the uprights and with straight arms hold it over your collarbone.

MOVEMENT

Keeping your shoulder blades together, lower the bar in a slow and controlled manner to your mid chest (just above your nipples).

FINISH

Pause briefly, then press the bar back to finish just over your collarbone. (Stop just short of locking out your elbows.)

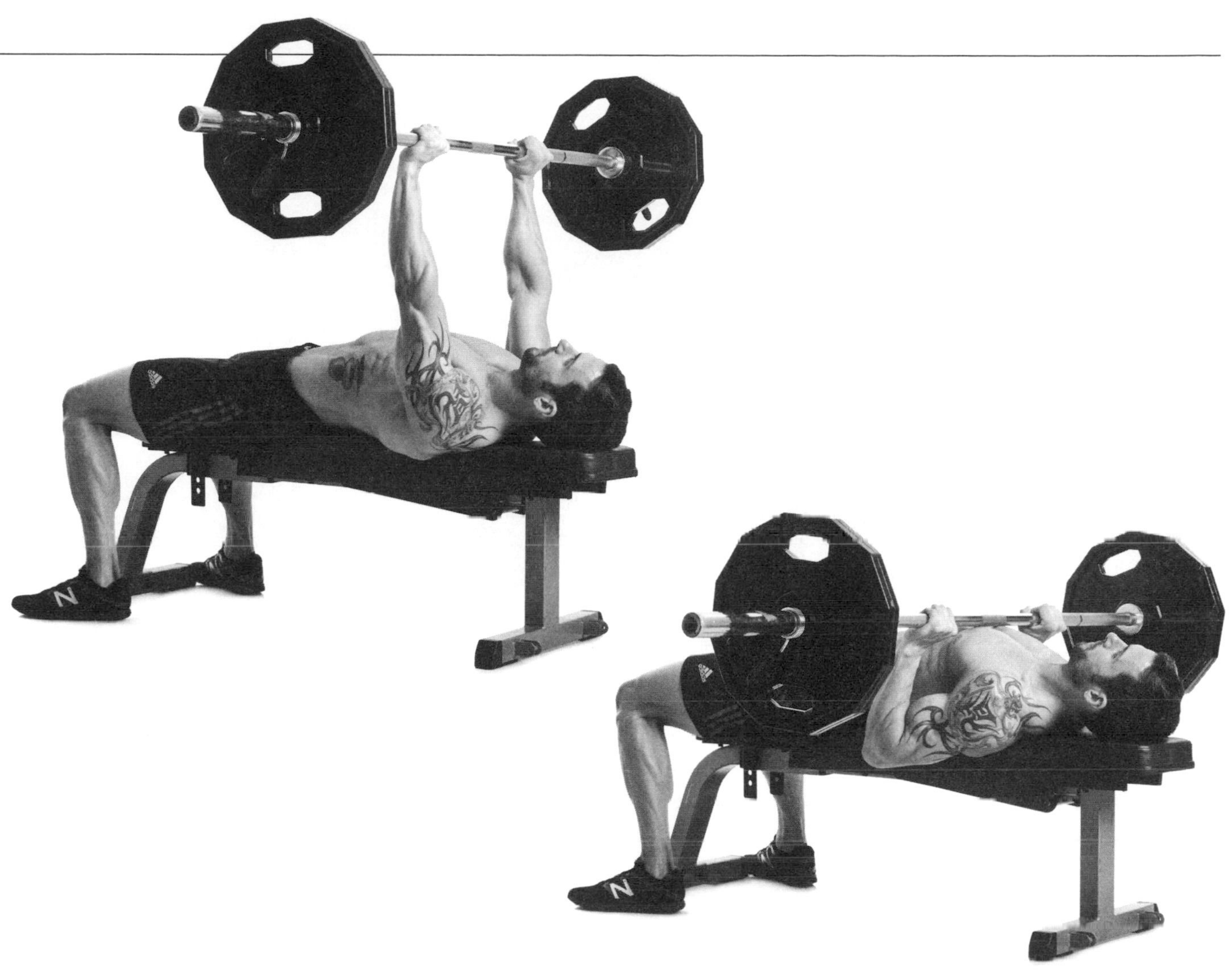

CLOSE-GRIP BENCH PRESS

PURPOSE

For overall chest development.

START

Lie on a bench with your head, torso, and hips pressed against the bench and keep your feet flat on the floor. Use an overhand grip, place your hands less than shoulder width apart (around 8 inches). Remove the bar from the uprights and with straight arms hold it over your collarbone.

MOVEMENT

Keeping your shoulder blades together, lower the bar in a slow and controlled manner to your mid chest (just above your nipples).

FINISH

Pause briefly, then press the bar back to finish just over your collarbone. (Stop just short of locking out your elbows.)

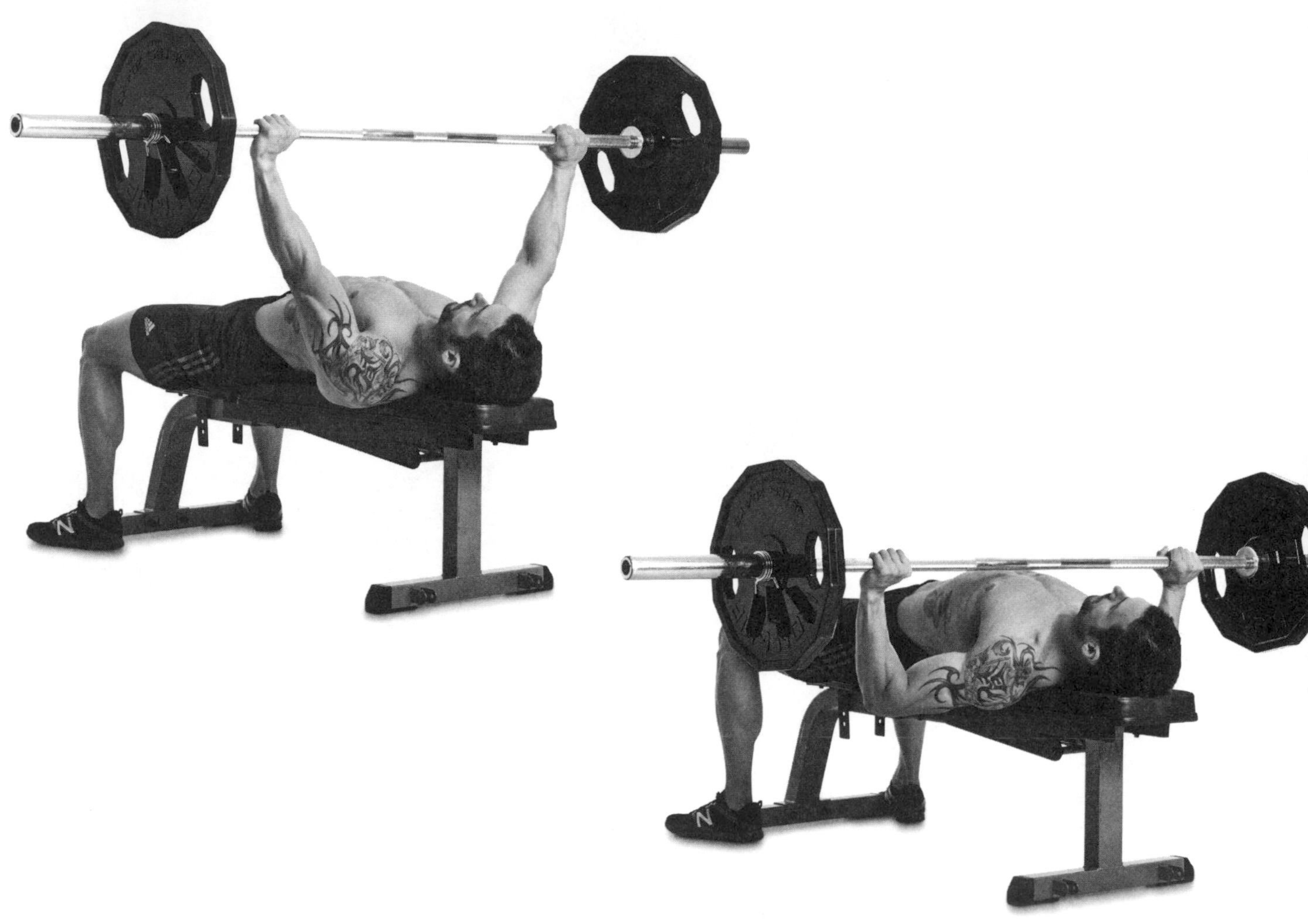

WIDE-GRIP BENCH PRESS

PURPOSE

For greater chest development by eliminating the use of the triceps and shoulders.

START

Lie on a bench with your head, torso, and hips pressed against the bench and keep your feet flat on the floor. Use an overhand grip and use a wide grip (twice that of shoulder width). Remove the bar from the uprights and with straight arms hold it over your collarbone.

MOVEMENT

Keeping your shoulder blades together, lower the bar in a slow and controlled manner to your mid chest (just above your nipples).

FINISH

Pause briefly, then press the bar back to finish just over your collarbone. (Stop just short of locking your elbows.)

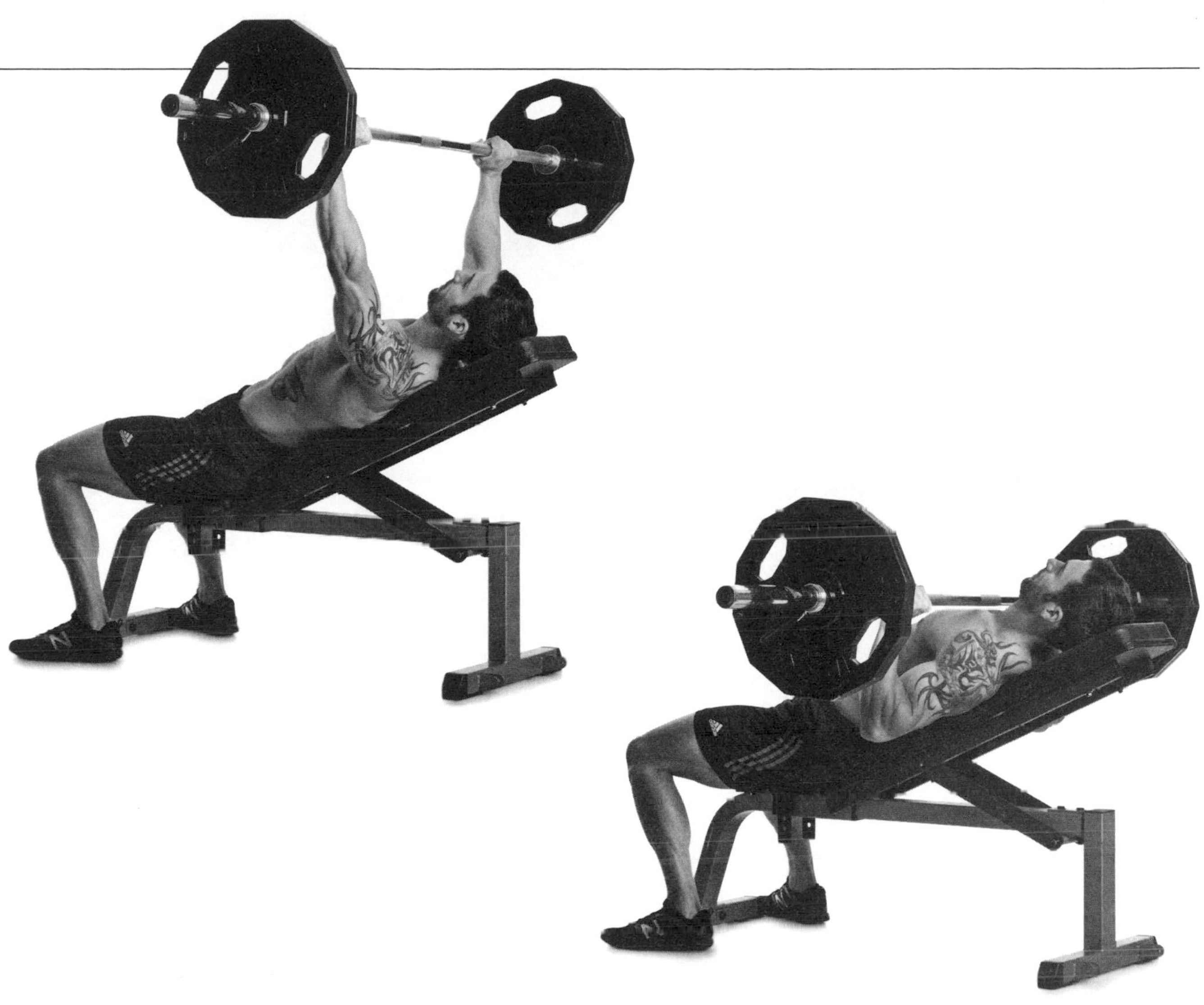

INCLINE BENCH PRESS

PURPOSE

Target the upper chest and handle greater resistance.

START

Set the incline to a 10- to 30-degree angle. (A steeper angle will put too much emphasis on the deltoids.) Keeping your torso, head, and hips pressed against the bench and feet flat on the floor, use an overhand grip slightly wider than shoulder width. Remove the bar from the uprights and with straight arms hold it over your chin.

MOVEMENT

Lower the barbell, in a controlled manner, to 1 to 2 inches from your collarbone.

FINISH

Pause briefly, then press the barbell back to finish above your chin.

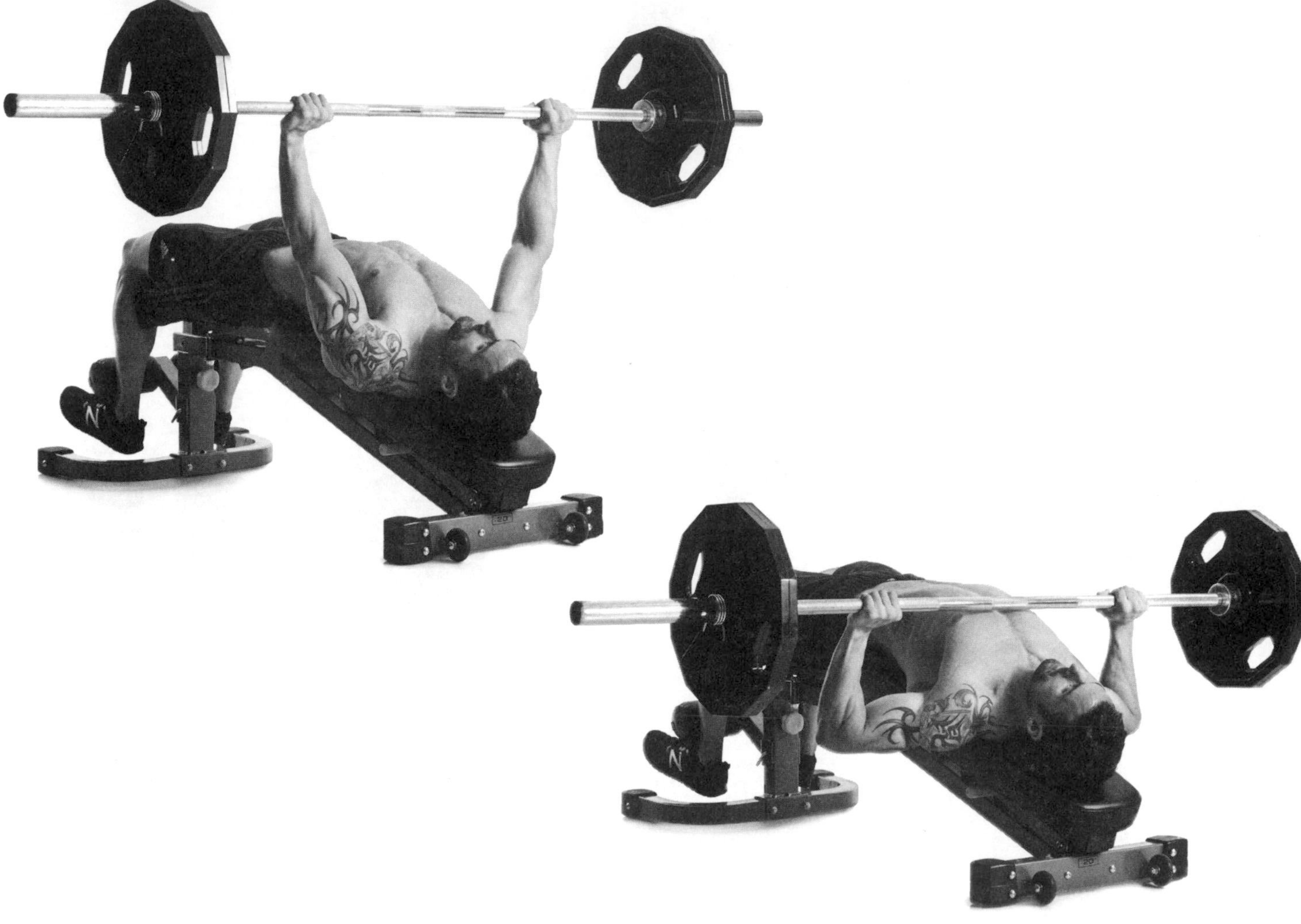

DECLINE BENCH PRESS

PURPOSE
Target the lower chest.

START
Lie on a decline bench with your shins hooked beneath the leg support. Hold the bar with an overhand grip and just outside your shoulders.

MOVEMENT
Start with the barbell over your lower chest. Lower the bar in a controlled pattern to touch your chest.

FINISH
Pause briefly, without resting the bar on your chest, then press the barbell back up.

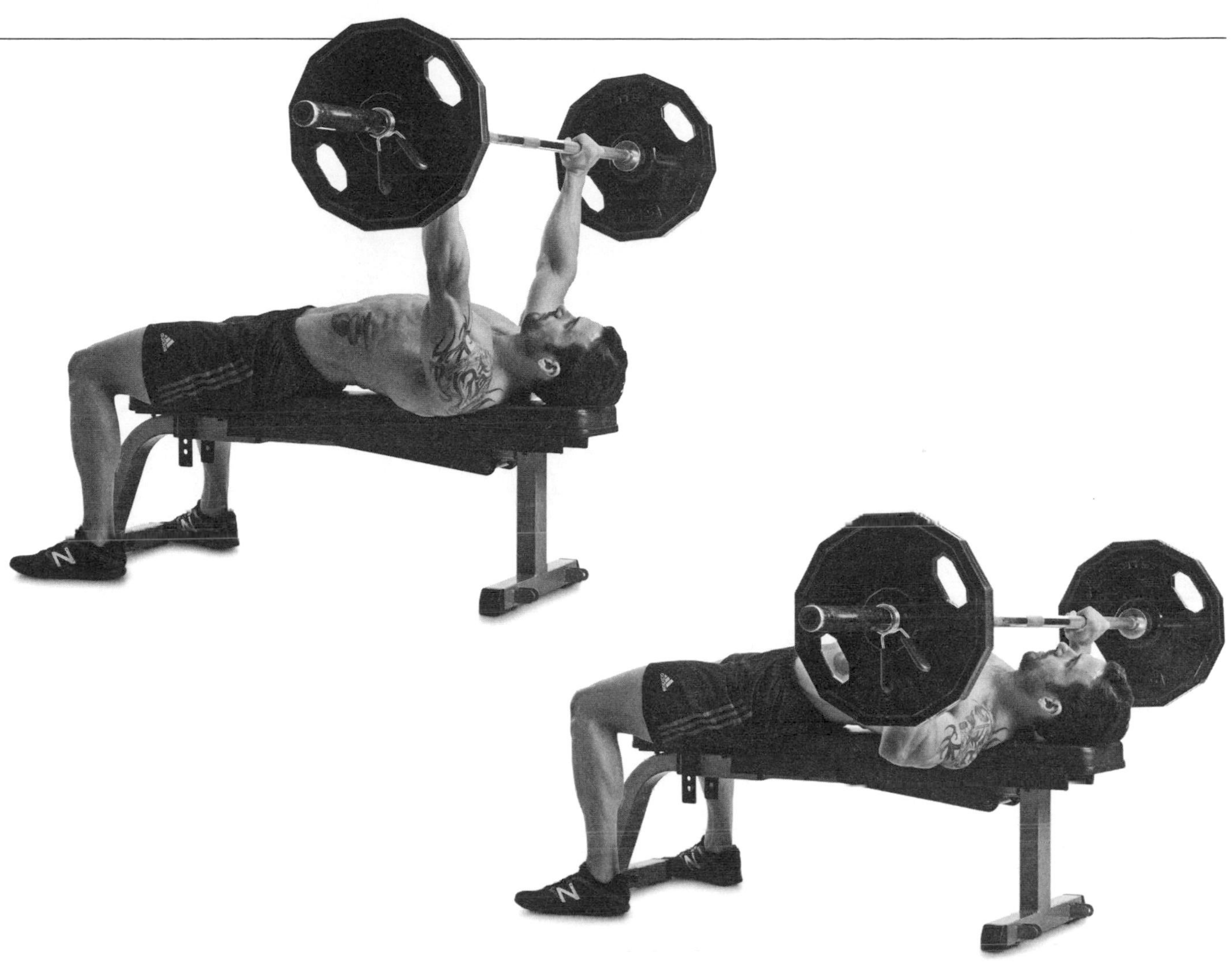

NECK BENCH PRESS

Note: For safety, always use a spotter when performing this exercise.

PURPOSE

For greater upper chest and anterior deltoid development.

START

Be sure to have an advanced lifter spot you on this movement. Lie on a bench with your head, torso, and hips pressed against the bench, while keeping your feet flat on the floor. Use an overhand grip (wrapping your thumbs around the barbell) and place your hands just outside your shoulders (slightly wider than shoulder width). Remove the bar from the uprights and with straight arms hold it over your collarbone.

MOVEMENT

Keeping your shoulder blades together, lower the bar in a slow and controlled manner to your upper chest, just above your collarbone and lower neck.

FINISH

Pause briefly, then press the bar back to finish just over your collarbone and neck. (Stop just short of locking your elbows.)

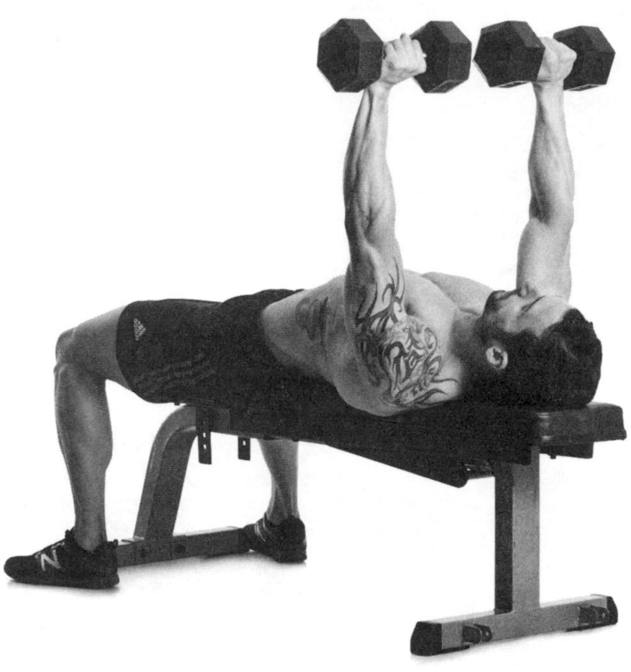

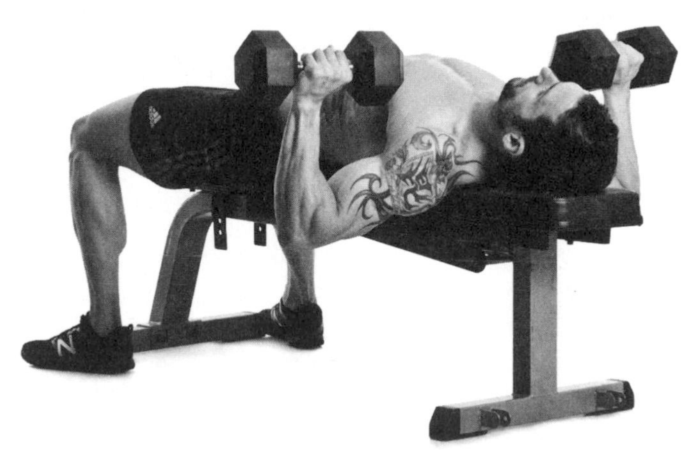

BENCH PRESS

PURPOSE

For overall chest development.

START

Lie on a flat bench holding two dumbbells over your mid chest using an overhand grip (wrapping your thumbs around the dumbbell).

MOVEMENT

Keeping your shoulder blades pinched, bend your elbows and lower the dumbbells until they are just outside your chest near your armpits—just off your chest.

FINISH

Pause, then press the dumbbells back to the starting position. (Do not clank the weights at the top, instead focus on flexing the chest.)

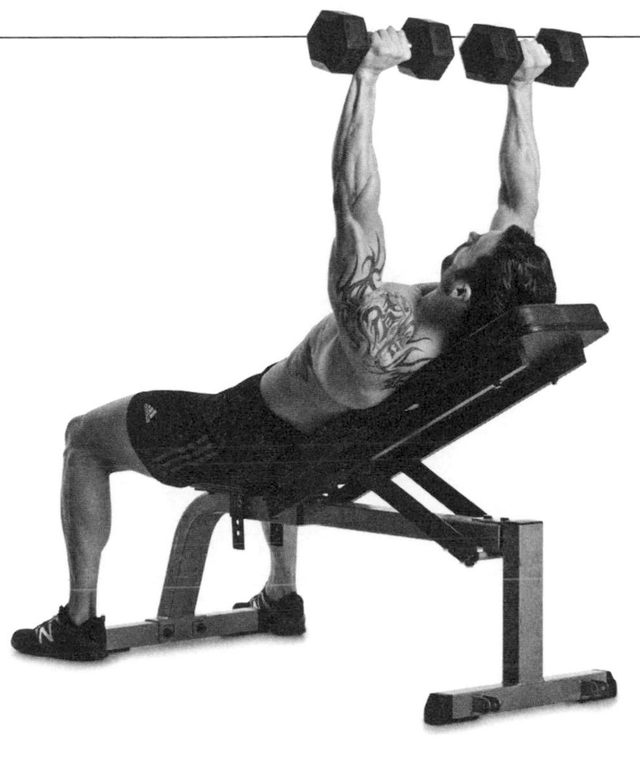

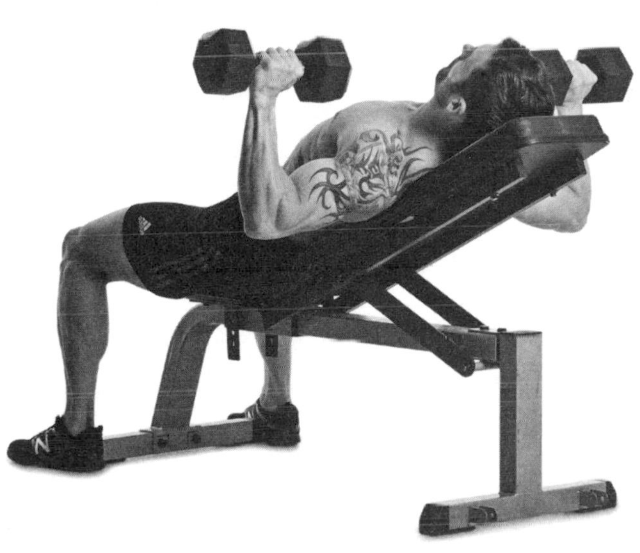

INCLINE BENCH PRESS

PURPOSE

For upper chest development.

START

Lie on an incline bench holding two dumbbells over your upper chest and collarbone area using an overhand grip.

MOVEMENT

Keeping your shoulder blades pinched, and your head, torso, and hips against the bench, bend your elbows and lower the dumbbells until they are just outside your chest near your armpits—just off your chest.

FINISH

Pause, then press the dumbbells back to the starting position above your collarbone. (Do not clank the weights at the top, instead focus on flexing the chest.)

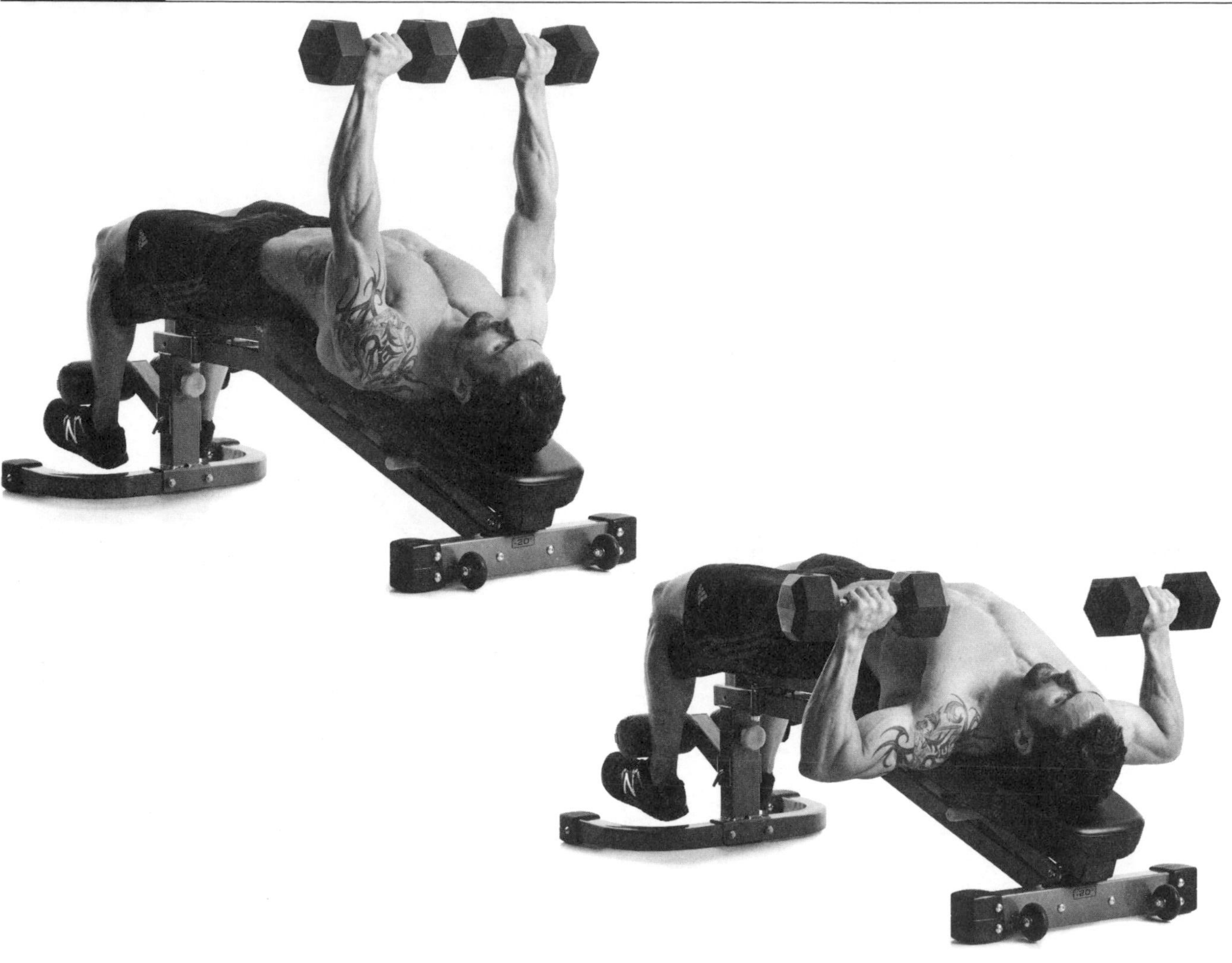

DECLINE BENCH PRESS

PURPOSE
Target the lower chest.

START
Lie on a decline bench with your shins hooked beneath the leg support. Hold the dumbbells with an overhand grip and just outside your shoulders.

MOVEMENT
Start with the dumbbells over your lower chest. Lower the dumbbells in a controlled pattern finishing an inch or two above your chest with your elbows outside the body.

FINISH
Pause briefly, then press the dumbbells back up.

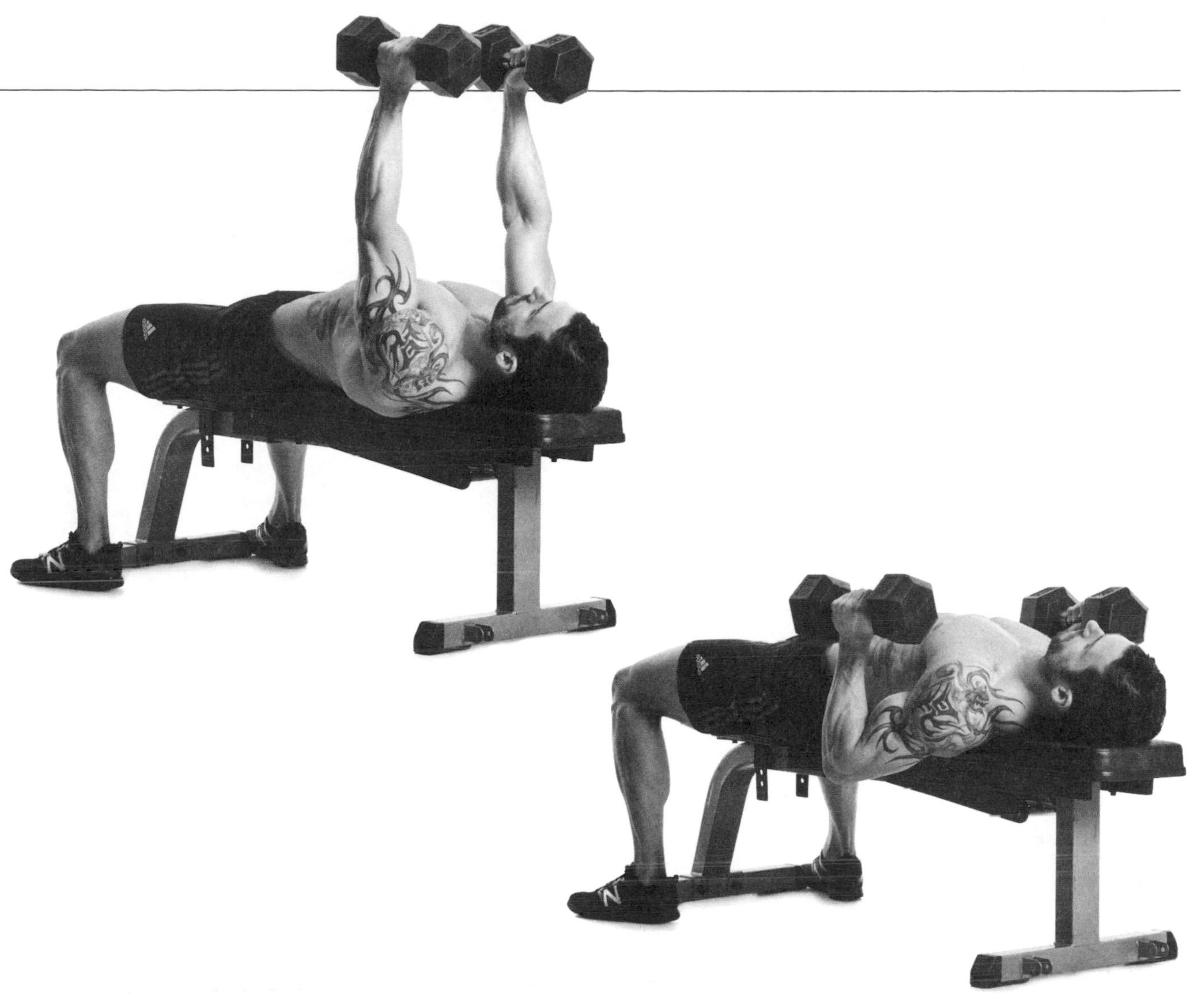

NEUTRAL-GRIP BENCH PRESS

PURPOSE
To work the chest with greater use from the triceps and less strain on the shoulders.

START
Grab a pair of dumbbells with a neutral grip (palms facing each other). This is also known as a hammer grip. Lie on a bench. Hold the dumbbells over your shoulders with arms extended.

MOVEMENT
Lower the weights straight down just outside your chest and allow your elbows to pass by your sides. Stop before the dumbbells can touch your chest.

FINISH
Pause, then return to the top by pressing.

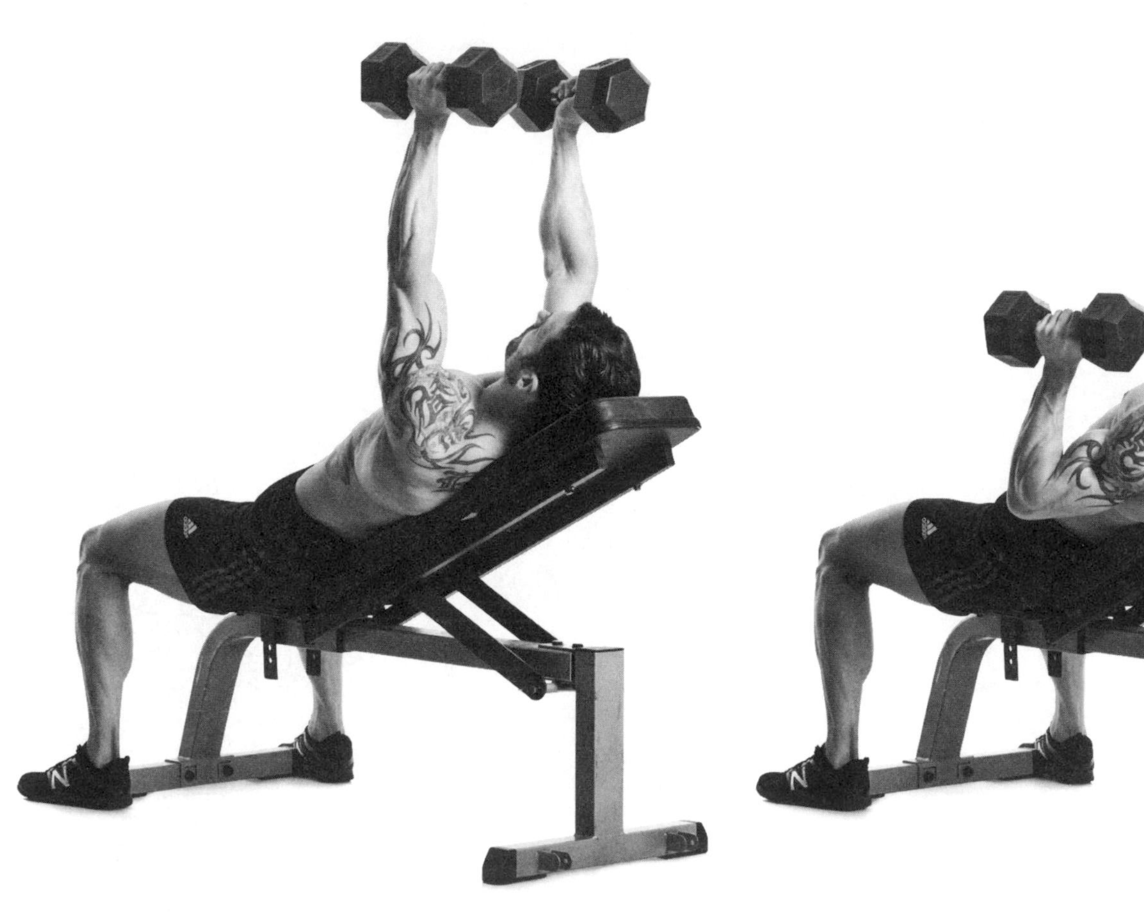

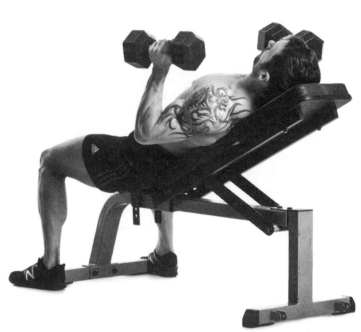

NEUTRAL-GRIP INCLINE BENCH PRESS

PURPOSE
To work the upper chest with greater use from the triceps and less strain on the shoulders.

START
Grab a pair of dumbbells with a neutral grip (palms facing each other). Lie on an incline bench. Hold the weights above your shoulders.

MOVEMENT
Lower the weights straight down just outside your chest and allow your elbows to pass by your sides. Stop before the dumbbells can touch your chest.

FINISH
Pause, then return to the top by pressing.

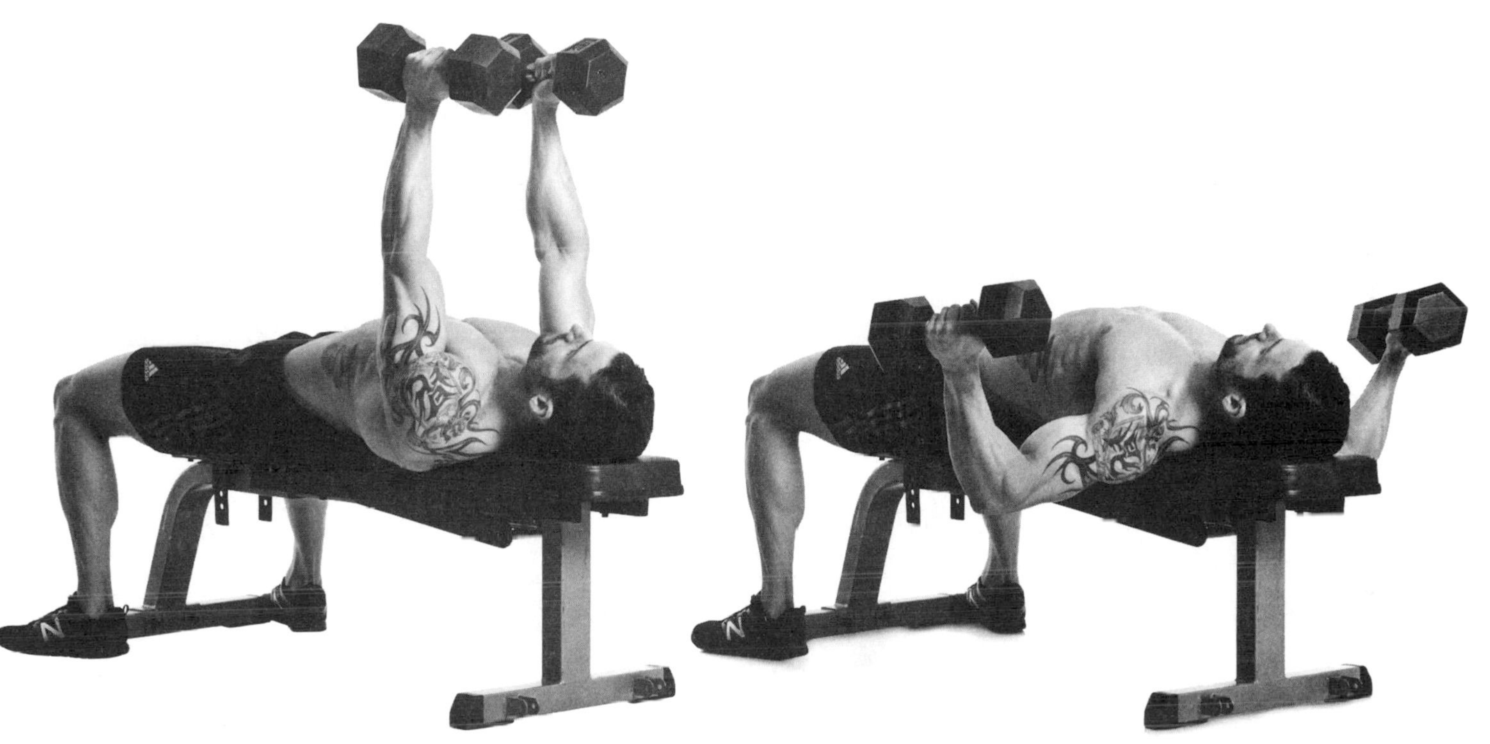

FLAT CHEST FLY

PURPOSE

To isolate and create better upper chest development.

START

Lie on a bench while holding a dumbbell in each hand. Start with your palms facing each other, arms straight, and the weights held over your upper chest.

MOVEMENT

Simultaneously lower the dumbbells to just outside your chest. Maintain a slight bend in the elbows.

FINISH

Flex your chest, and in a slight "hugging" pattern, bring the dumbbells back to the starting position over the top of your chest.

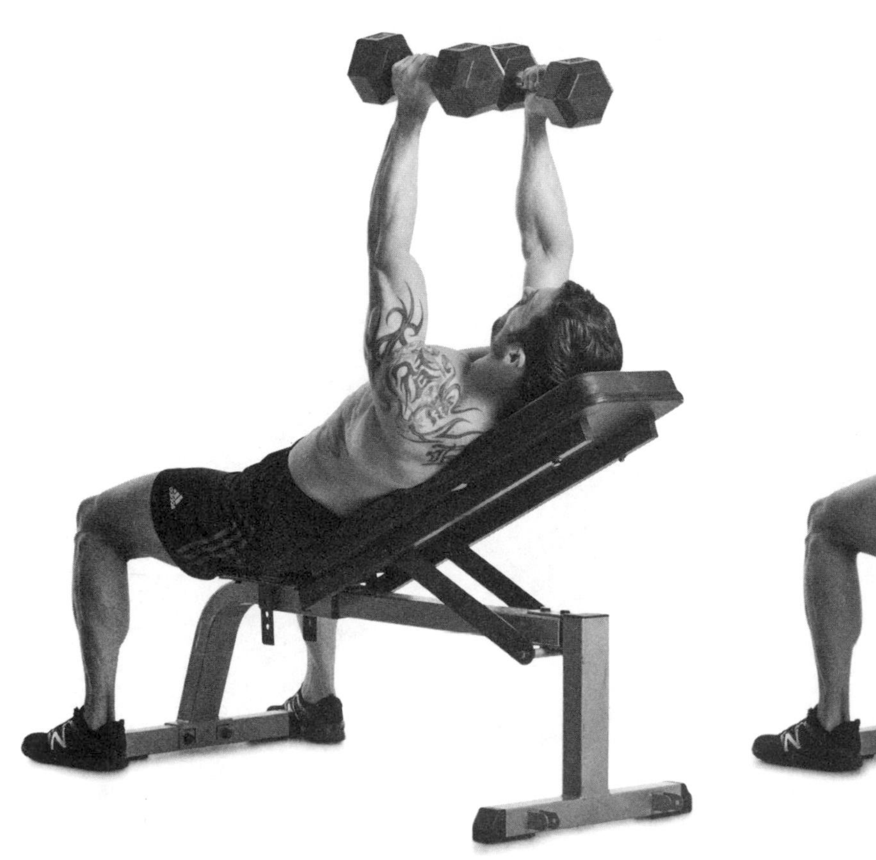

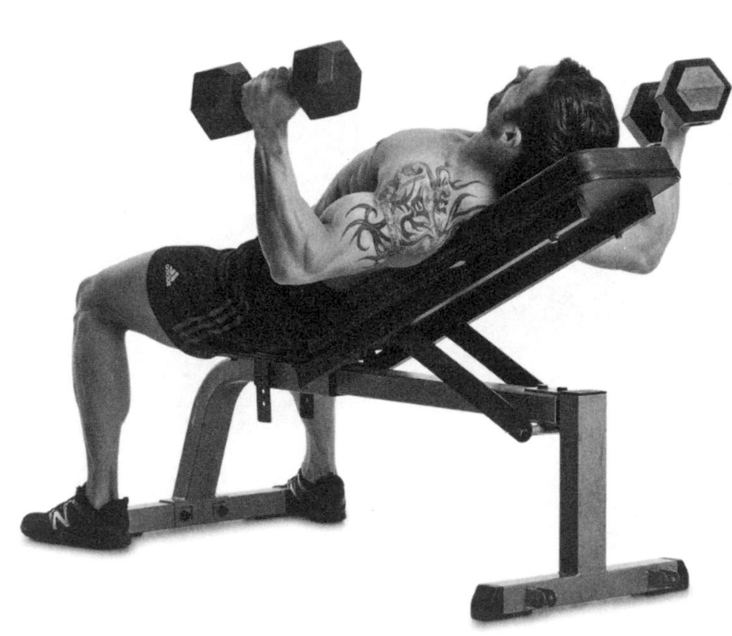

INCLINE FLY

PURPOSE

To isolate and create better chest development.

START

Lie on an incline bench while holding a dumbbell in each hand. Start with your palms facing each other and the weights over your chest.

MOVEMENT

Simultaneously lower the dumbbells to just outside your chest. Maintain a slight bend in the elbows.

FINISH

Flex your chest, and in a slight "hugging" motion, bring the dumbbells back to the starting position just over the center of your chest.

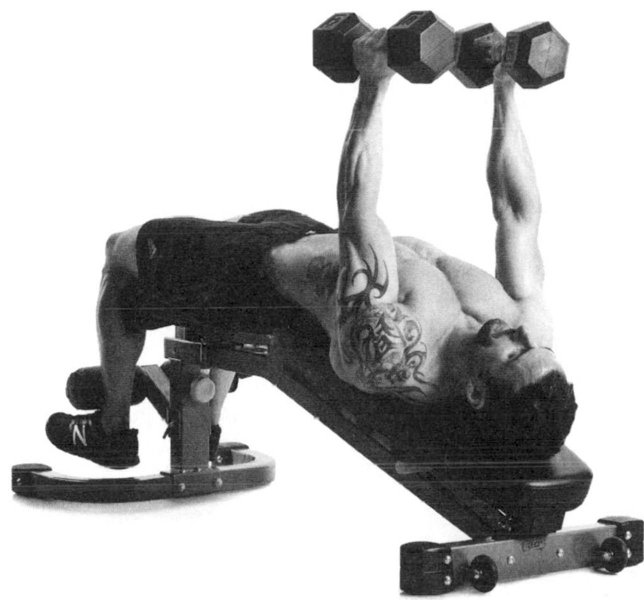

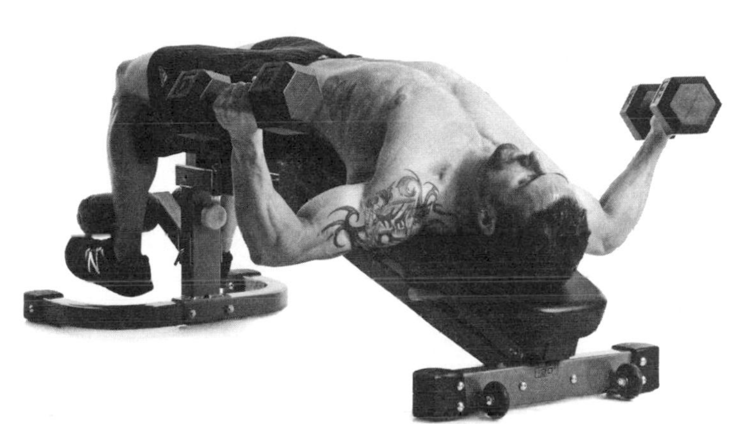

DECLINE FLY

PURPOSE

To isolate and create better lower chest development.

START

Lie on a decline bench while holding a dumbbell in each hand. Start with your palms facing each other and the weights over your chest.

MOVEMENT

Simultaneously lower the dumbbells to just outside your chest. Maintain a slight bend in the elbows.

FINISH

Flex your chest, and in a slight "hugging" motion, bring the dumbbells back to the starting position.

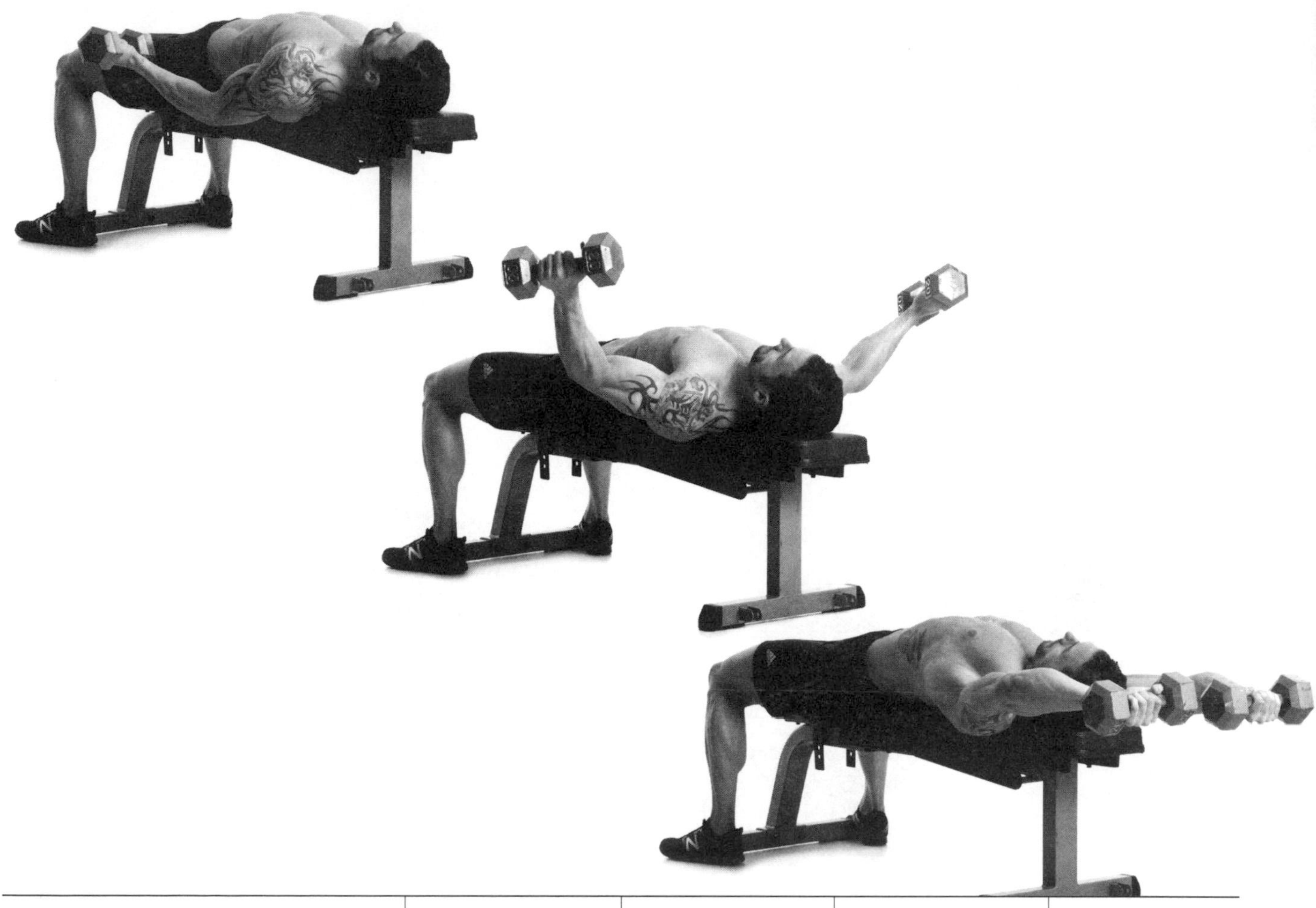

AROUND THE WORLD

PURPOSE
To isolate the chest.

START
Start by lying on a bench and holding two dumbbells with your palms facing up just outside your hips.

MOVEMENT
In circular pattern lift the dumbbells simultaneously from your hips along your side to just over the top of your shoulders.

FINISH
Follow the reverse pattern back to your starting position outside your hips.

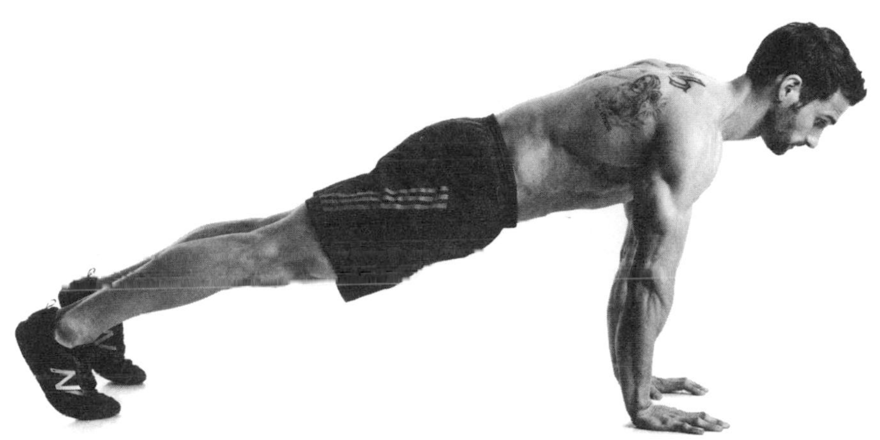

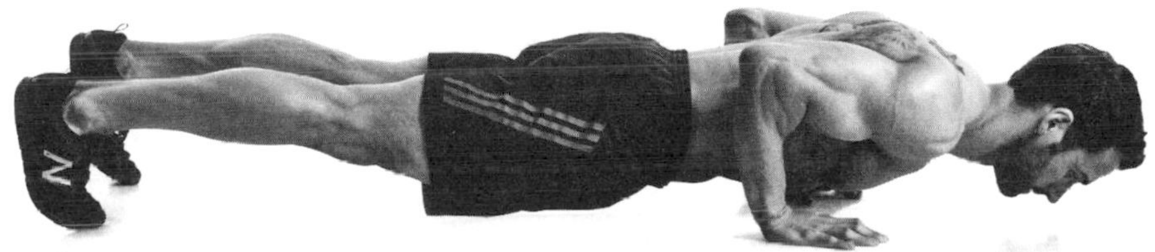

PUSHUP

PURPOSE

To gain better overall chest development and stability of the chest and shoulders.

START

Place your hands just outside your chest. Brace your core, fully extend your arms, and keep your feet shoulder width apart while creating a plank position.

MOVEMENT

Keeping your elbows in, lower your body to the floor, pushing through your palms and bracing your core.

FINISH

Pause at the bottom, then return to the top position.

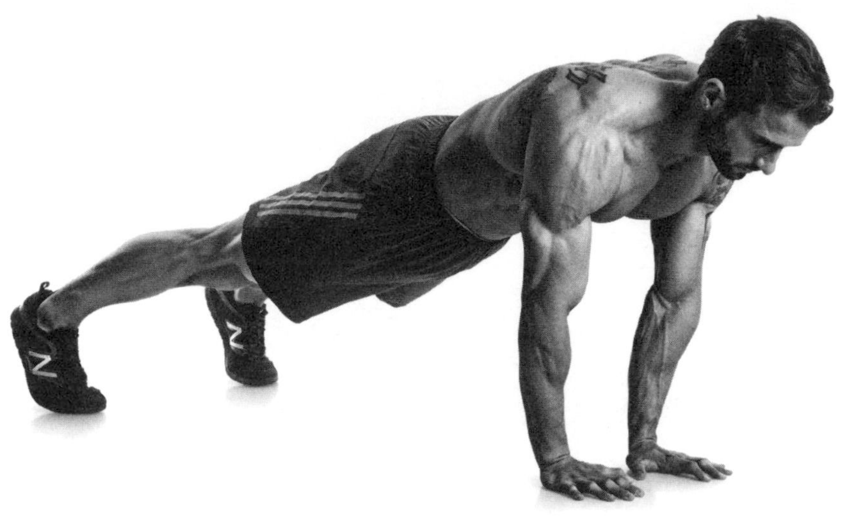

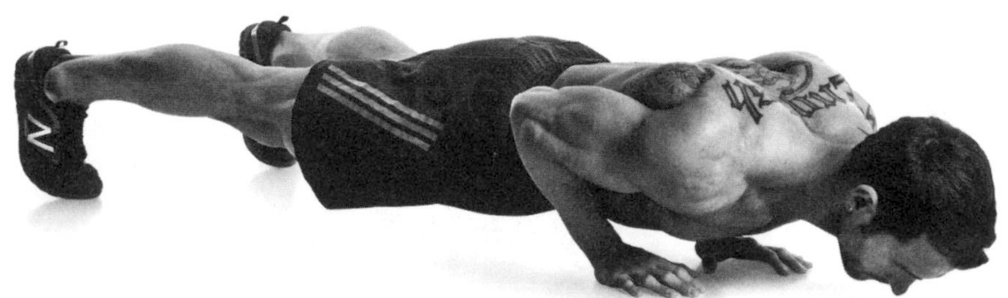

CLOSE-GRIP PUSHUP

PURPOSE
To use more of the triceps during a typical chest exercise.

START
Place your hands underneath your chest and inside your shoulders. Place your feet shoulder width apart and your body at the top pushup position.

MOVEMENT
Keeping your back flat and core braced, lower your body to the floor, pushing through your palms.

FINISH
Pause at the bottom, then push through your palms to return to the top pushup position.

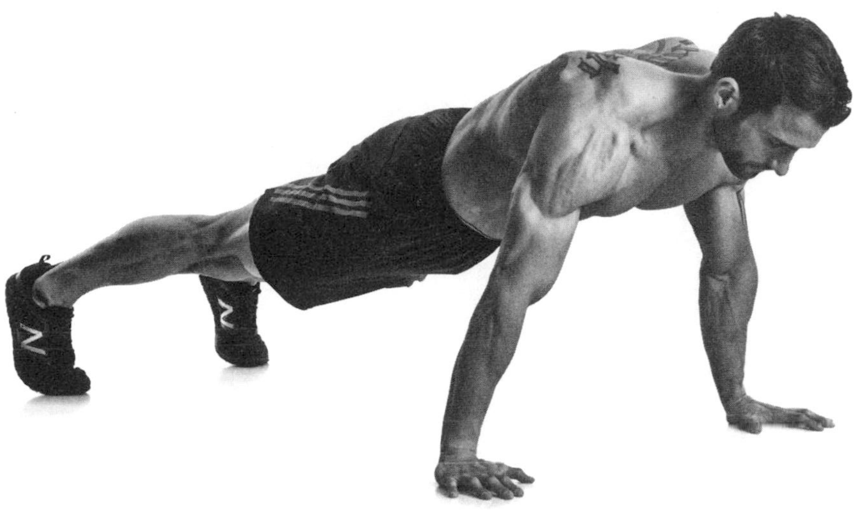

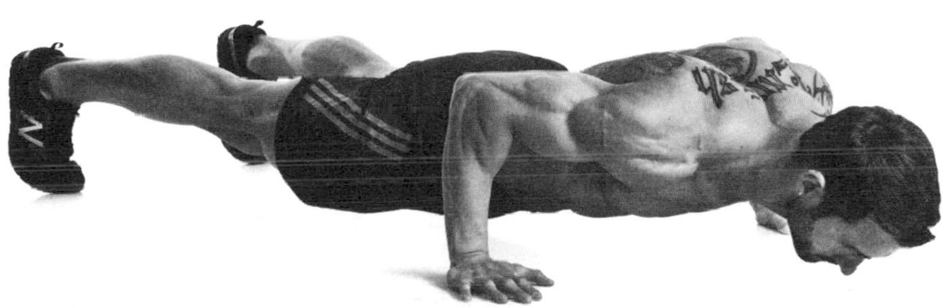

WIDE-GRIP PUSHUP

PURPOSE
To add a greater stretch to the muscle fibers of the chest.

START
Place your hands 3 to 4 inches outside the chest, just below shoulder height. Place your feet shoulder width apart and extend your arms straight.

MOVEMENT
Keeping your elbows in as much as possible, lower your chest and body simultaneously to the floor.

FINISH
Pause at the bottom, then push through your palms to return to the top pushup position.

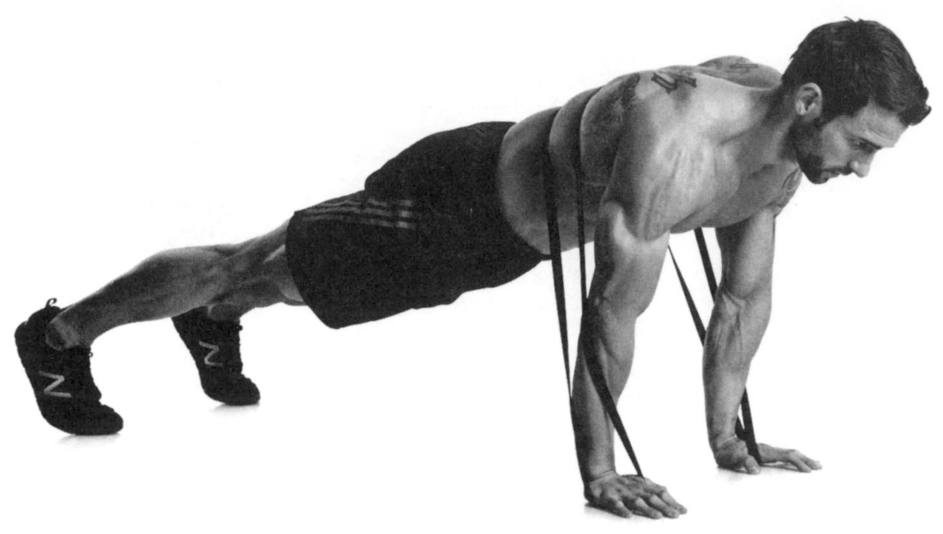

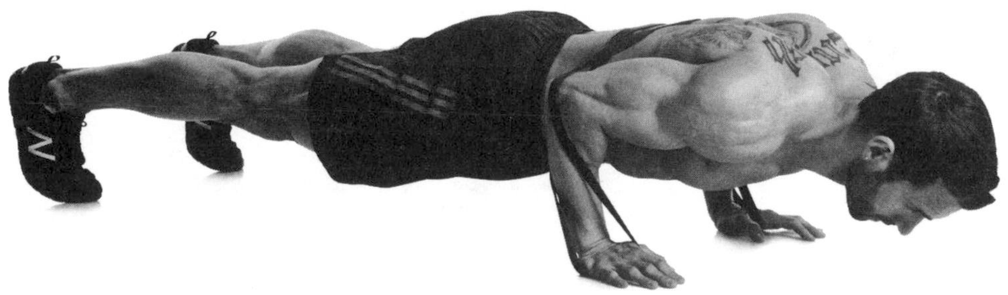

WEIGHTED PUSHUP (BAND, CHAIN, OR PLATE)

PURPOSE
To add a greater level of resistance on your pushup.

START
Wrap an exercise band around your back and secure it under your hands. Assume a top pushup position with feet shoulder width apart.

MOVEMENT
Lower your body toward the floor until your chest is $\frac{1}{2}$ inch to 1 inch off the floor.

FINISH
Push through your palms and brace your core to return to the top position.

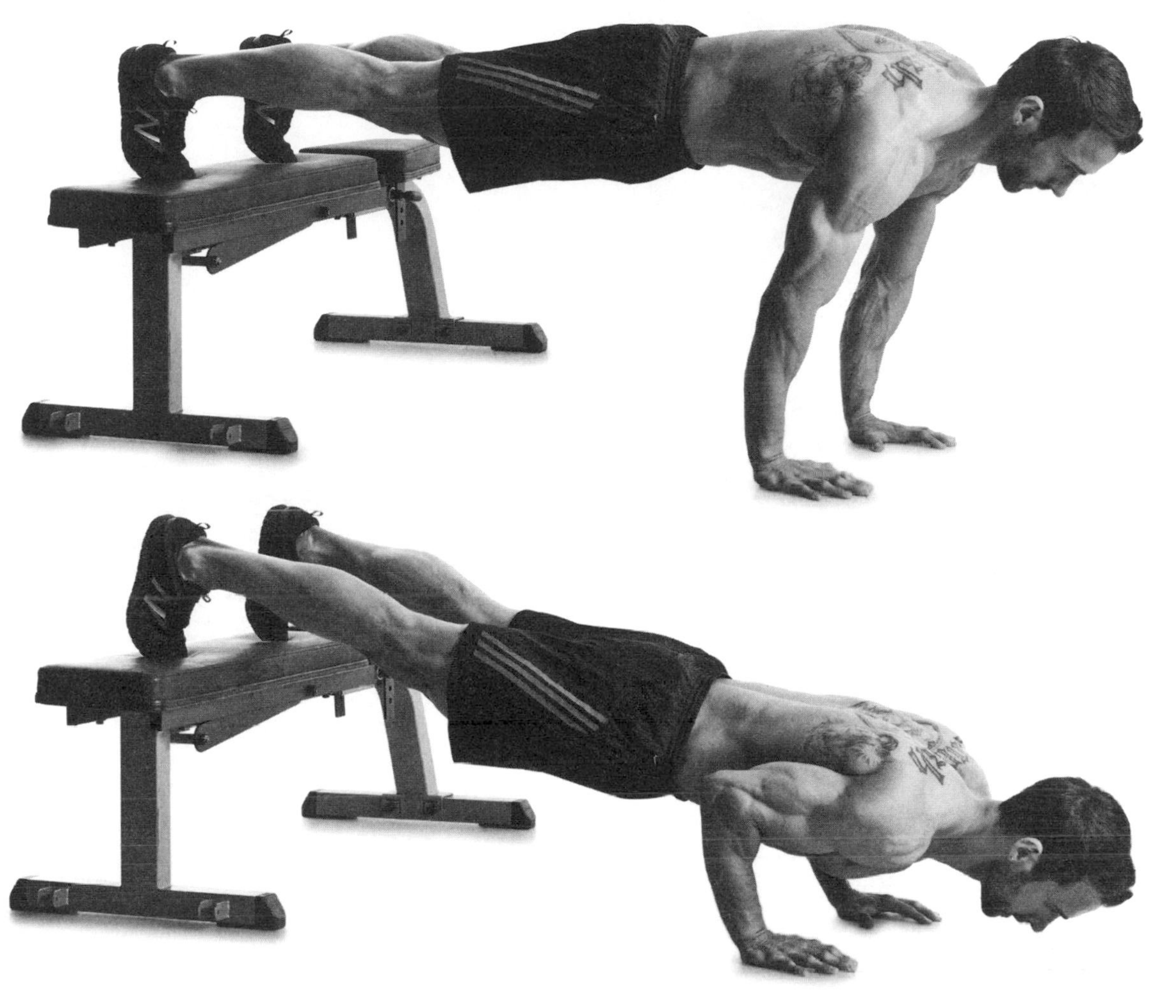

FEET-ELEVATED PUSHUP

PURPOSE
To place a greater emphasis on your core and lower pectorals.

START
In a pushup position, brace your core and place the balls of your feet on a bench.

MOVEMENT
Maintaining good posture and a strong core, lower your body toward the floor.

FINISH
Push through your palms, brace your core, and finish at the top position.

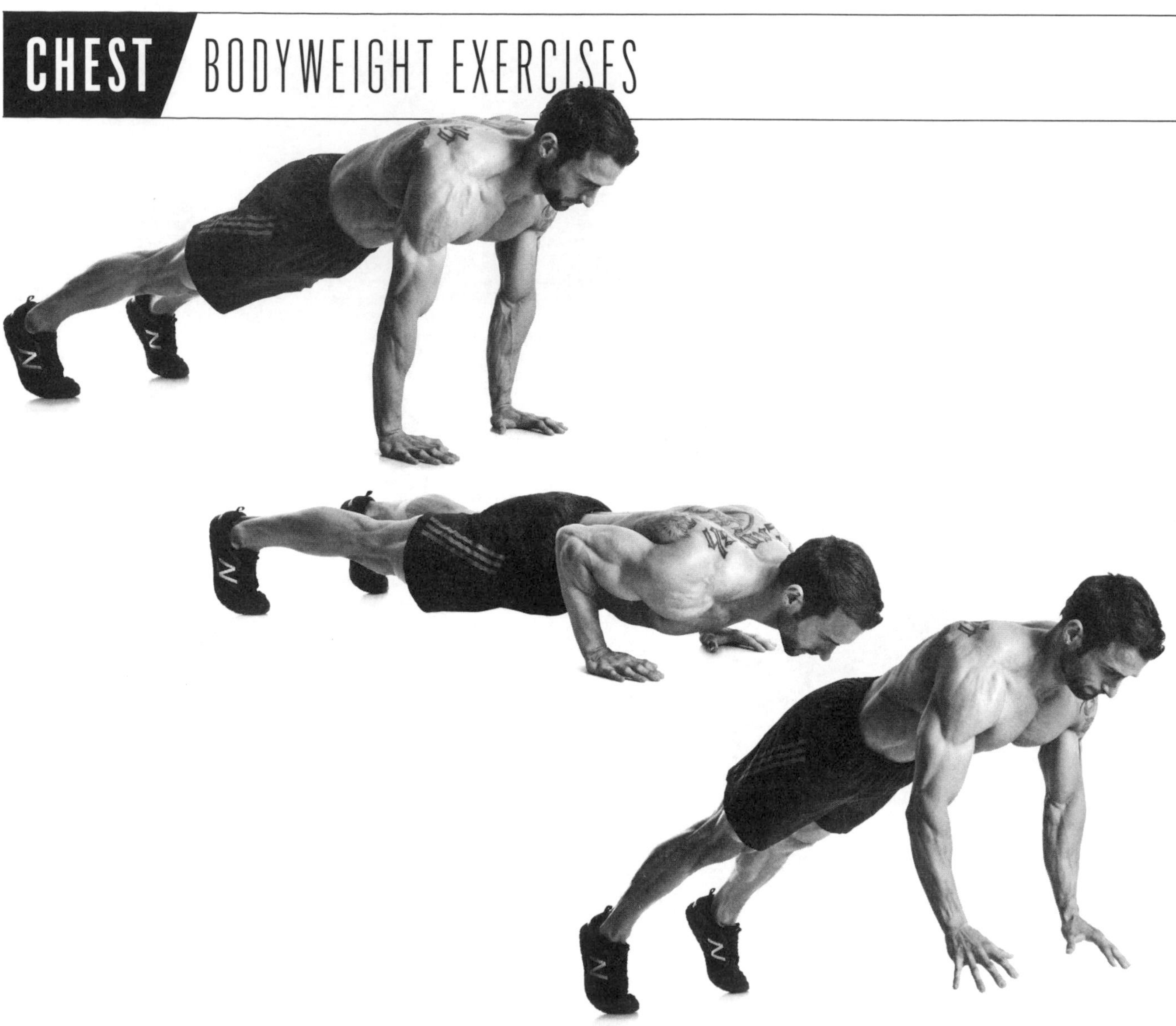

PLYOMETRIC PUSHUP

PURPOSE

Target the fast-twitch fibers in your chest.

START

With your hands just outside your chest, your feet shoulder width apart, start in the top position of a pushup. Brace your core.

MOVEMENT

Lower yourself to the floor while keeping your elbows in. Once you reach your lowest point, $\frac{1}{2}$ inch to 1 inch off the ground, push your body up in a fast, explosive manner, creating a space between your hands and the floor.

FINISH

Return to your starting position.

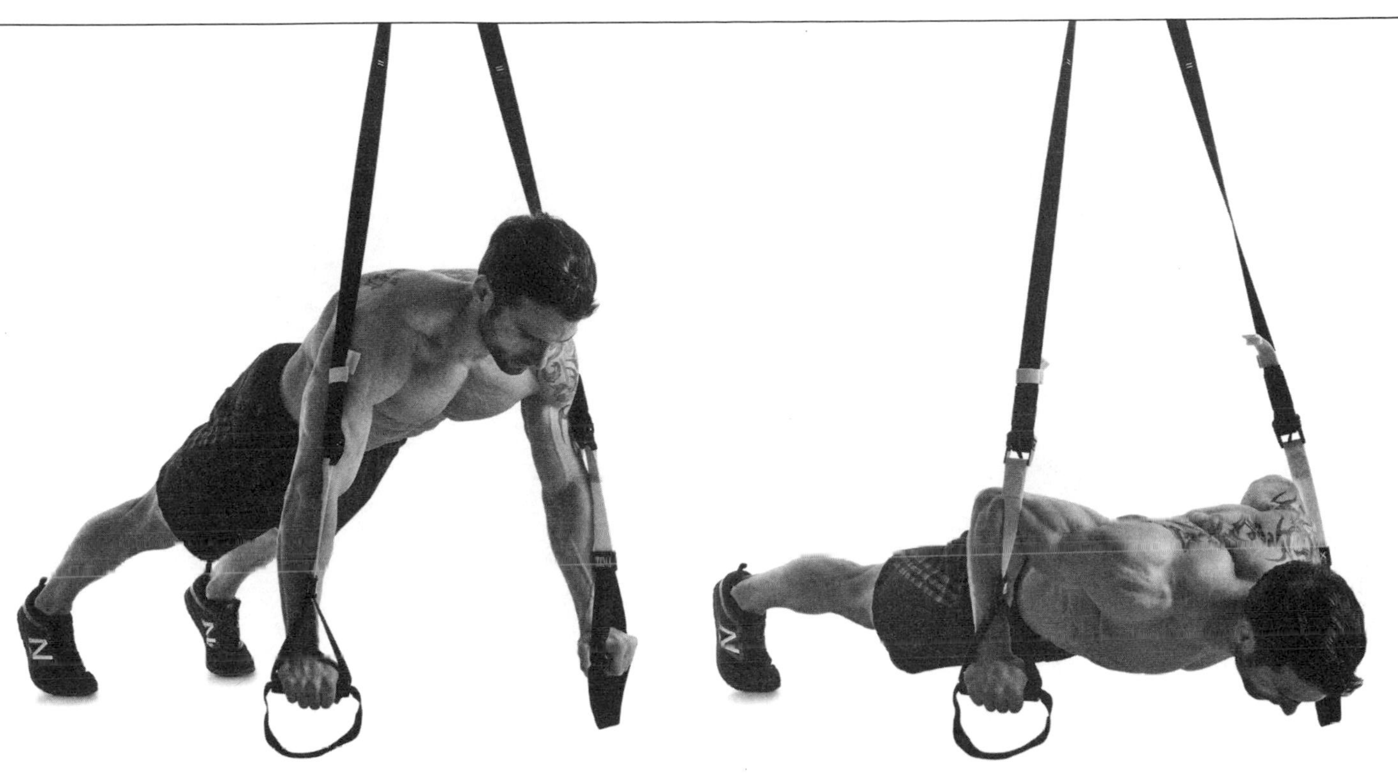

SUSPENDED PUSHUP (TRX/BLAST STRAP)

PURPOSE

To strengthen the smaller stabilizing muscles of the arms and give the chest muscles a more intense workout.

START

Grab the handles of a TRX strap and extend your arms in front of your chest. Your feet should be shoulder width apart and your body anywhere from parallel to 45 degrees to the floor.

MOVEMENT

Lower your body toward the floor until your hands end up just outside your shoulders. Keep your elbows in and your head in a neutral position as you lower. Brace your core throughout the movement.

FINISH

Push your body back up to the starting position.

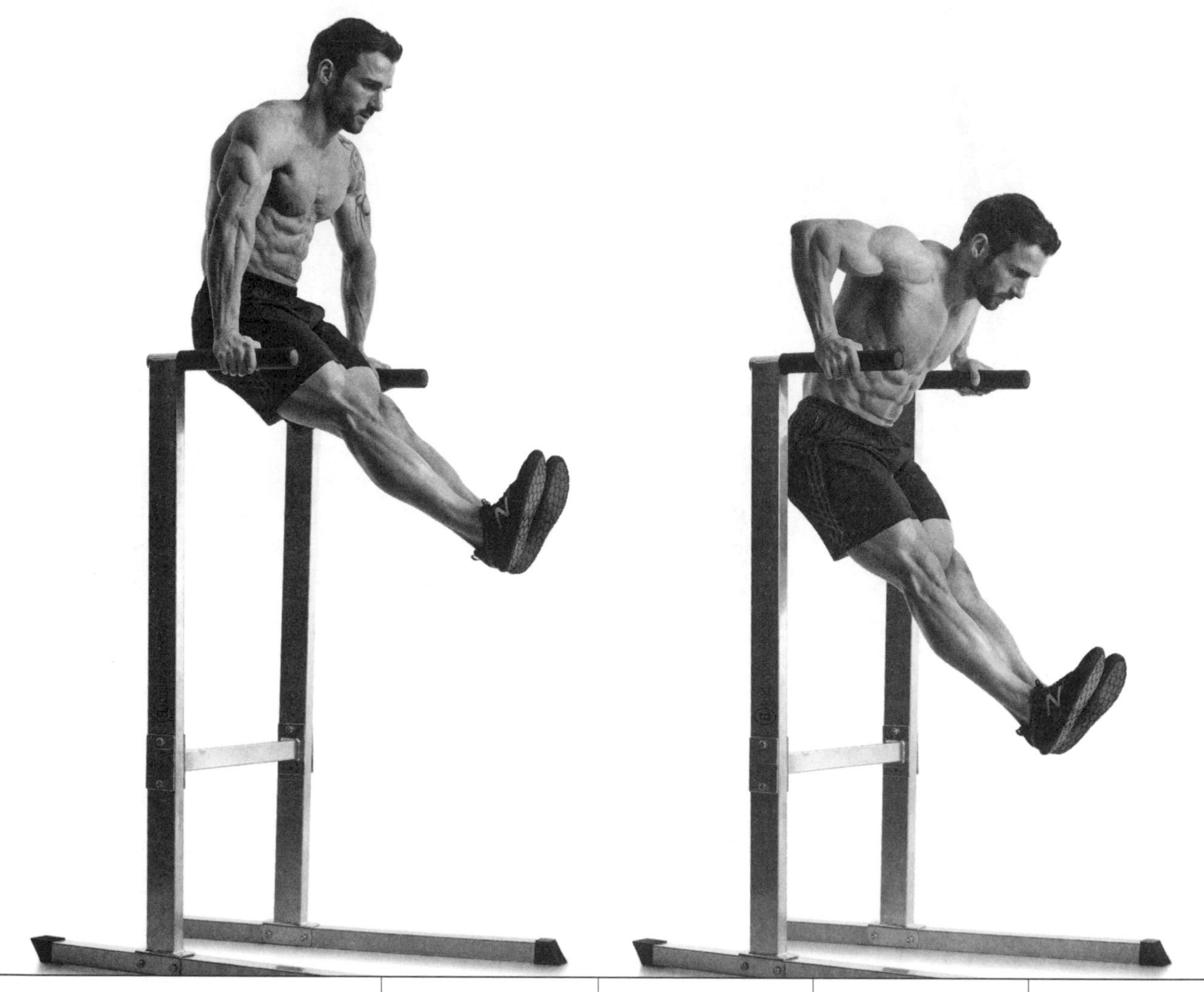

ELBOW-OUT PARALLEL DIP

PURPOSE
To isolate the pectorals during a dip movement.

START
Place your hands on a parallel bar to hold your body up. Bow your elbows out and place your legs in front of your torso.

MOVEMENT
Lower your body between the bars, keeping your elbows out.

FINISH
Push yourself back to the top position.

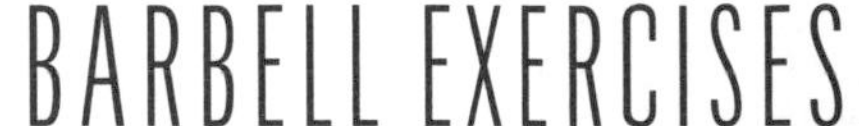

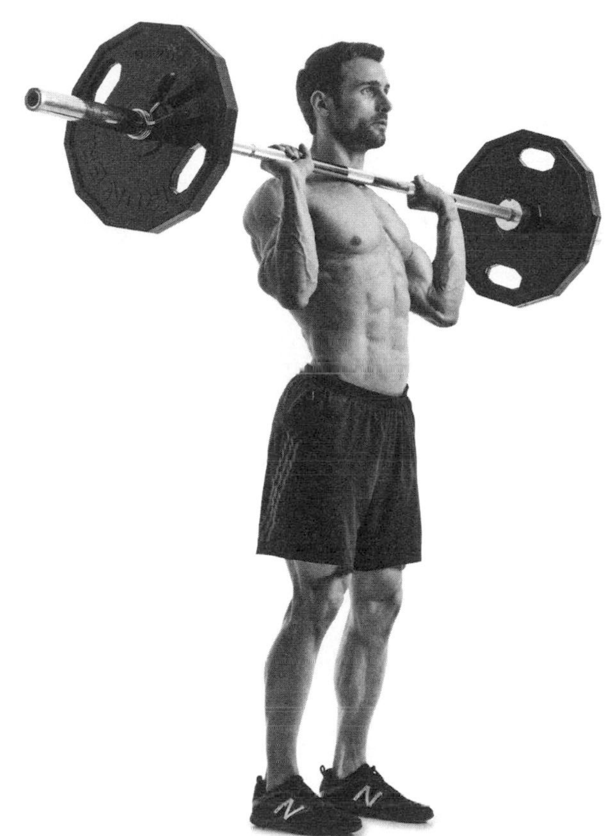

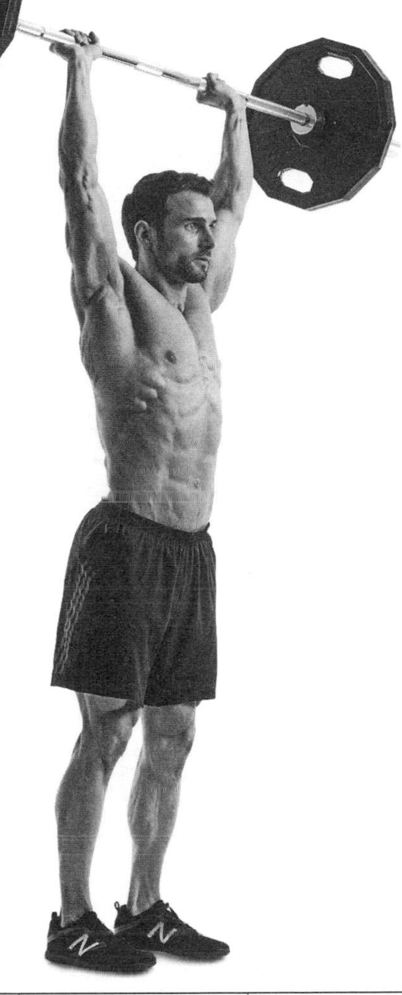

STANDING MILITARY PRESS

PURPOSE

Target your front deltoids and triceps.

START

Grab a barbell with an overhand grip, just beyond shoulder width, and place it in front of your shoulders. Keep your feet shoulder width apart. Brace your core and keep a slight bend to your knees.

MOVEMENT

Push the barbell straight overhead by keeping your head back slightly but your torso upright. Your arms should finish completely straight.

FINISH

Pause, then slowly lower your arms back to the starting position.

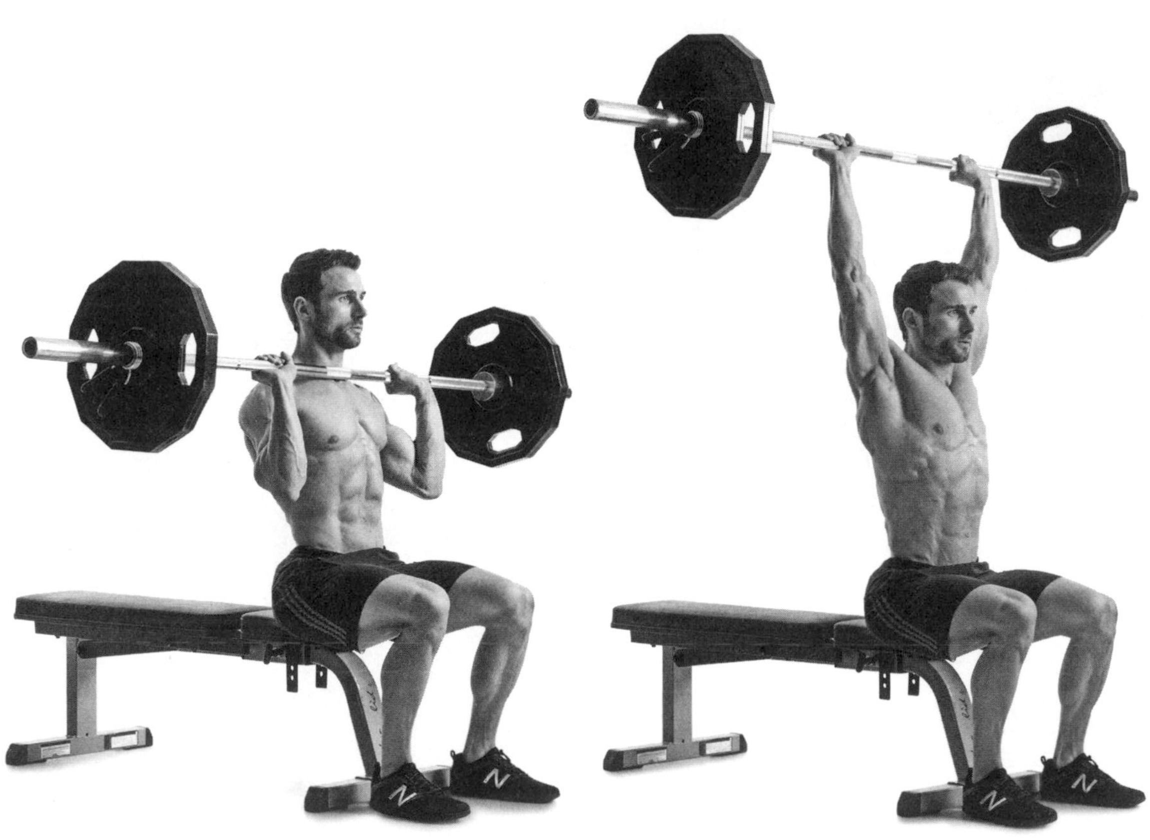

SEATED MILITARY PRESS

PURPOSE

Target your deltoids.

START

Sit at the end of a bench, with your torso upright and a natural arch to your back. Position a barbell, held with an overhand grip, in front of your shoulders.

MOVEMENT

Press the barbell directly over your shoulders.

FINISH

Pause, then slowly lower the barbell to the starting position.

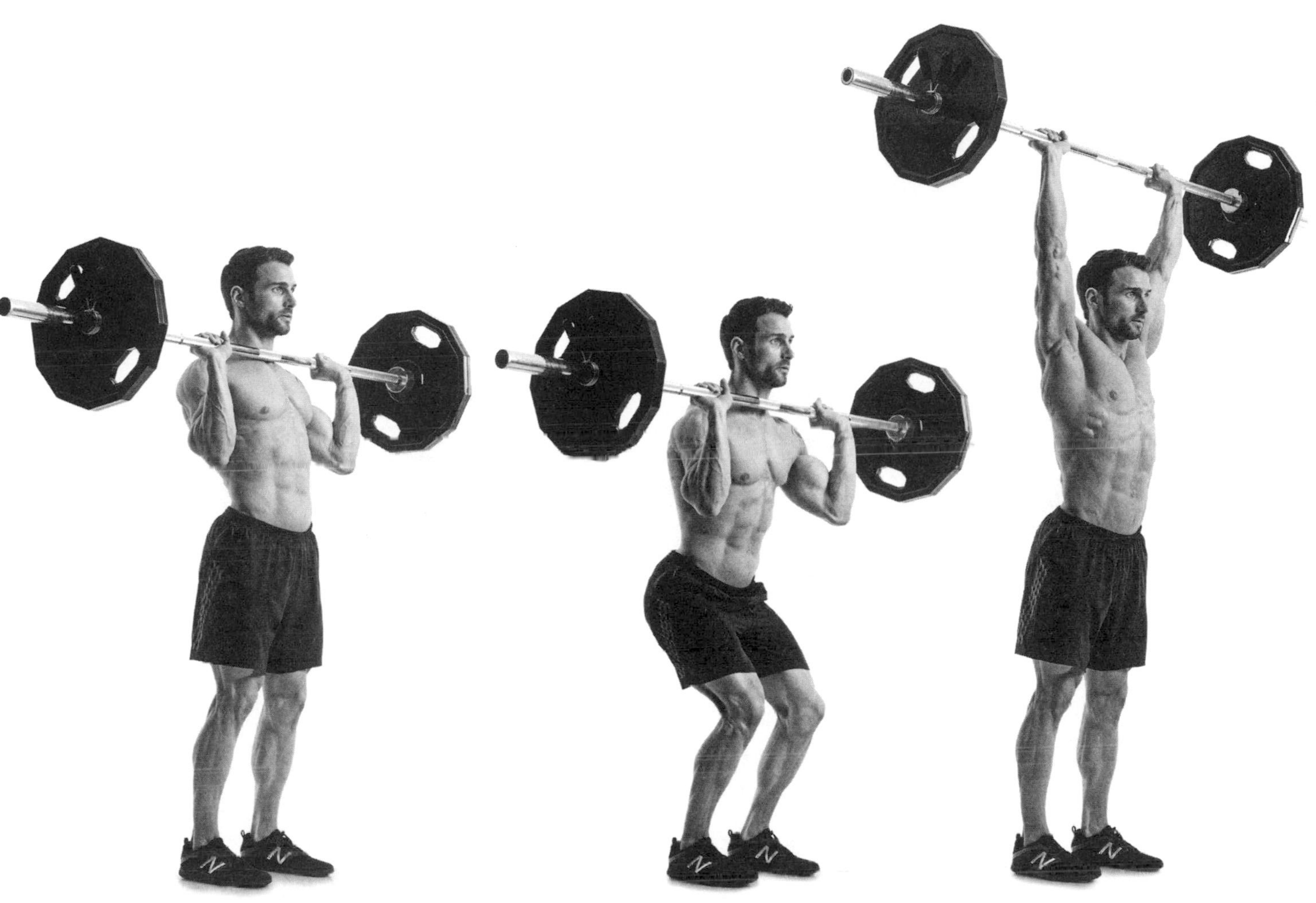

PUSH PRESS

PURPOSE
Target your front deltoids and triceps.

START
Grab a barbell with an overhand grip, just beyond shoulder width, and place it in front of your shoulders. Keep your feet shoulder width apart. Brace your core and keep a slight bend to your knees.

MOVEMENT
Use a slight hip bend and dip to your knees to push the barbell straight overhead by keeping your head back slightly but your torso upright. Your arms should finish completely straight.

FINISH
Pause briefly, then slowly lower your arms back to the starting position.

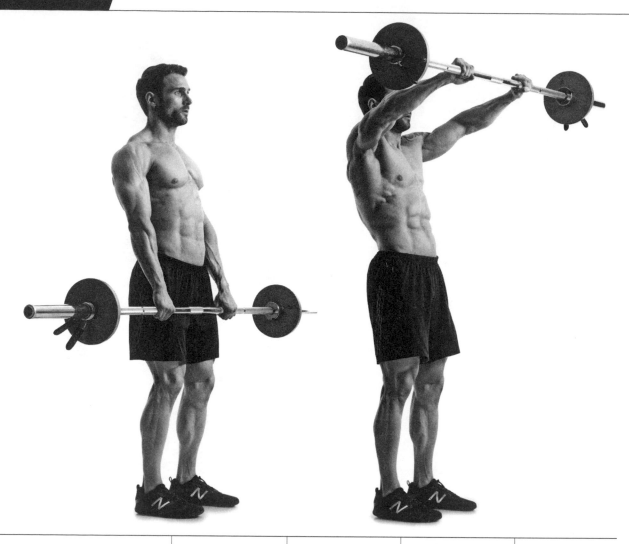

STANDING FRONT RAISE

PURPOSE

Target your front deltoids and triceps.

START

Grab a barbell with an overhand grip, just beyond shoulder width, and place it in front of your body at your hips. Brace your core and keep your knees slightly bent.

MOVEMENT

Raise the barbell to shoulder height.

FINISH

Pause, then slowly lower your arms back to the starting position.

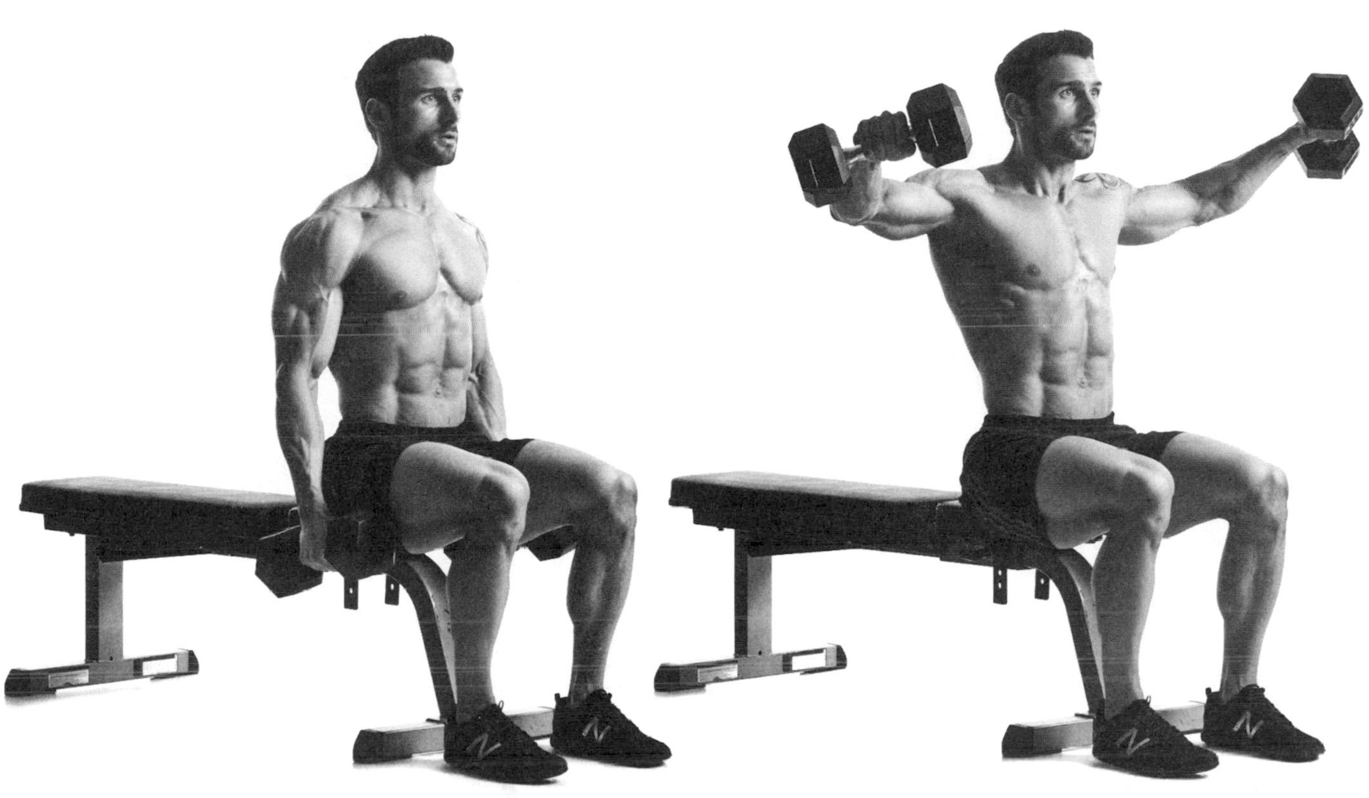

SEATED SIDE RAISE

PURPOSE
Target your anterior deltoids.

START
Sit on the end of a bench with a pair of dumbbells and let them hang at arm's length at your sides, with your palms facing each other.

MOVEMENT
Raise your arms straight out on the sides of your body until they are parallel to the floor.

FINISH
Pause briefly, then slowly lower your arms to the starting position.

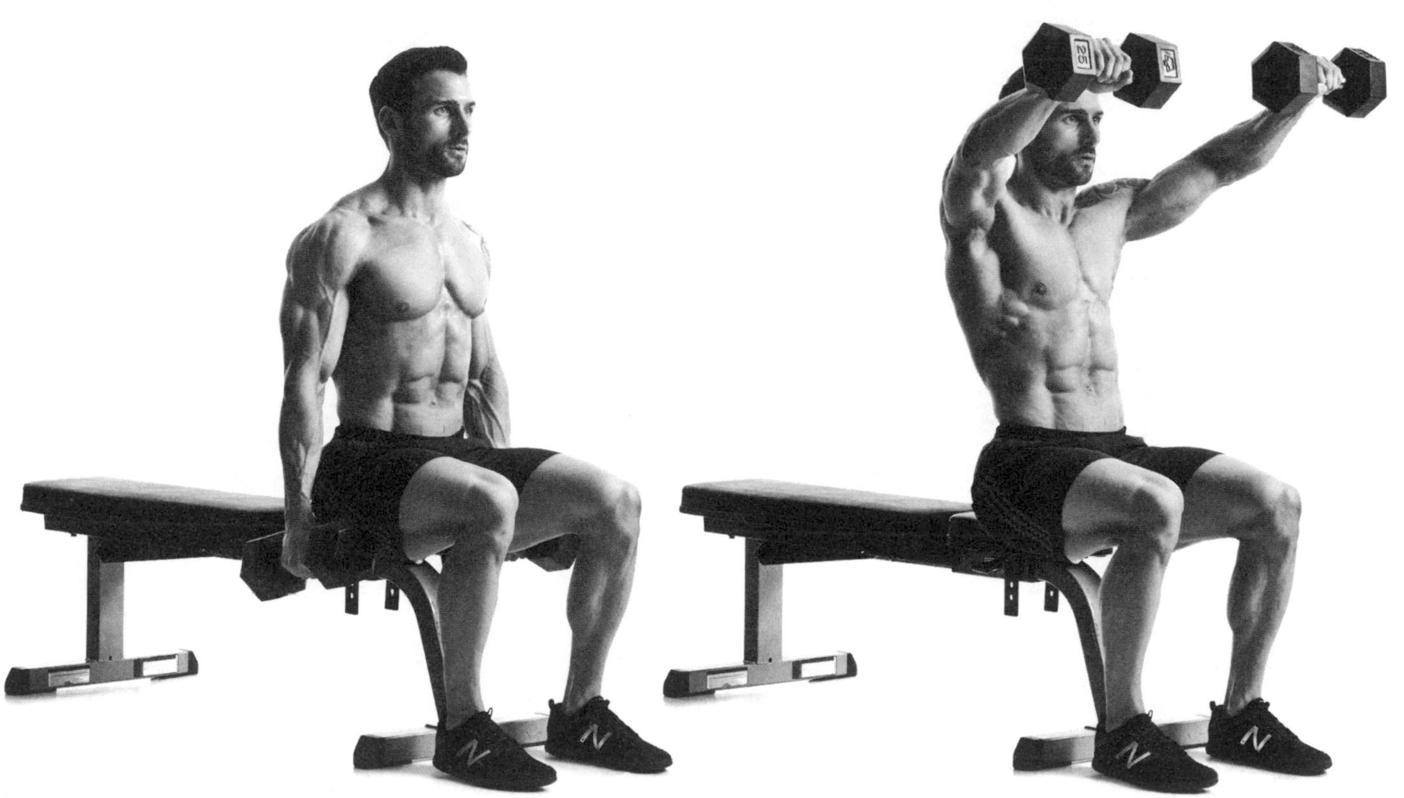

SEATED FRONT RAISE

PURPOSE
Target your anterior deltoids.

START
Sit on the end of a bench with a pair of dumbbells and let them hang at arm's length at your sides, with your palms facing each other.

MOVEMENT
Turn your wrists to point palms down as you raise your arms straight in front of your body until they are parallel to the floor and perpendicular to your torso.

FINISH
Pause briefly, then slowly lower your arms to the starting position.

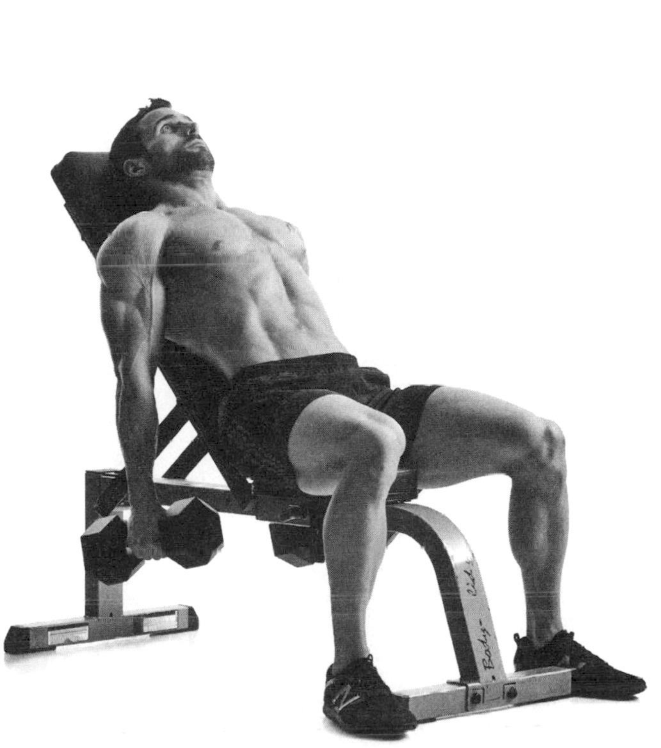

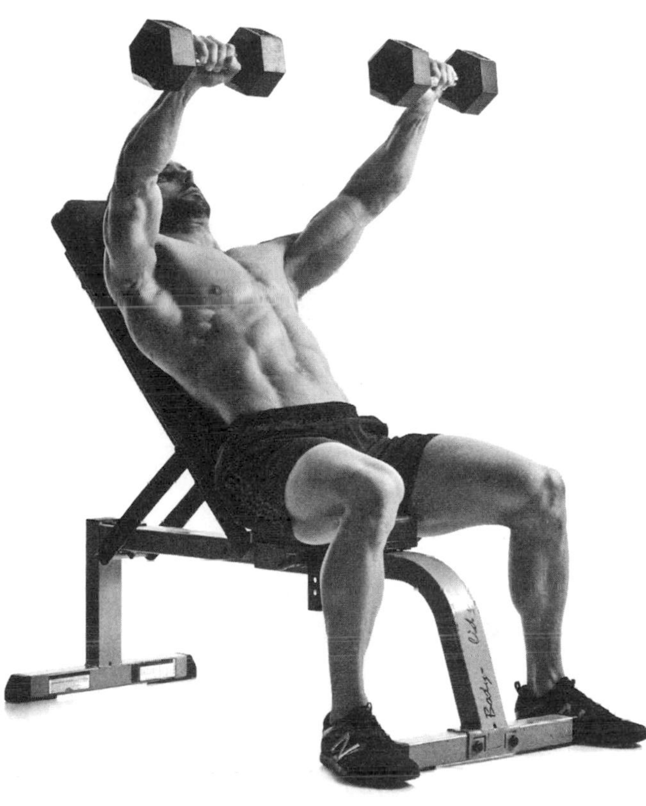

INCLINE FRONT RAISE

PURPOSE

Target your anterior deltoids.

START

Grab a pair of dumbbells and lie on an incline bench. Let the dumbbells hang at arm's length at your sides with your palms facing each other.

MOVEMENT

Raise your arms straight in front of your body until they are higher than parallel to the floor and perpendicular to your torso.

FINISH

Pause briefly, then slowly lower your arms to the starting position.

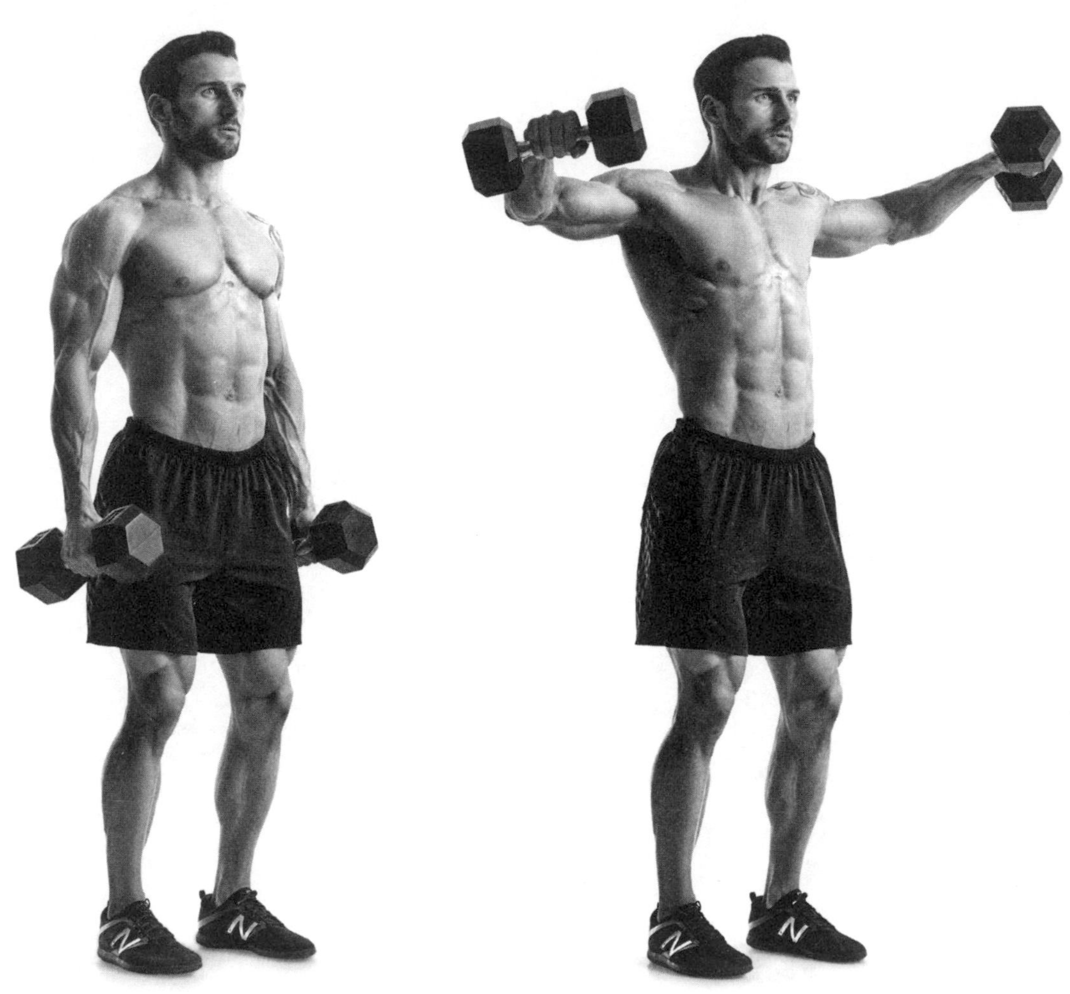

LATERAL RAISE

PURPOSE
Target your anterior deltoids.

START
Grab a pair of dumbbells and let them hang at arm's length at your sides, with your palms facing each other.

MOVEMENT
Raise your arms straight out on the sides of your body until they are parallel to the floor.

FINISH
Pause briefly, then slowly lower your arms to the starting position.

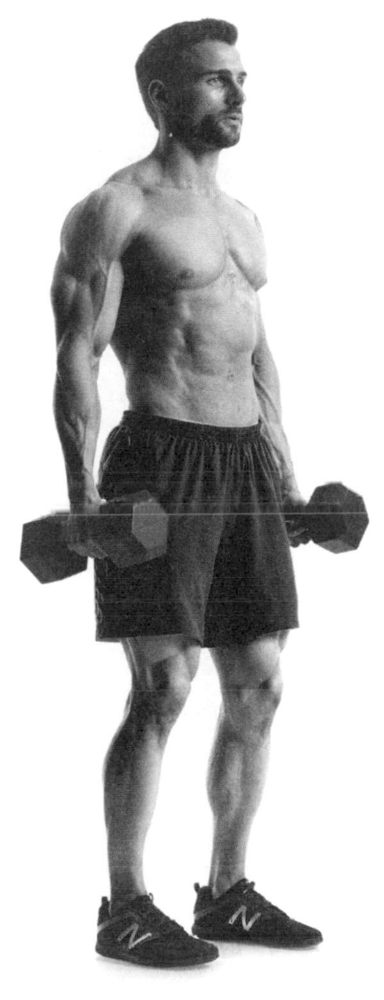

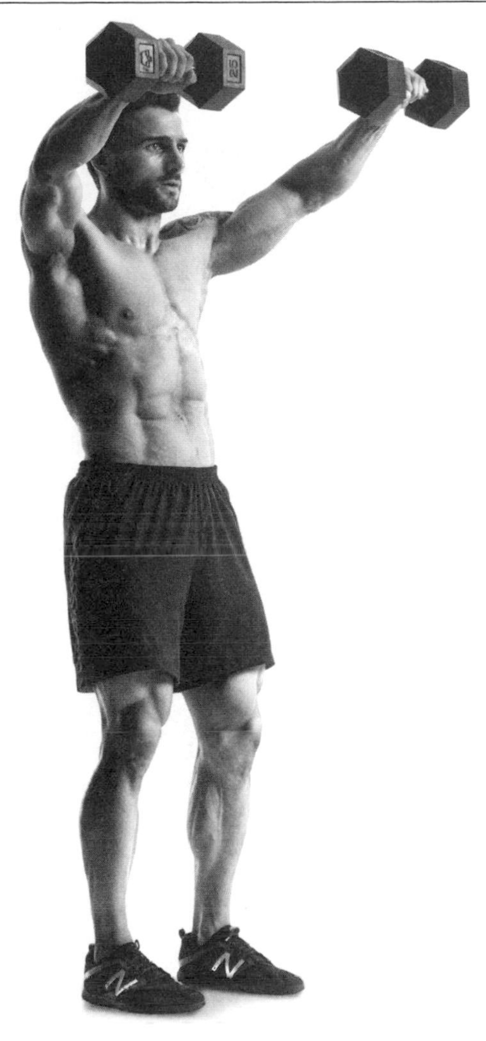

FRONT RAISE

PURPOSE
Target your anterior deltoids.

START
Grab a pair of dumbbells and let them hang at arm's length at your sides, with your palms facing each other.

MOVEMENT
Turn your hands palms down as you raise your arms straight in front of your body until they are parallel to the floor and perpendicular to your torso.

FINISH
Pause briefly, then slowly lower your arms to the starting position.

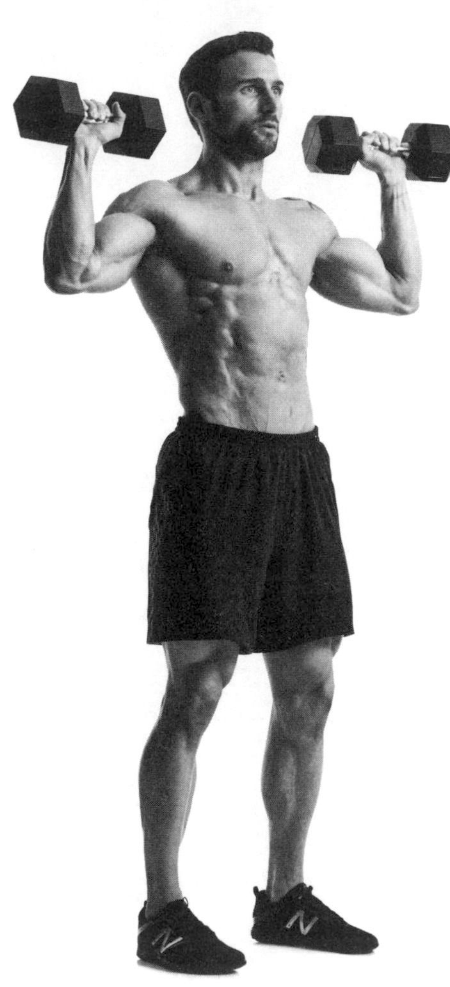

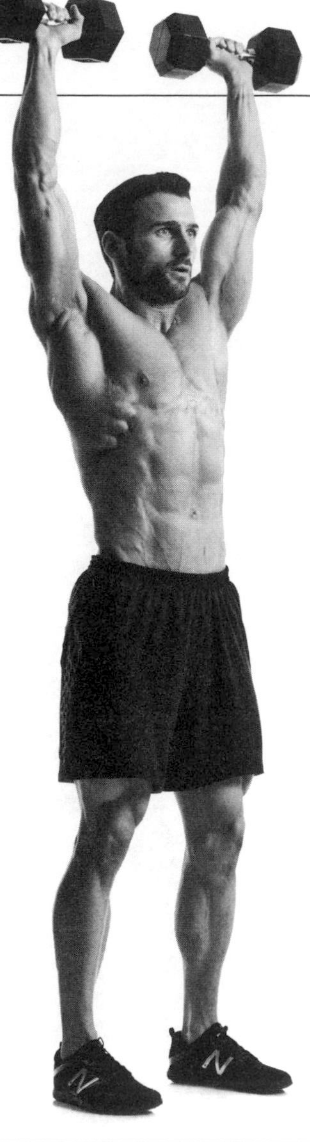

STANDING PRESS

PURPOSE

Target your front deltoids and triceps.

START

Grab a pair of dumbbells with an overhand grip, just beyond shoulder width, and place them just over your shoulders. Keep your feet shoulder width apart. Brace your core and keep a slight bend to your knees.

MOVEMENT

Push the dumbbells straight overhead by keeping your head back slightly but your torso upright. Your arms should finish completely straight.

FINISH

Pause briefly, then slowly lower your arms back to the starting position.

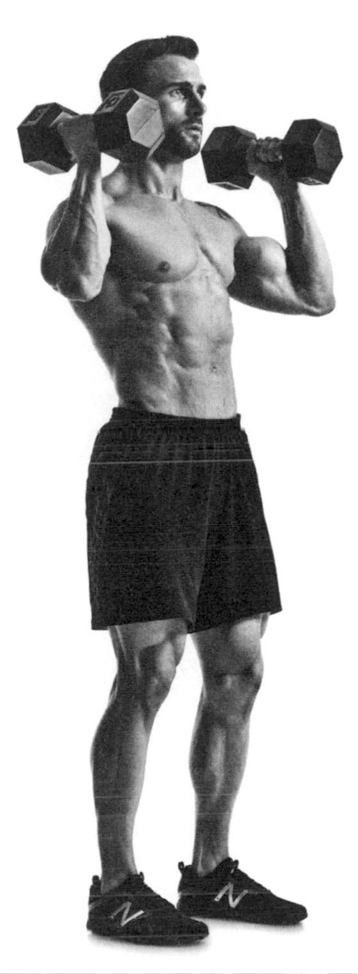
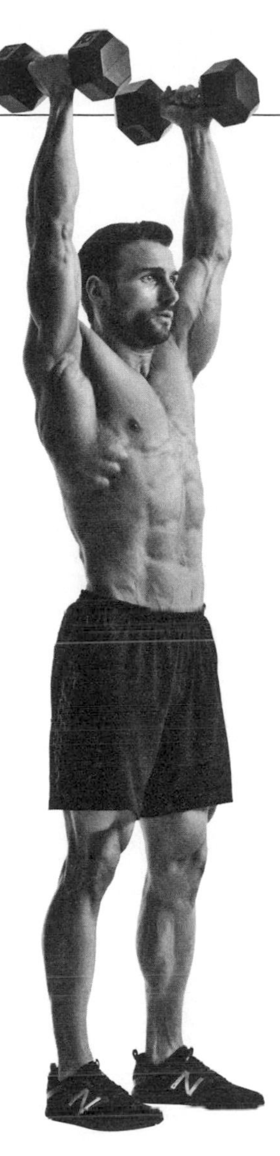

NEUTRAL-GRIP STANDING PRESS

PURPOSE

Target your front deltoids and triceps.

START

Grab a pair of dumbbells with a neutral grip and hold them just over your shoulders. Keep your feet shoulder width apart. Brace your core and keep a slight bend to your knees.

MOVEMENT

Push the dumbbells straight overhead by keeping your head back slightly but your torso upright. Your arms should finish completely straight.

FINISH

Pause briefly, then slowly lower your arms back to the starting position.

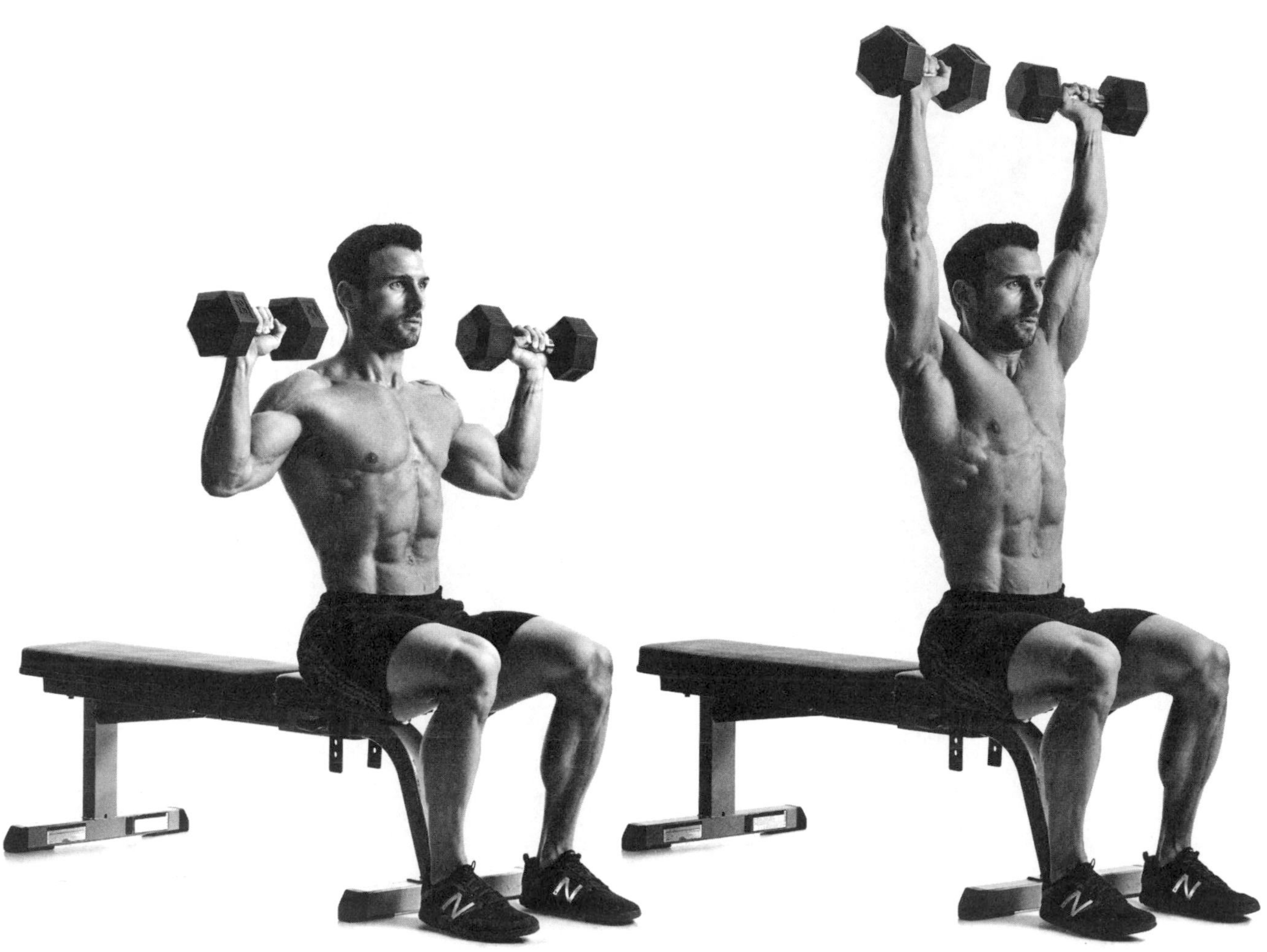

SEATED PRESS

PURPOSE

Target your front deltoids and triceps.

START

Sitting on the end of a bench, grab a pair of dumbbells with an overhand grip, and hold them just over your shoulders. Keep your feet shoulder width apart. Brace your core and keep a slight bend to your knees.

MOVEMENT

Push the dumbbells straight overhead by keeping your head back slightly but your torso upright. Your arms should finish completely straight.

FINISH

Pause briefly, then slowly lower your arms back to the starting position.

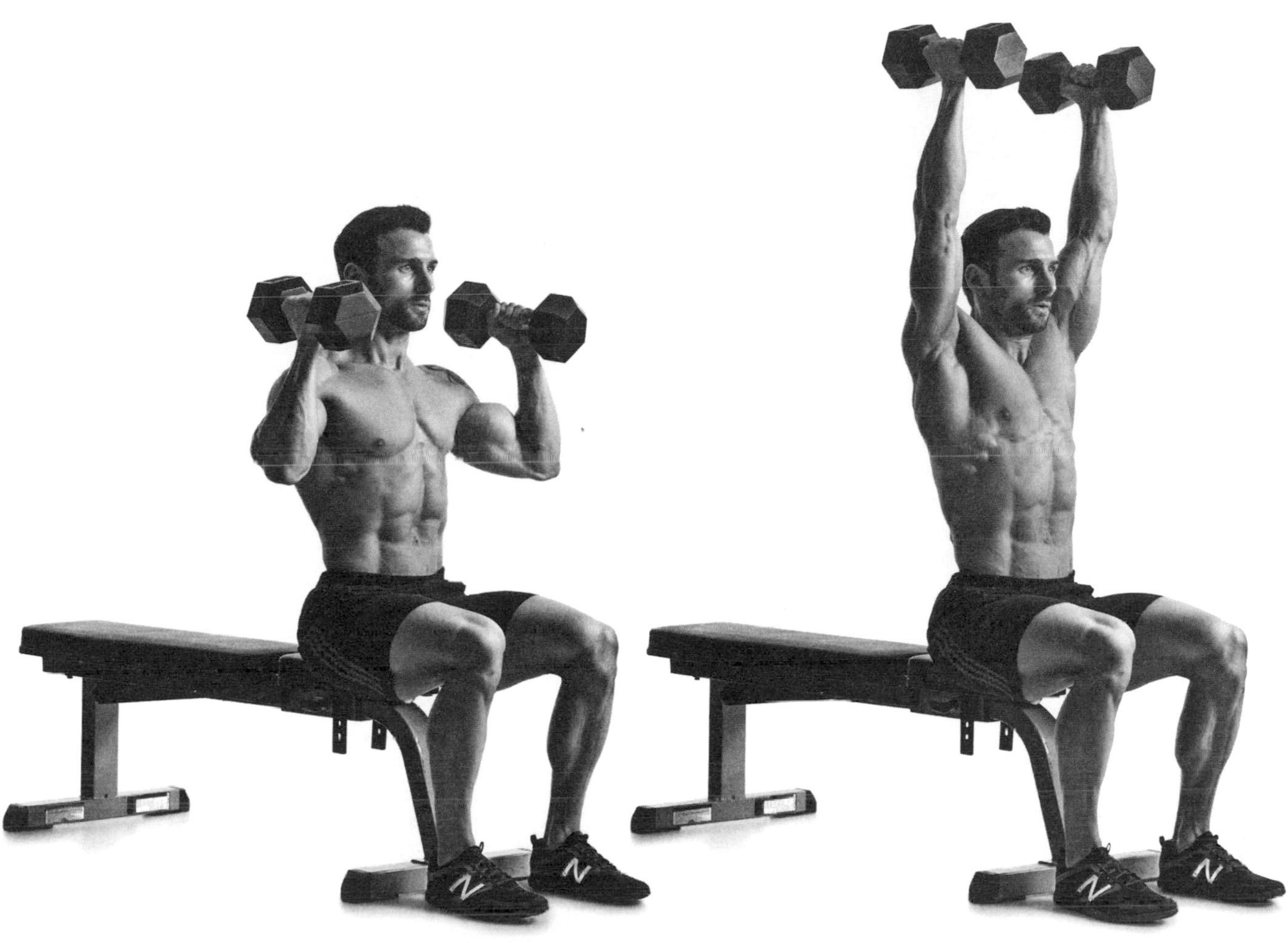

NEUTRAL-GRIP SEATED PRESS

PURPOSE

Target your front deltoids and triceps.

START

Sitting on the end of a bench, grab a pair of dumbbells with a neutral grip, and hold them just over your shoulders. Keep your feet shoulder width apart. Brace your core and keep a slight bend to your knees.

MOVEMENT

Push the dumbbells straight overhead with your palms facing in. Keep your head back slightly and your torso upright. Your arms should finish completely straight.

FINISH

Pause briefly, then slowly lower your arms back to the starting position.

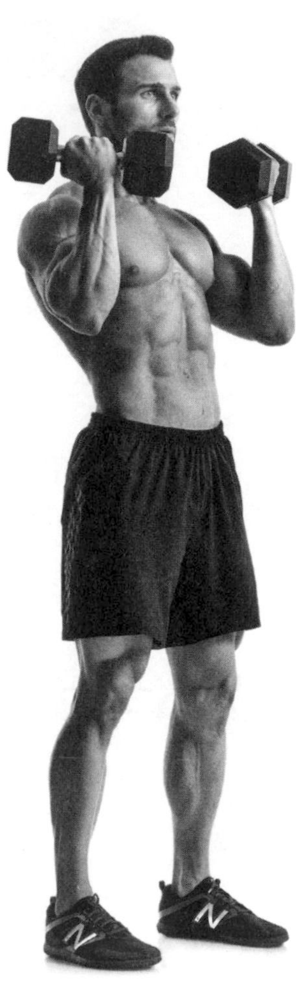

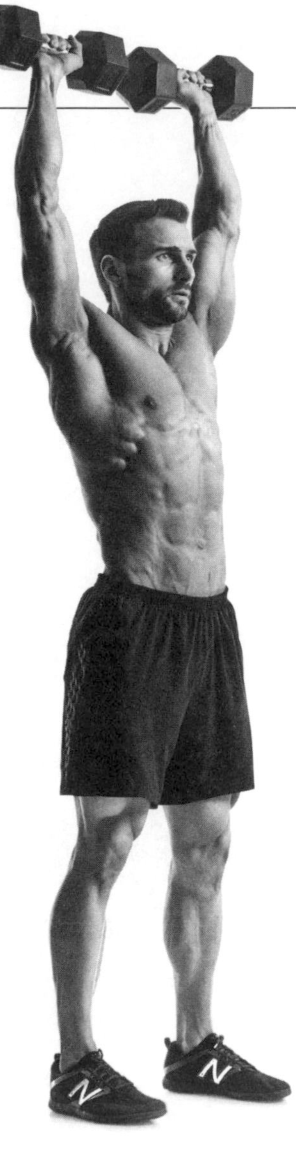

ARNOLD PRESS

PURPOSE

Target your front deltoids and triceps.

START

Stand holding a pair of dumbbells with an overhand grip and rotate the dumbbells so your palms are facing your chest. Keep the dumbbells at shoulder width and place them in front of your body. Keep your feet shoulder width apart. Brace your core and keep a slight bend to your knees.

MOVEMENT

Begin to push the dumbbells straight overhead while rotating your palms forward and keeping your head back slightly but your torso upright. Your arms should finish completely straight with your palms forward.

FINISH

Pause briefly, then slowly lower the dumbbells back to the starting position with the exact opposite pattern.

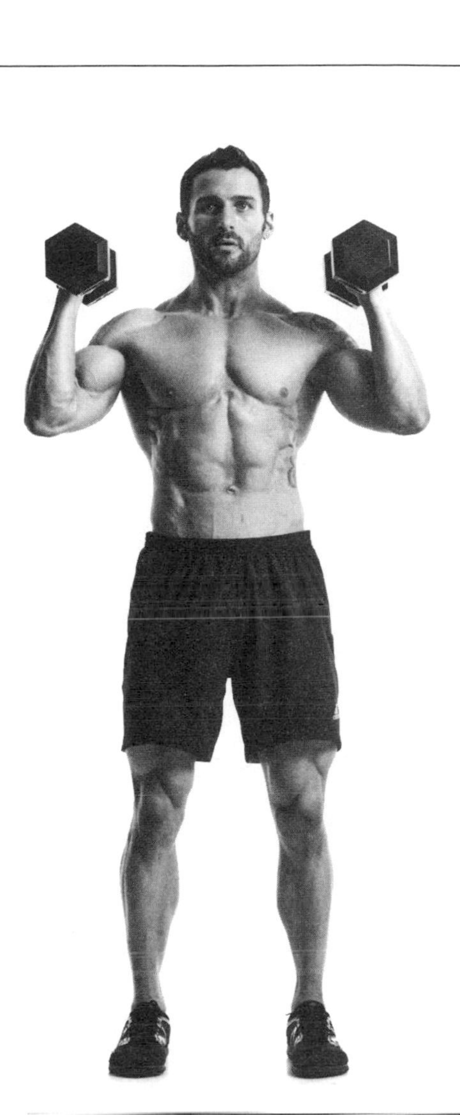

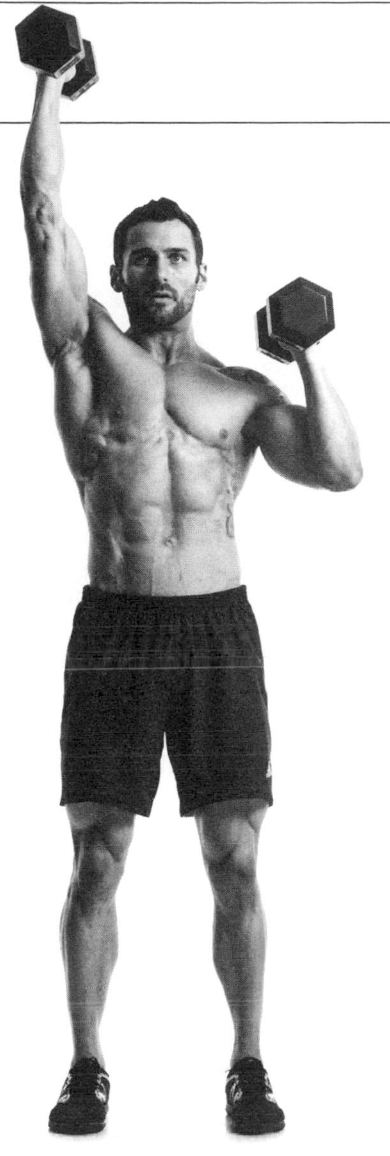

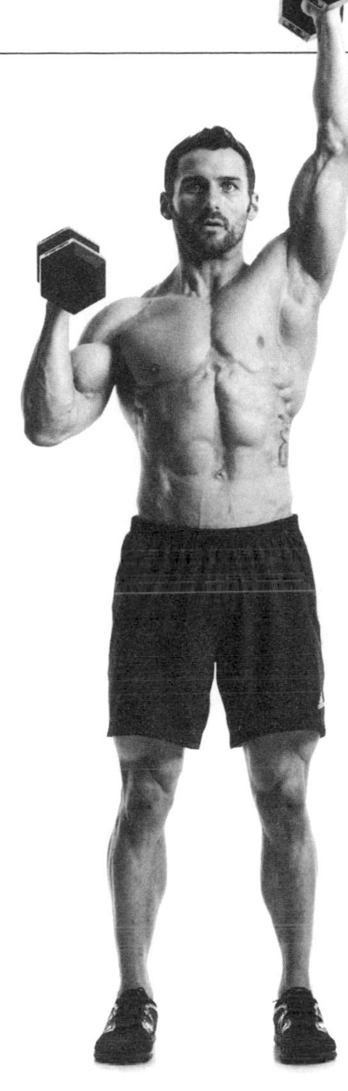

SEESAW PRESS

PURPOSE

Target your front deltoids and triceps.

START

Stand holding a pair of dumbbells with an overhand grip, just beyond shoulder width and place them above your shoulders. Keep your feet shoulder width apart. Brace your core and keep a slight bend to your knees.

MOVEMENT

Push one dumbbell straight overhead by keeping your head back slightly but your torso upright. Your arm should finish completely straight.

FINISH

Pause briefly, then slowly lower the dumbbell and alternate sides continuously.

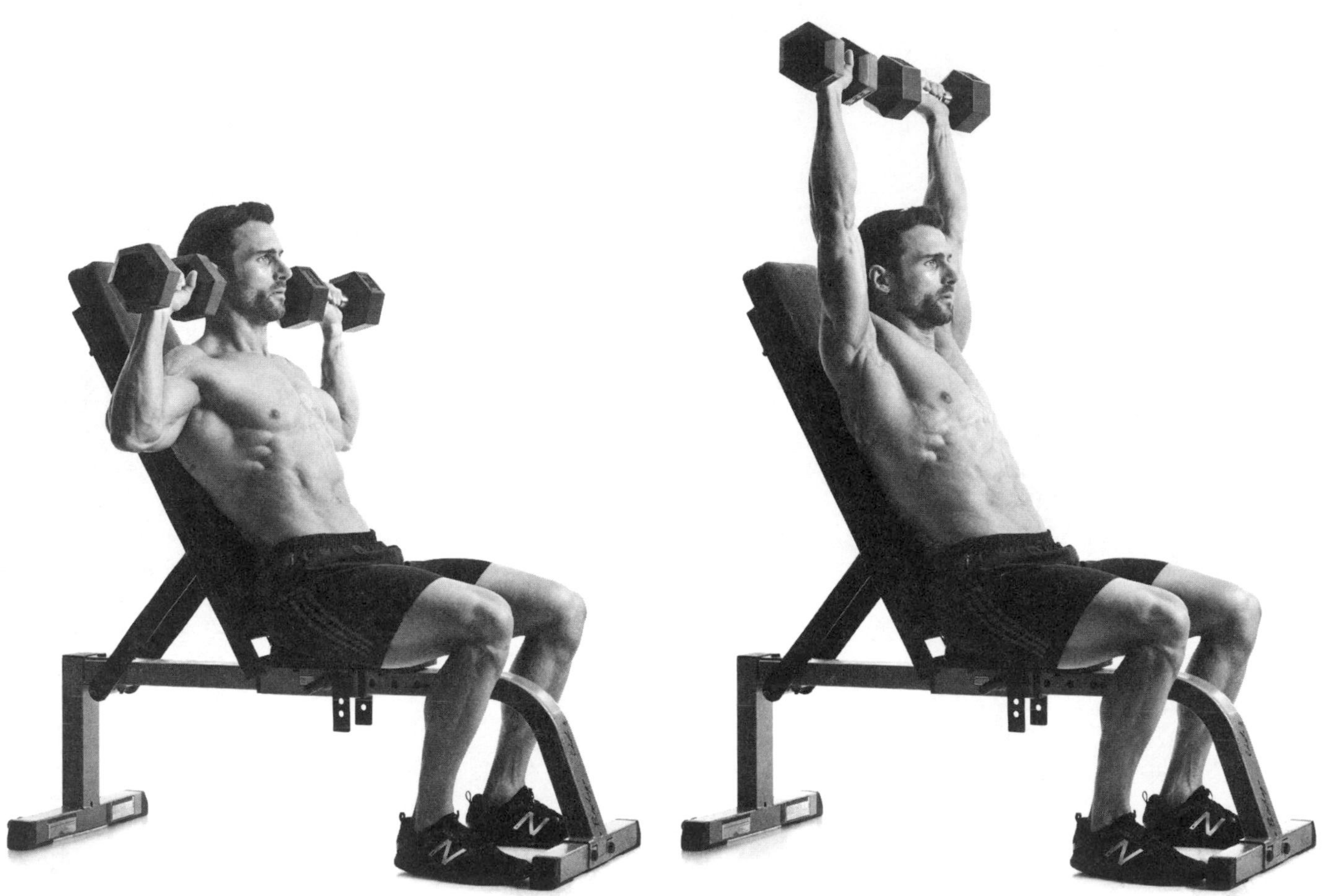

INCLINE SHOULDER PRESS

PURPOSE

Target your front deltoids and triceps.

START

Sitting on an incline bench set to 75 degrees, grab a pair of dumbbells with a overhand grip, and hold them above your shoulders. Brace your core and keep your feet shoulder width apart and flat on the ground.

MOVEMENT

Push the dumbbells straight overhead keeping your head back slightly and your torso upright. Your arms should finish completely straight.

FINISH

Pause briefly, then slowly lower your arms back to the starting position.

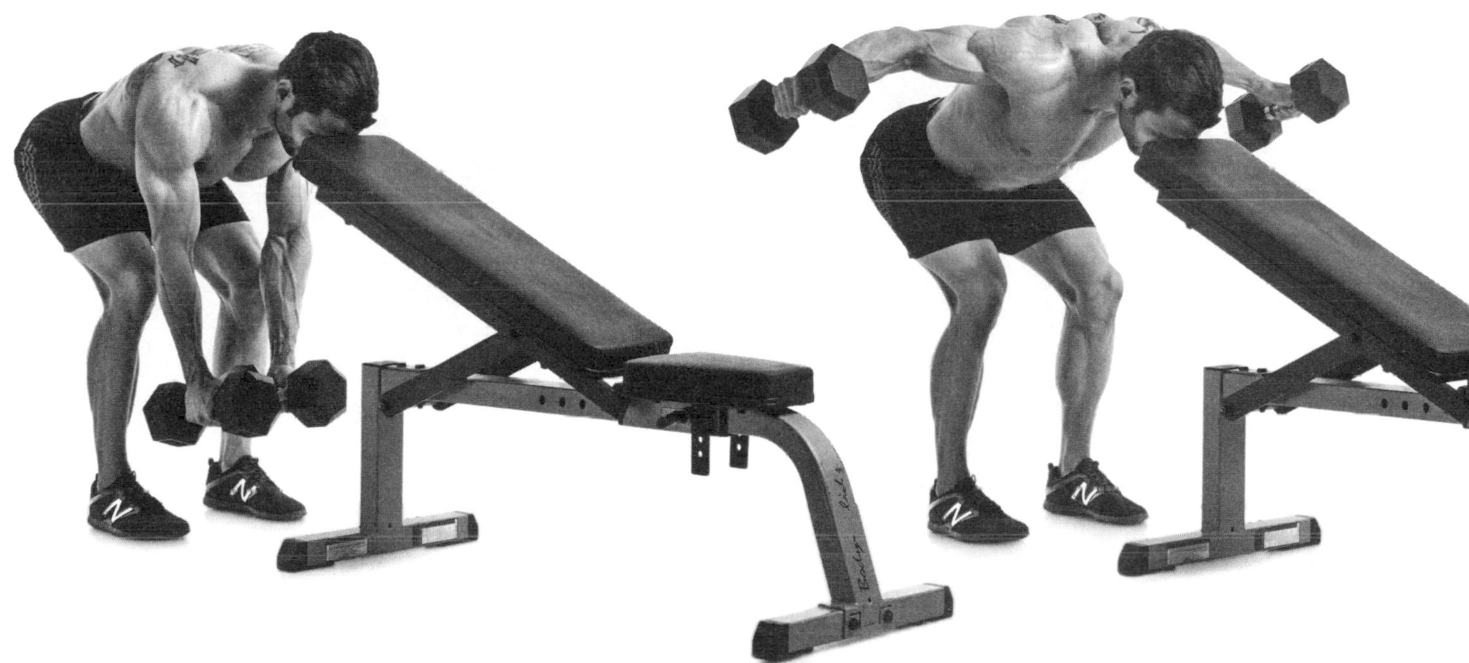

BENT-OVER REAR DELTOID RAISE (HEAD ON BENCH)

PURPOSE

Target your posterior deltoids.

START

Grab a pair of dumbbells and stand with your forehead resting on the top of an incline bench. Keep your lower back naturally arched and your palms facing each other.

MOVEMENT

Raise your arms straight out to your sides.

FINISH

Pause briefly, then slowly lower your arms back to the starting position.

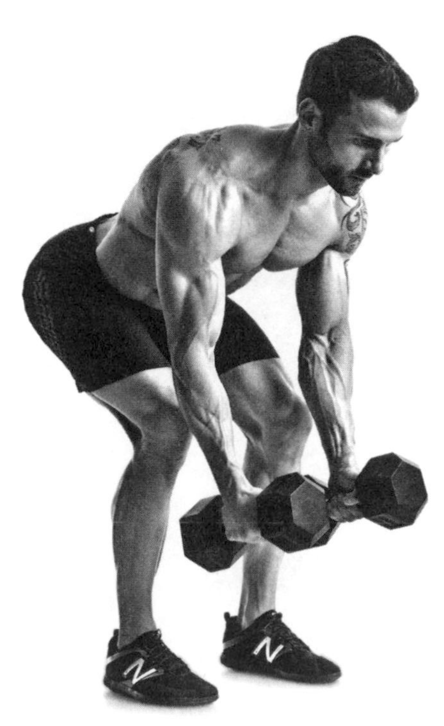

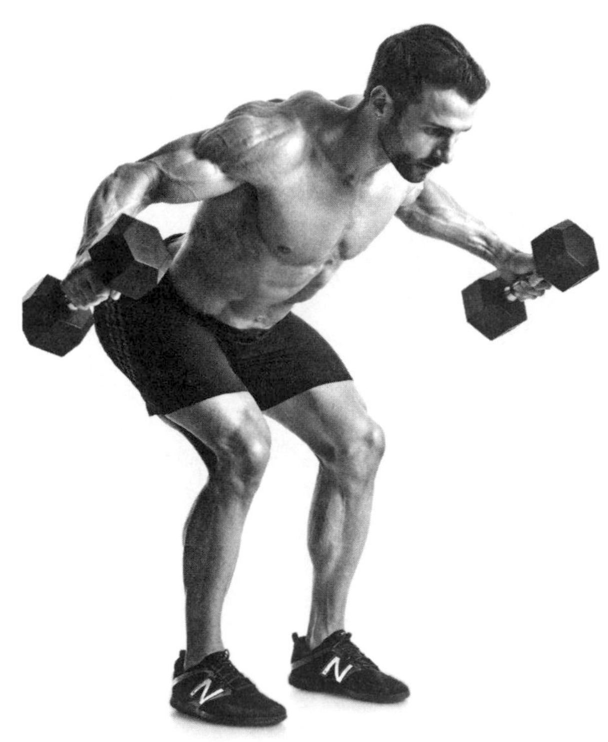

BENT-OVER REAR DELTOID RAISE

PURPOSE

Target your posterior deltoids.

START

Grab a pair of dumbbells and bend forward at your hips (hinge) until your torso is almost parallel to the floor. Keep your lower back naturally arched and your palms facing each other. Maintain a slight bend in your arms.

MOVEMENT

Raise your arms straight out to your sides without changing the bend in your elbows. Keep your torso as still as possible.

FINISH

Pause briefly, then slowly lower your arms back to the starting position.

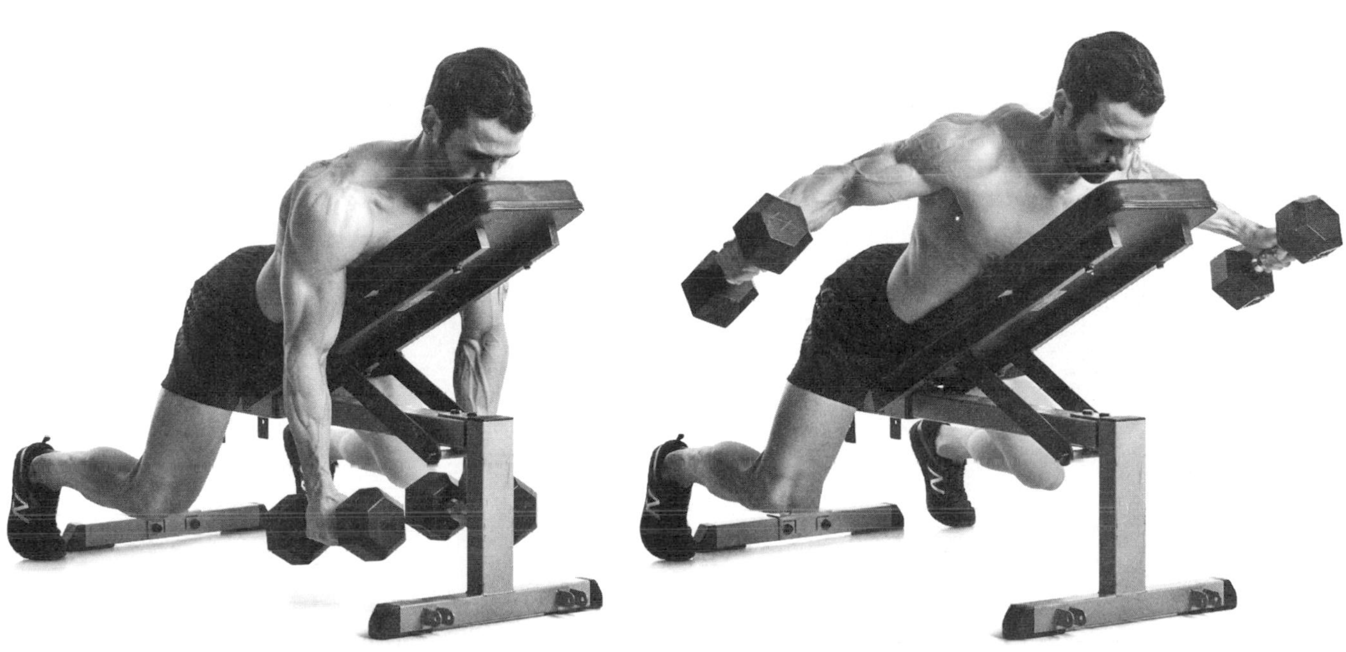

LYING INCLINE REAR LATERAL RAISE

PURPOSE

Target your posterior deltoids.

START

Lie with your chest down on an incline bench set to 10 to 30 degrees. Grab a pair of dumbbells and keep your lower back naturally arched and your palms facing each other.

MOVEMENT

Raise your arms straight out to your sides while keeping your chest up.

FINISH

Pause briefly, then slowly lower your arms back to the starting position.

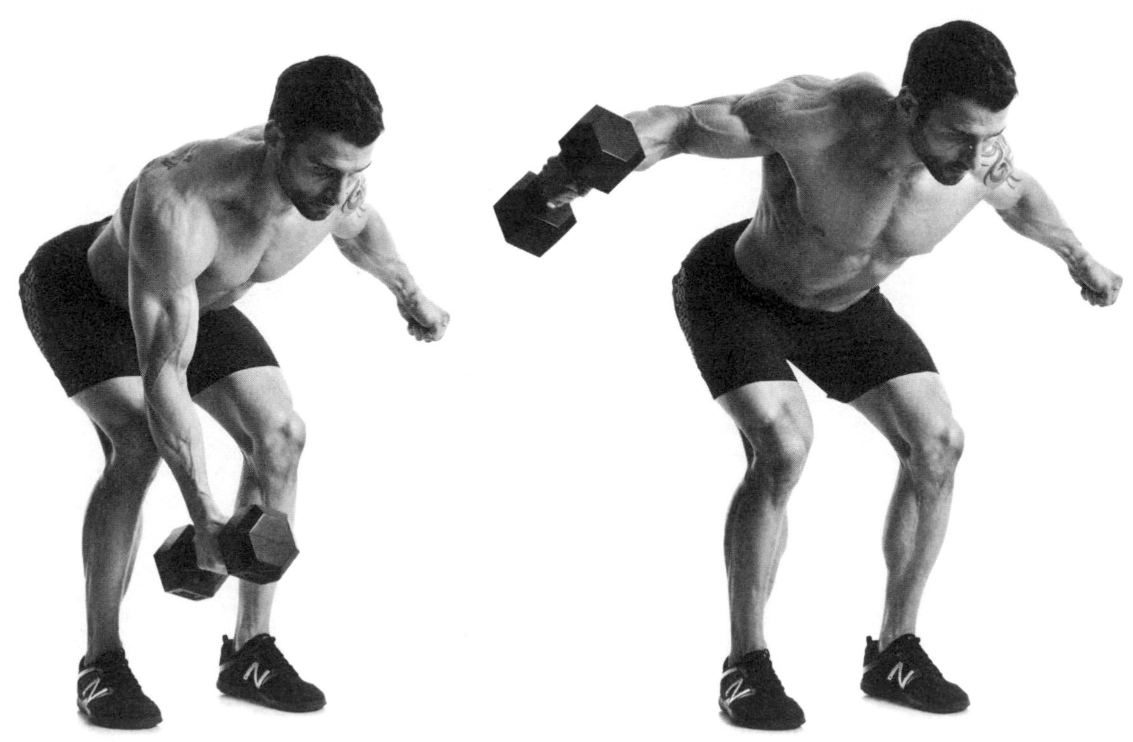

SINGLE-ARM REAR LATERAL RAISE

PURPOSE

Target your posterior deltoids.

START

Grab a dumbbell in one hand with a neutral grip. Bend forward at your hips (hinge) until your torso is almost parallel to the floor. Keep your lower back naturally arched and maintain a slight bend in your arm.

MOVEMENT

Raise your arm straight out to your side without changing the bend in your elbow. Keep your torso as still as possible.

FINISH

Pause briefly, then slowly lower your arm back to the starting position.

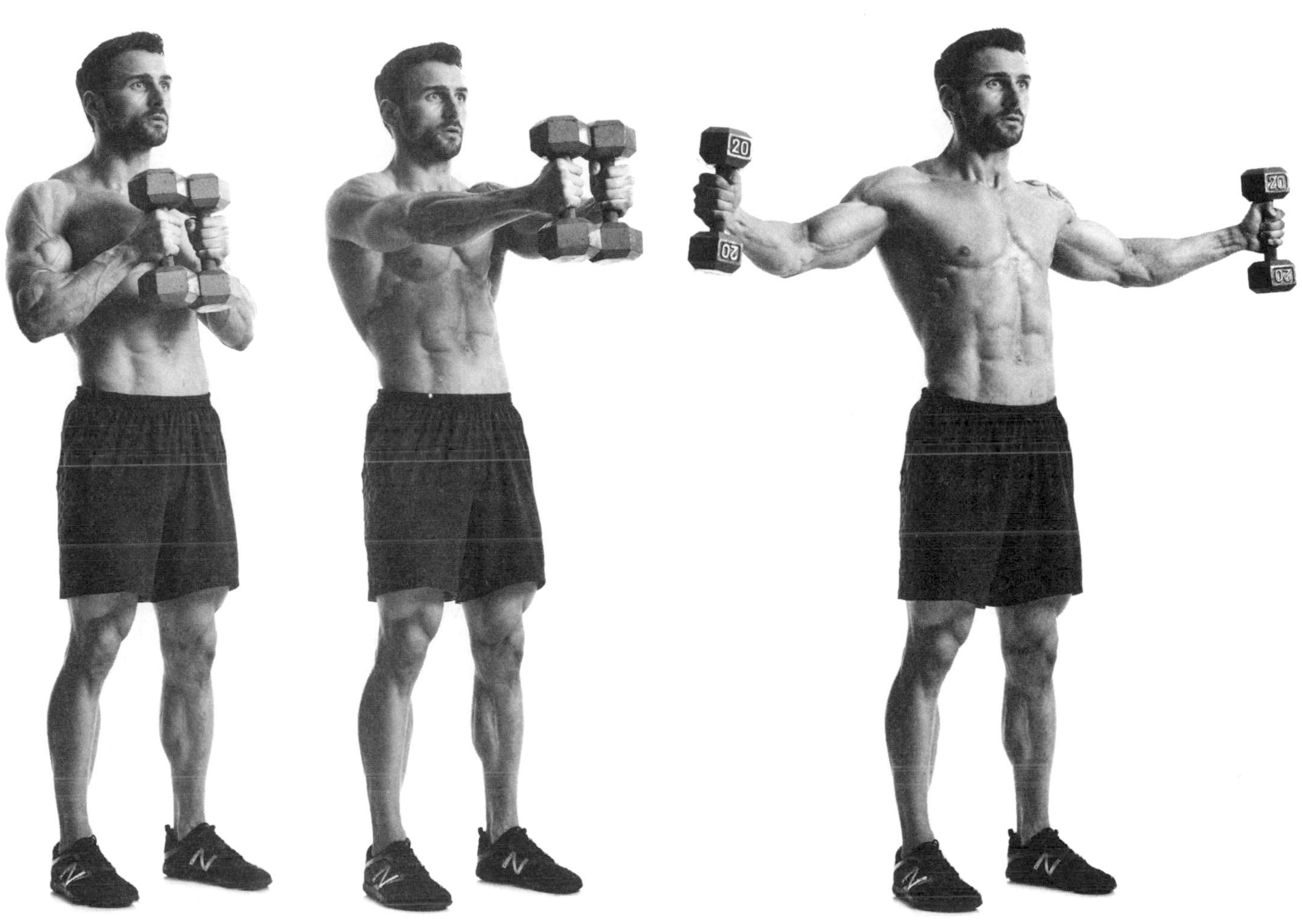

IRON CROSS

PURPOSE

Target your deltoids.

START

Stand holding a pair of dumbbells with your hands in the center of your chest and your palms facing each other.

MOVEMENT

Push the dumbbells out in front of your body until your arms are straight. Next, pull the dumbbells out to the sides of your body at shoulder height.

FINISH

Return the dumbbells to the front of your body and pull them back to your chest.

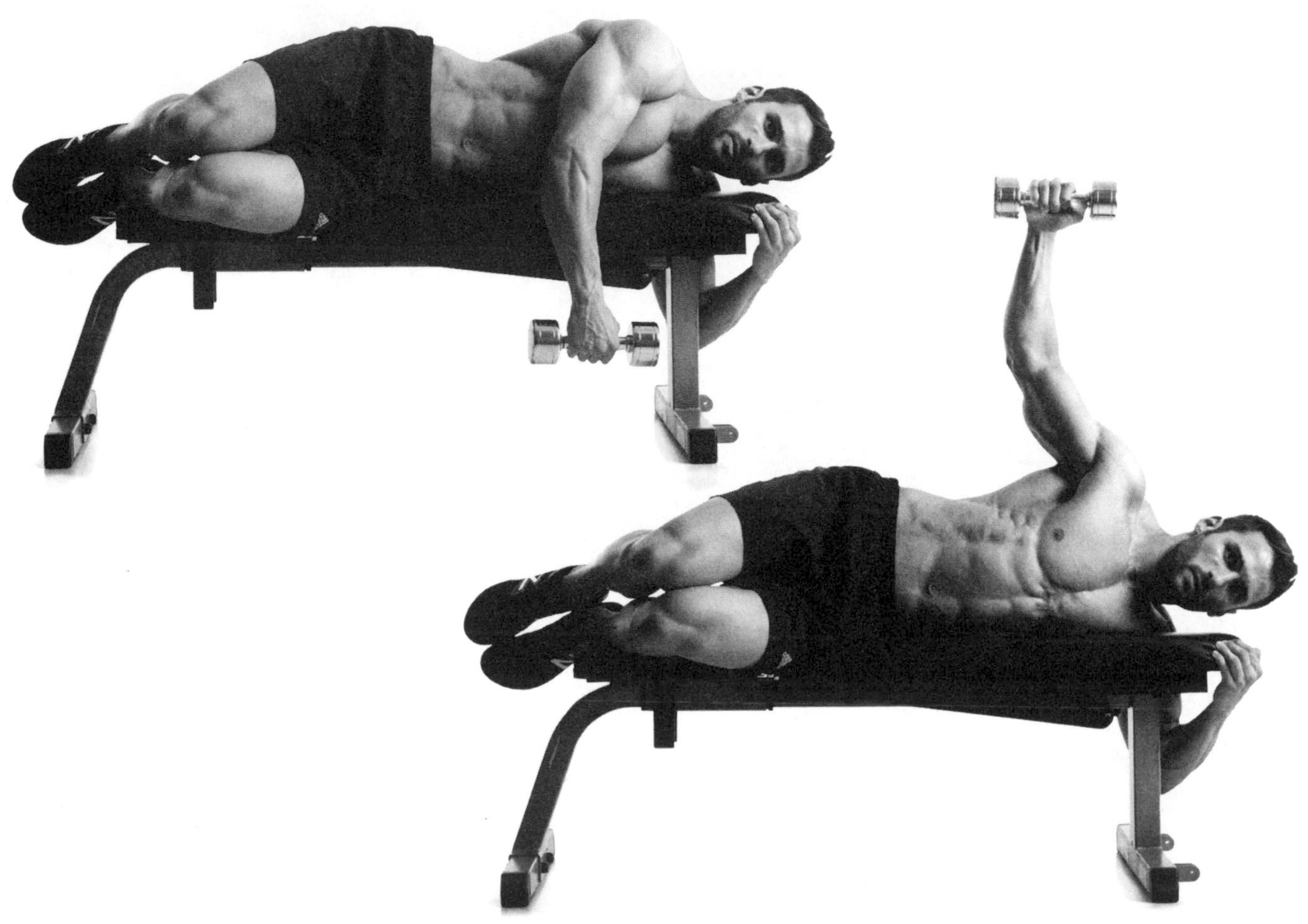

SIDE-LYING ONE-ARM LATERAL RAISE

PURPOSE

Target your posterior deltoids.

START

Lie on your left side on a flat bench. Grab a dumbbell with your right hand and let your right arm hang straight down so it's perpendicular to the floor and your palm is facing back. Keep a slight bend in your elbow.

MOVEMENT

Raise your arm in an arc straight above your shoulder.

FINISH

Pause, then slowly lower your arm back to the starting position.

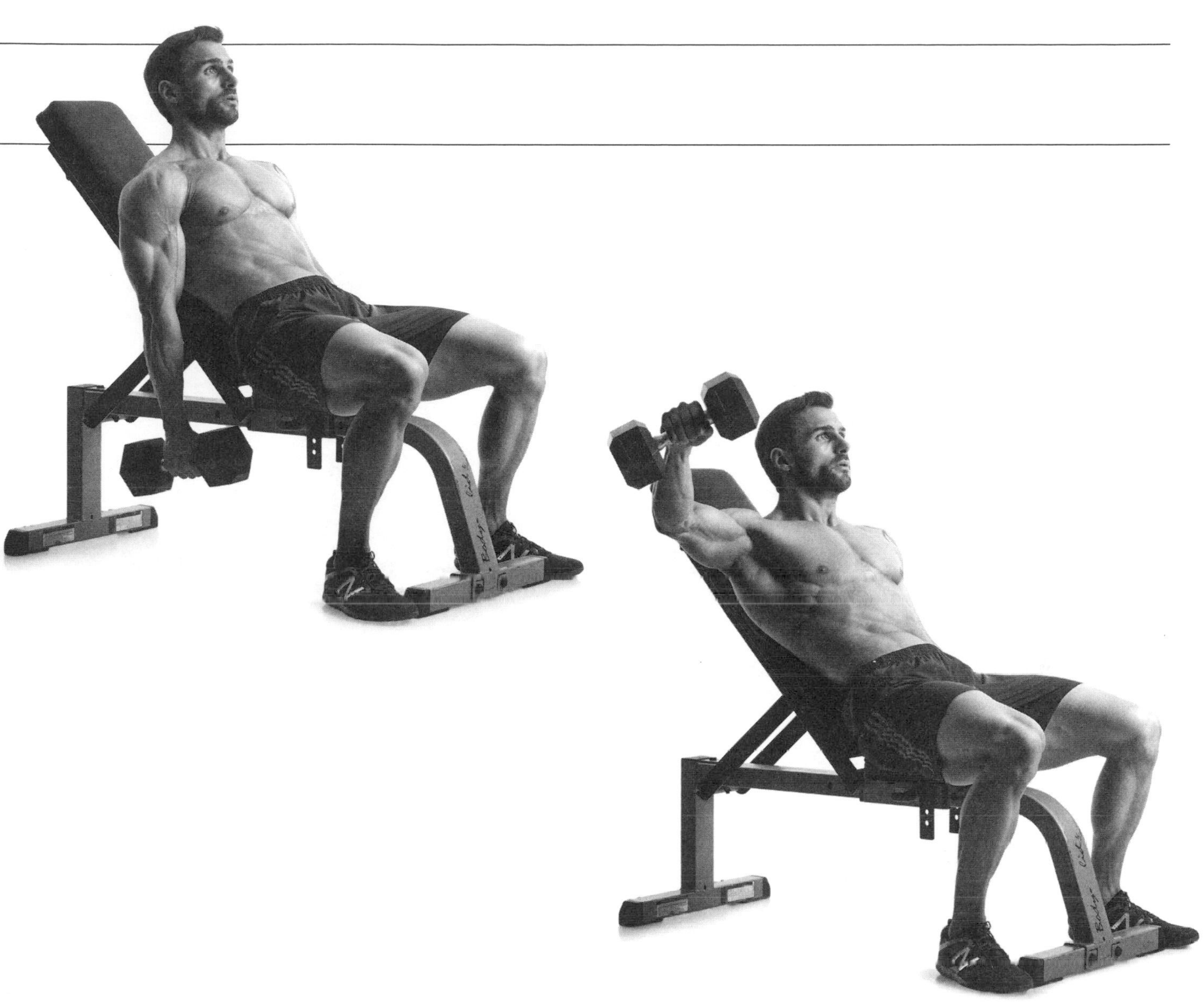

ONE-ARM INCLINE LATERAL RAISE

PURPOSE
Target your posterior deltoids.

START
Sit on an incline bench set to 10 to 30 degrees. Grab a dumbbell and allow your arm to rest straight down at your side, with your palm facing in. Keep your lower back naturally arched.

MOVEMENT
Raise your arm straight out to your side while keeping your chest up.

FINISH
Pause briefly, then slowly lower your arm back to the starting position.

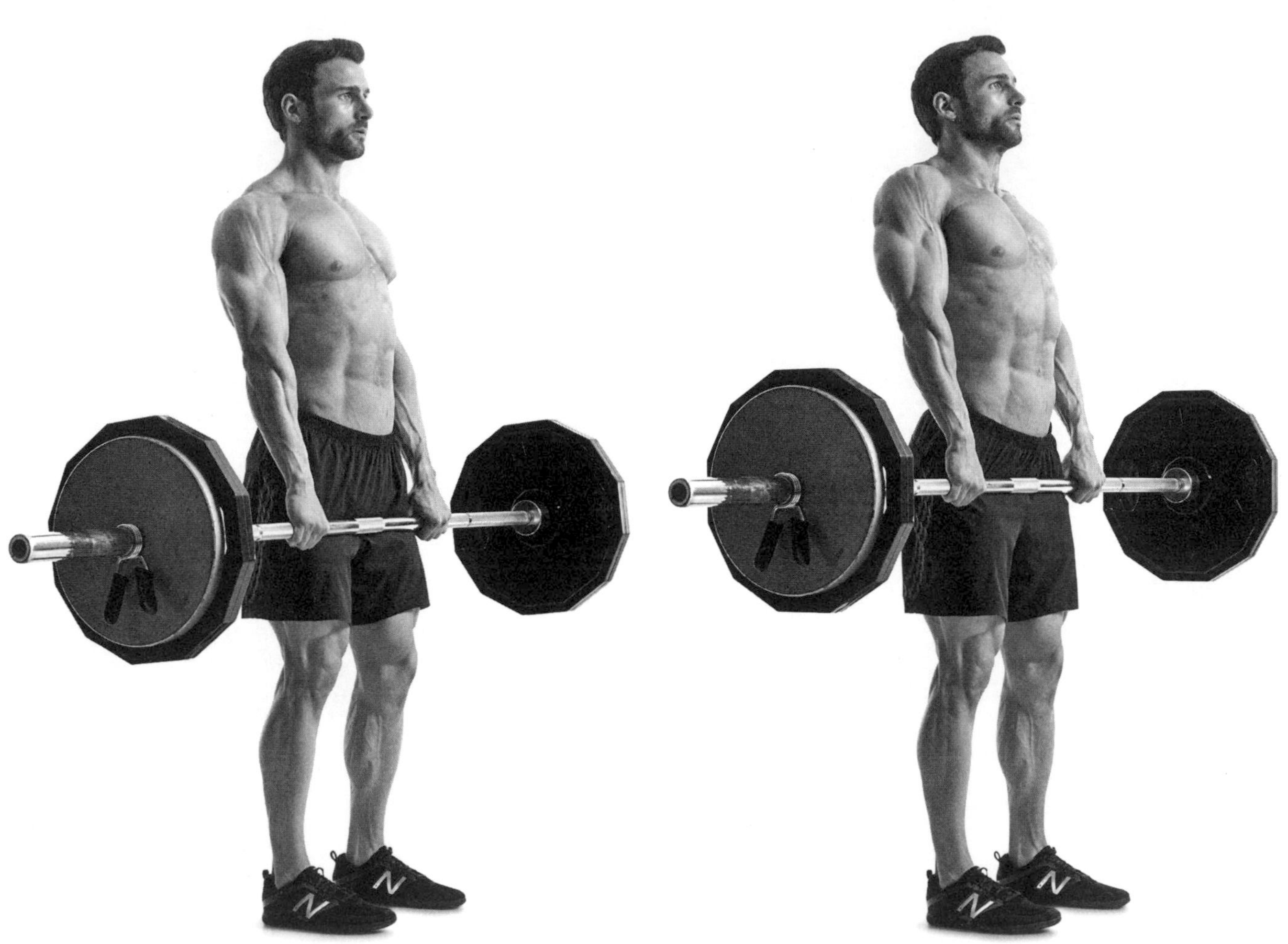

SHRUG

PURPOSE

Work the upper traps and levator scapulae muscle at the sides and back of the neck.

START

Grab a barbell with an overhand grip that's just beyond shoulder width. Let the bar hang at arm's length in front of your hips. Place your feet shoulder width apart.

MOVEMENT

Lean forward at your hips (just slightly). Bend your knees slightly and shrug your shoulders as high as you can. (Raise the top of your shoulders toward your ears while your arms remain straight.)

FINISH

Pause, then lower the bar back to the starting position.

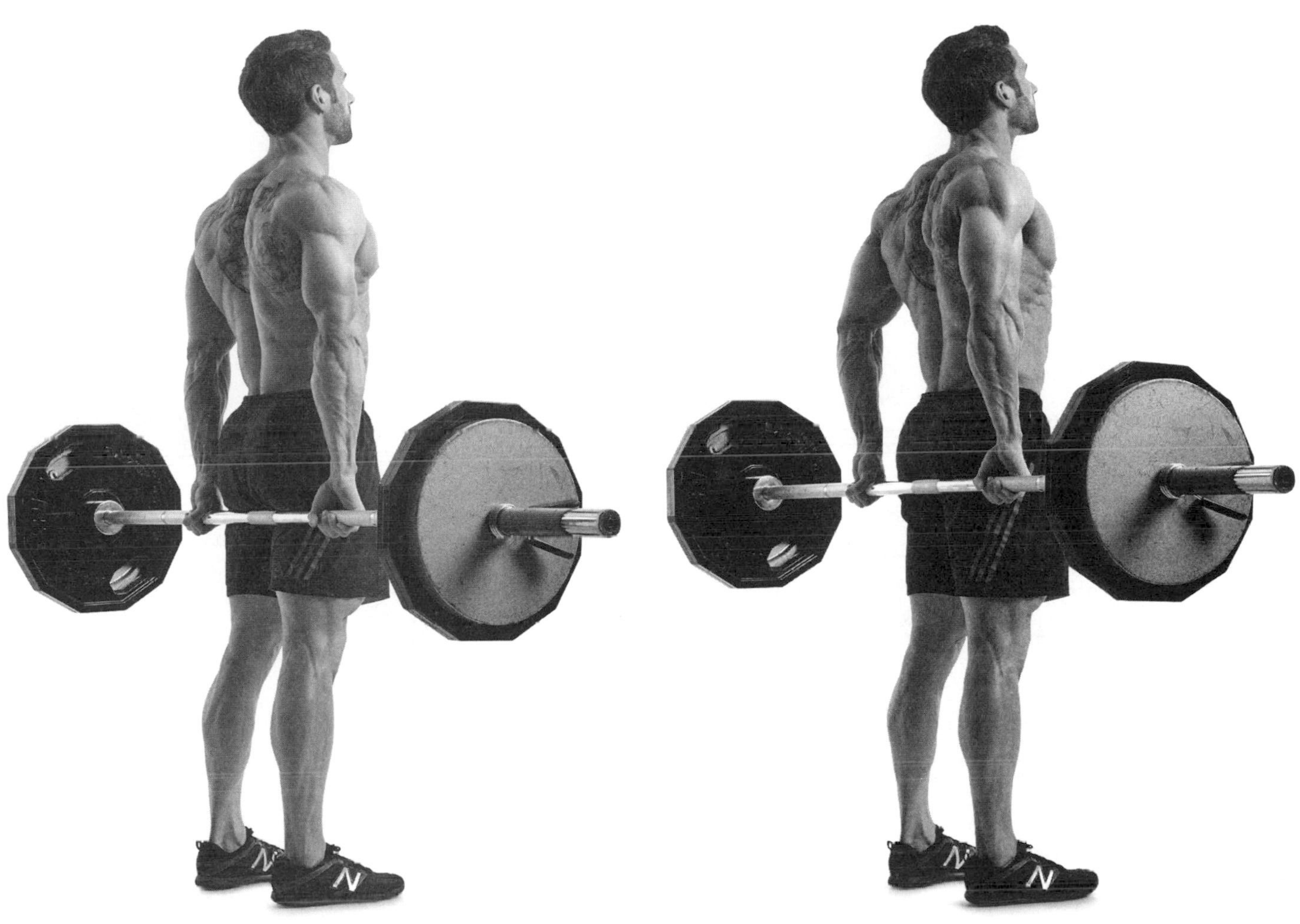

BEHIND-THE-BACK SHRUG

PURPOSE

Work the upper traps, middle traps, and levator scapulae.

START

Grab a barbell behind your backside with an overhand grip that's just beyond shoulder width. Let the bar hang at arm's length behind you. Place your feet shoulder width apart.

MOVEMENT

Lean forward at your hips (just slightly). Bend your knees slightly and shrug your shoulders as high as you can. (Raise the top of your shoulders toward your ears while your arms remain straight.)

FINISH

Pause, then lower the bar back to the starting position.

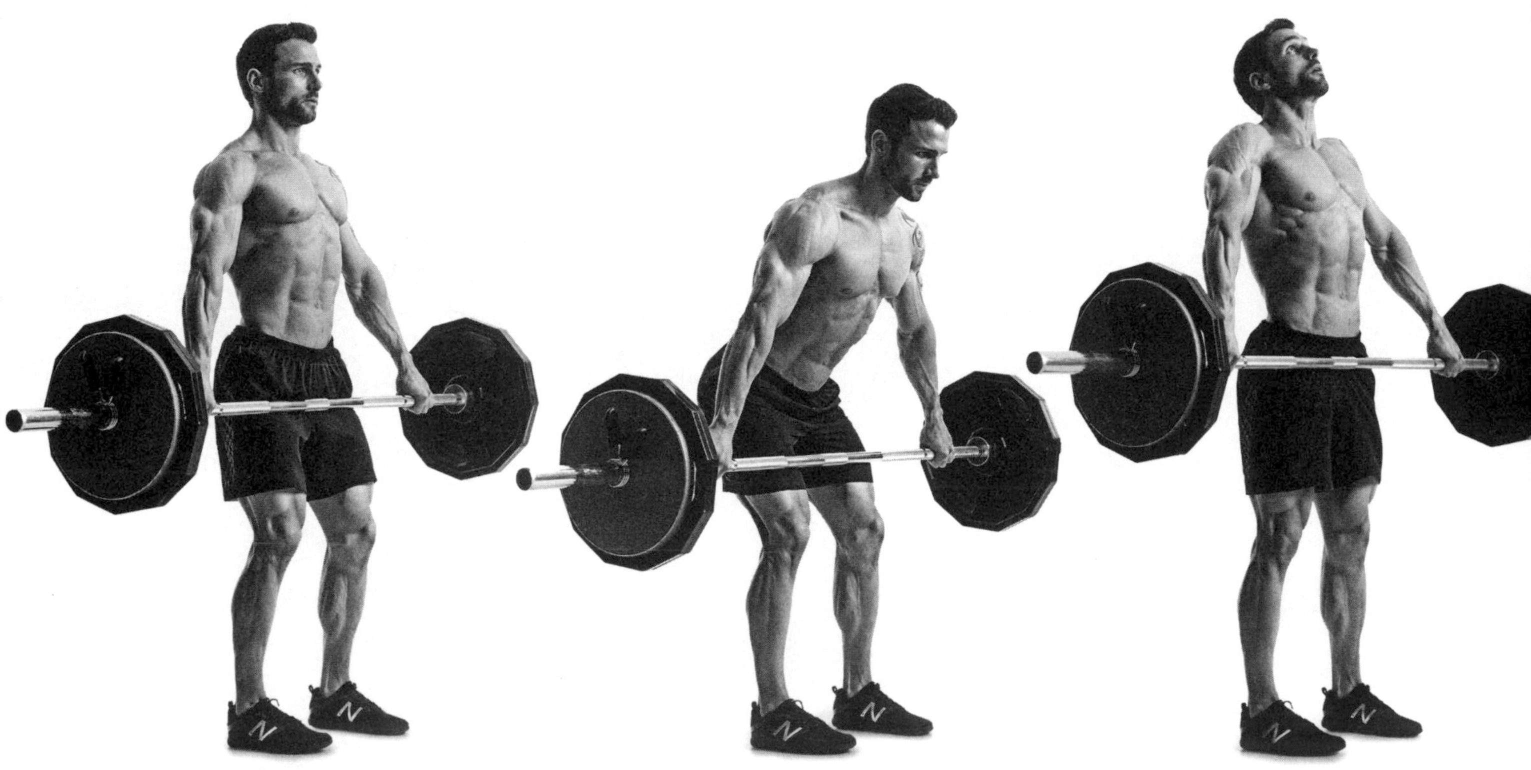

SNATCH SHRUG

PURPOSE

Work the upper traps, middle traps, rhomboids, and levator scapulae.

START

Grab a barbell with an overhand grip that's twice shoulder width. Let the bar hang at arm's length in front of your hips. Keep your feet shoulder width apart.

MOVEMENT

Lean forward at your hips (just slightly). Bend your knees slightly and shrug your shoulders as high as you can. (Raise the top of your shoulders toward your ears while your arms remain straight.)

FINISH

Pause, then lower the bar back to the starting position.

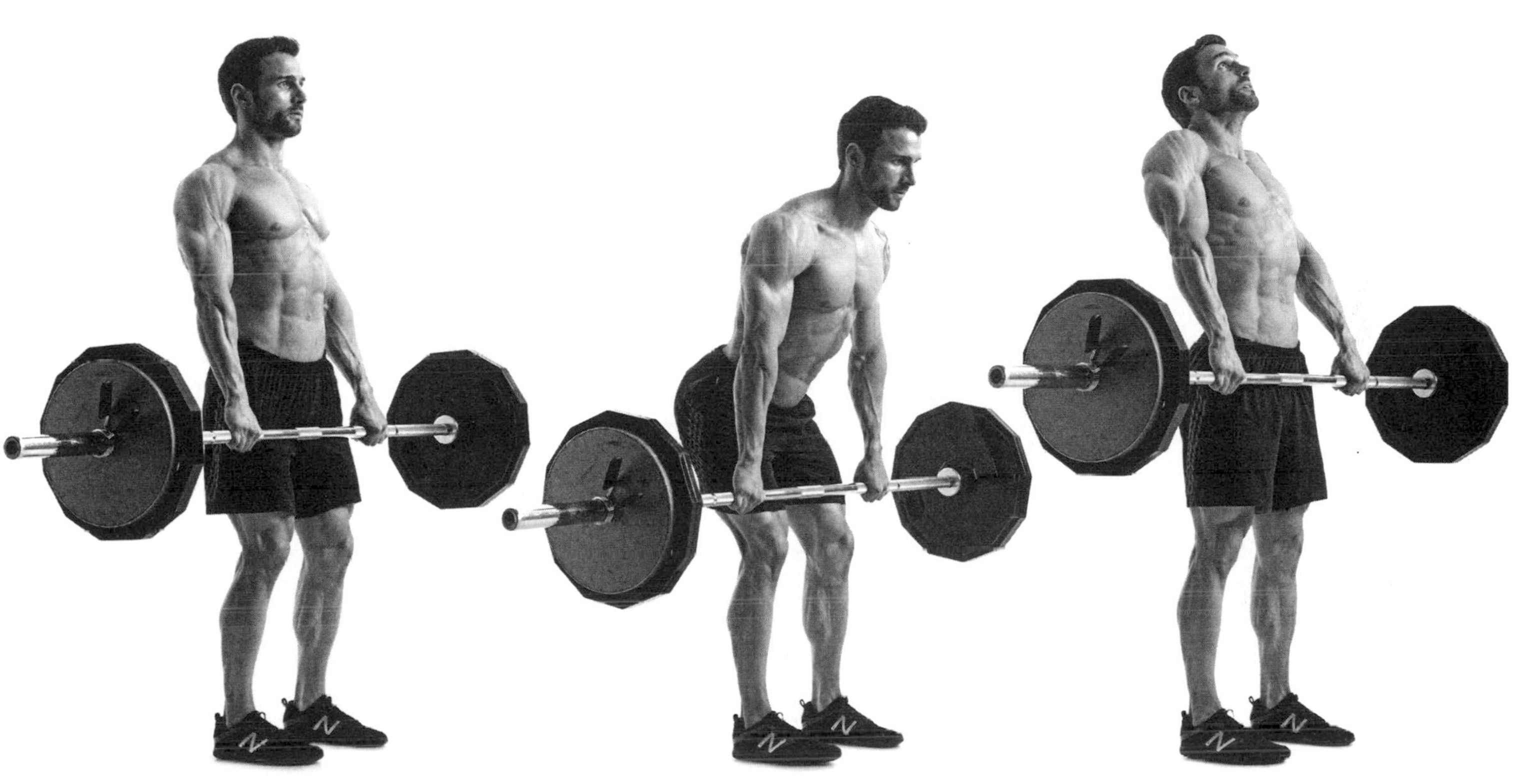

POWER-CLEAN SHRUG

PURPOSE

Work the upper traps and levator scapulae.

START

Grab a barbell with an overhand grip that's just beyond shoulder width. Let the bar hang at arm's length in front of your hips. Keep your feet shoulder width apart.

MOVEMENT

Lean forward at your hips (just slightly). Bend your knees slightly and using a slight hip hinge and dip to your knees, shrug your shoulders as high as you can. (Raise the top of your shoulders toward your ears while your arms remain straight.)

FINISH

Pause, then lower the bar back to the starting position.

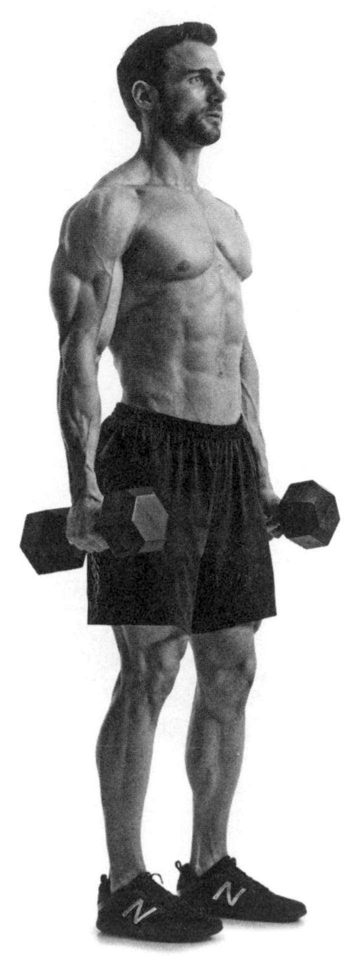

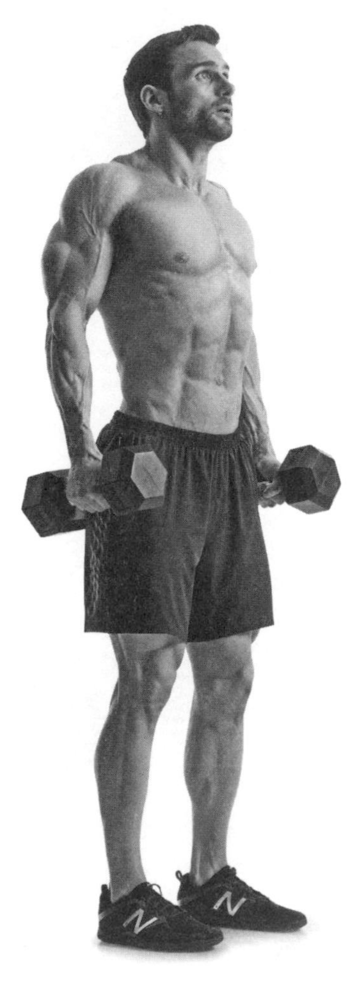

SHRUG

PURPOSE

Work the upper traps and levator scapulae.

START

Grab a pair of dumbbells with a neutral grip. Hold them at arm's length by your sides, palms facing each other. Place your feet shoulder width apart.

MOVEMENT

Stand tall and bend your knees slightly and shrug your shoulders as high as you can. (Raise the top of your shoulders toward your ears while your arms remain straight.)

FINISH

Pause, then lower the dumbbells back to the starting position.

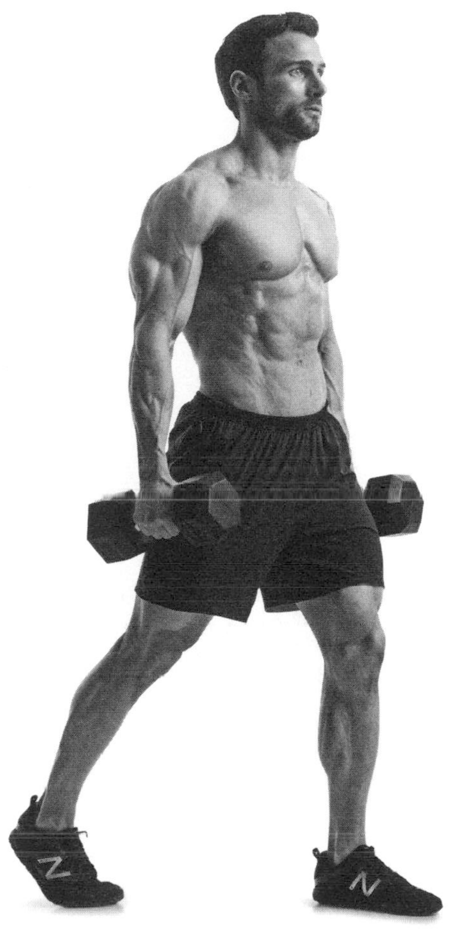

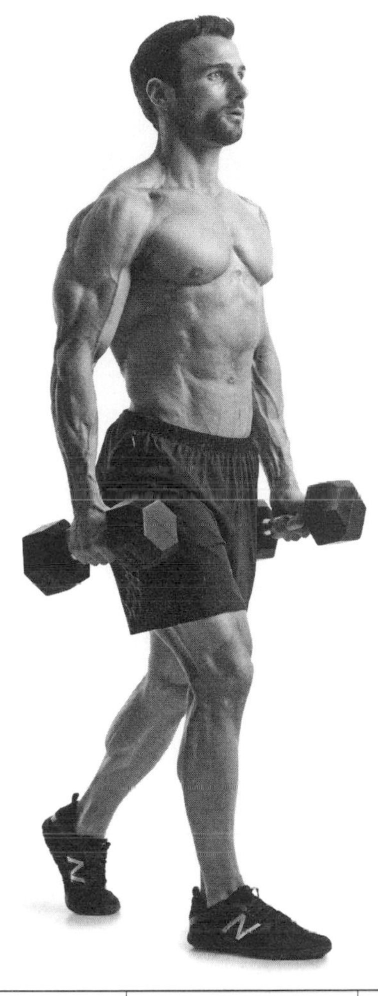

FARMER'S WALK

PURPOSE
Work the upper traps and levator scapulae.

START
Grab a pair of dumbbells with a neutral grip. Hold them at arm's length by your sides, palms facing each other.

MOVEMENT
Lean forward at your hips (just slightly). Bend your knees slightly and walk maintaining a controlled posture and braced core.

FINISH
Stop, then lower the weights to the floor.

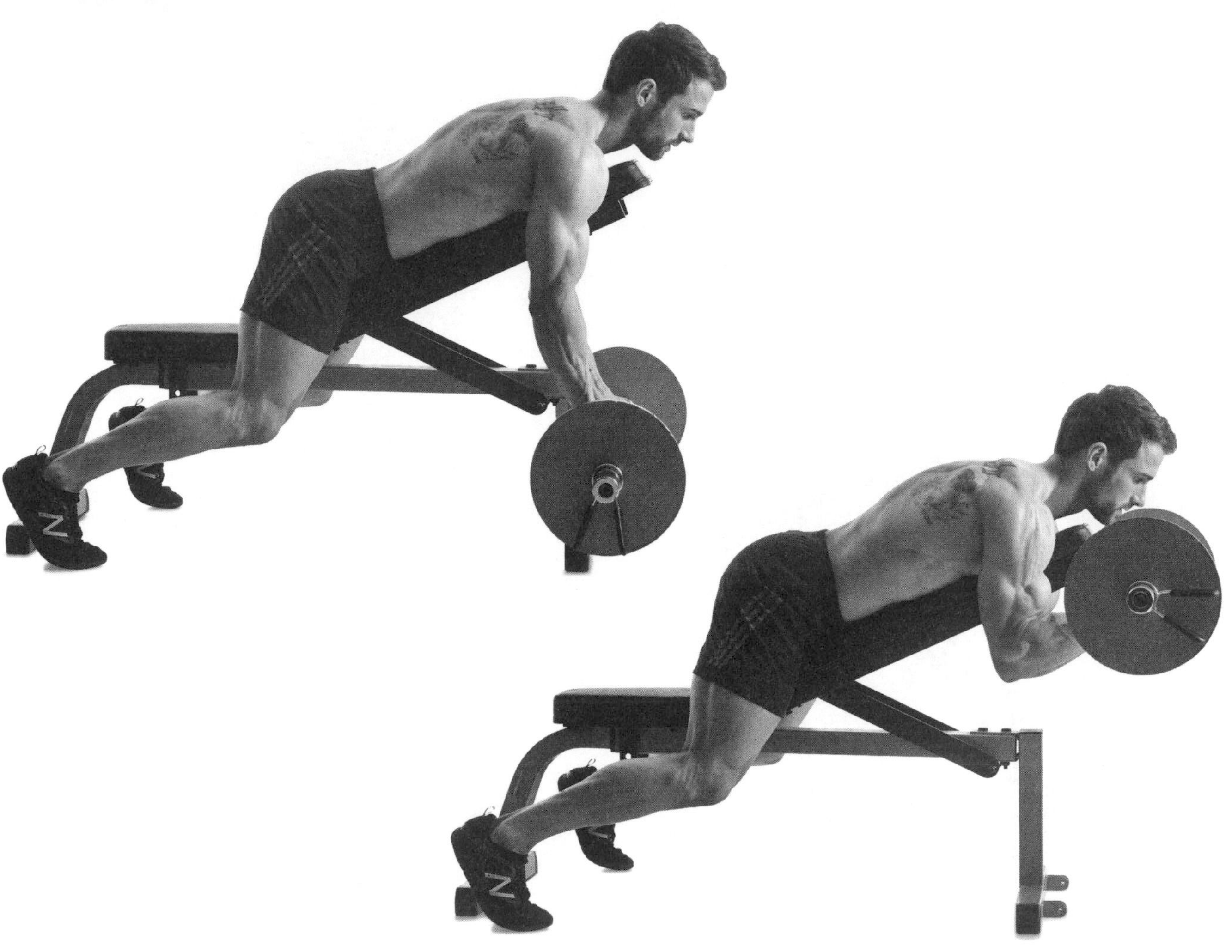

CHEST-SUPPORTED SPIDER CURL

PURPOSE

Target your biceps.

START

Lie with your chest against an incline bench set to 10 to 30 degrees. Keep the balls of your feet on the ground. Grab a barbell with an underhand grip that is shoulder width apart and allow the barbell to hang out in front of your chest.

MOVEMENT

Do not move your upper arms as you bend your elbows and curl the bar as high as you can.

FINISH

Pause briefly, then lower the weight back to the starting position.

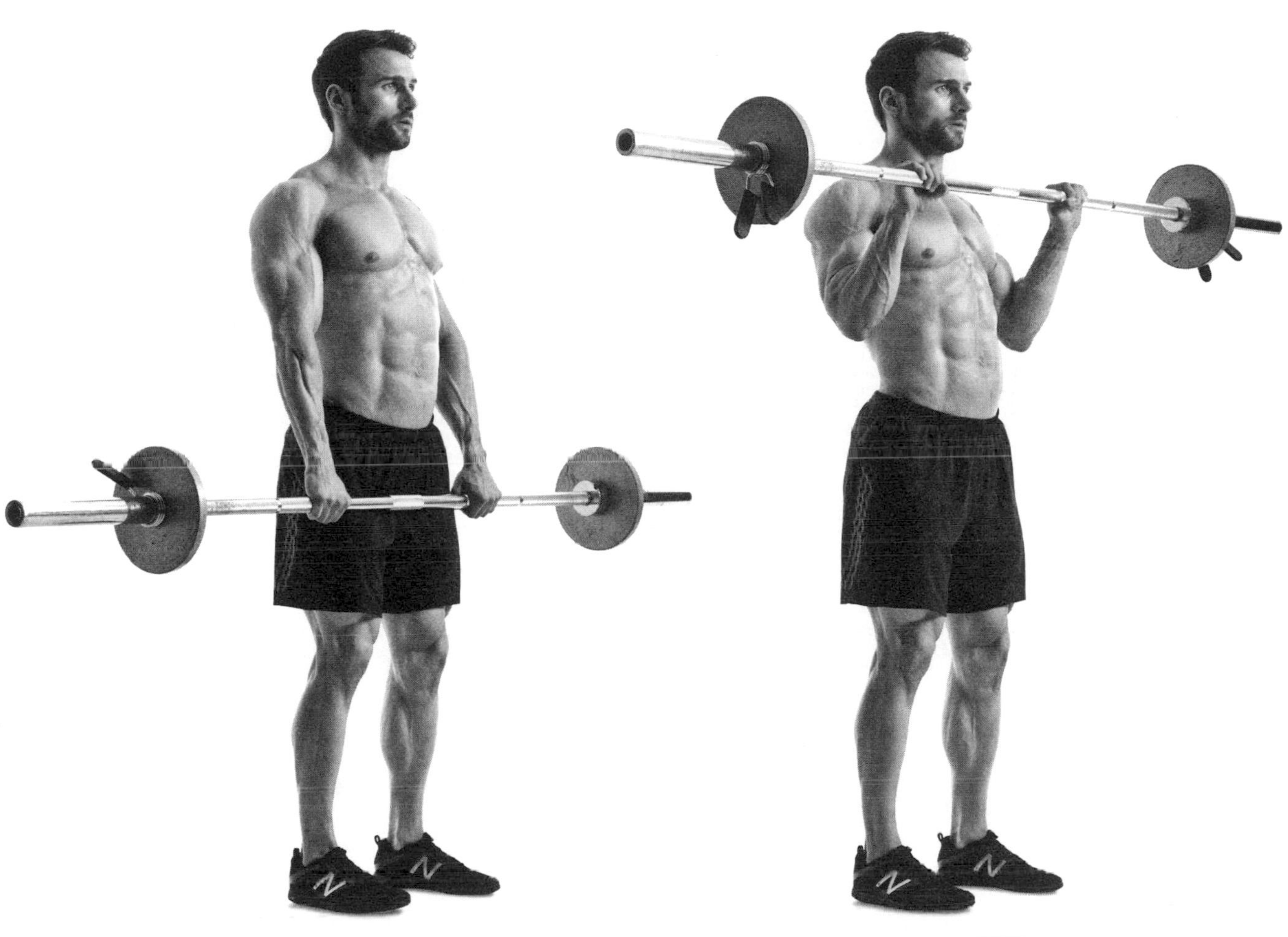

REVERSE-GRIP CURL

PURPOSE
Target your biceps.

START
Grab a barbell with an overhand grip that is shoulder width apart and allow the bar to hang at arm's length in front of your hips.

MOVEMENT
Do not move your upper arms as you bend your elbows and curl the bar as high as you can.

FINISH
Pause briefly, then lower the weight back to the starting position.

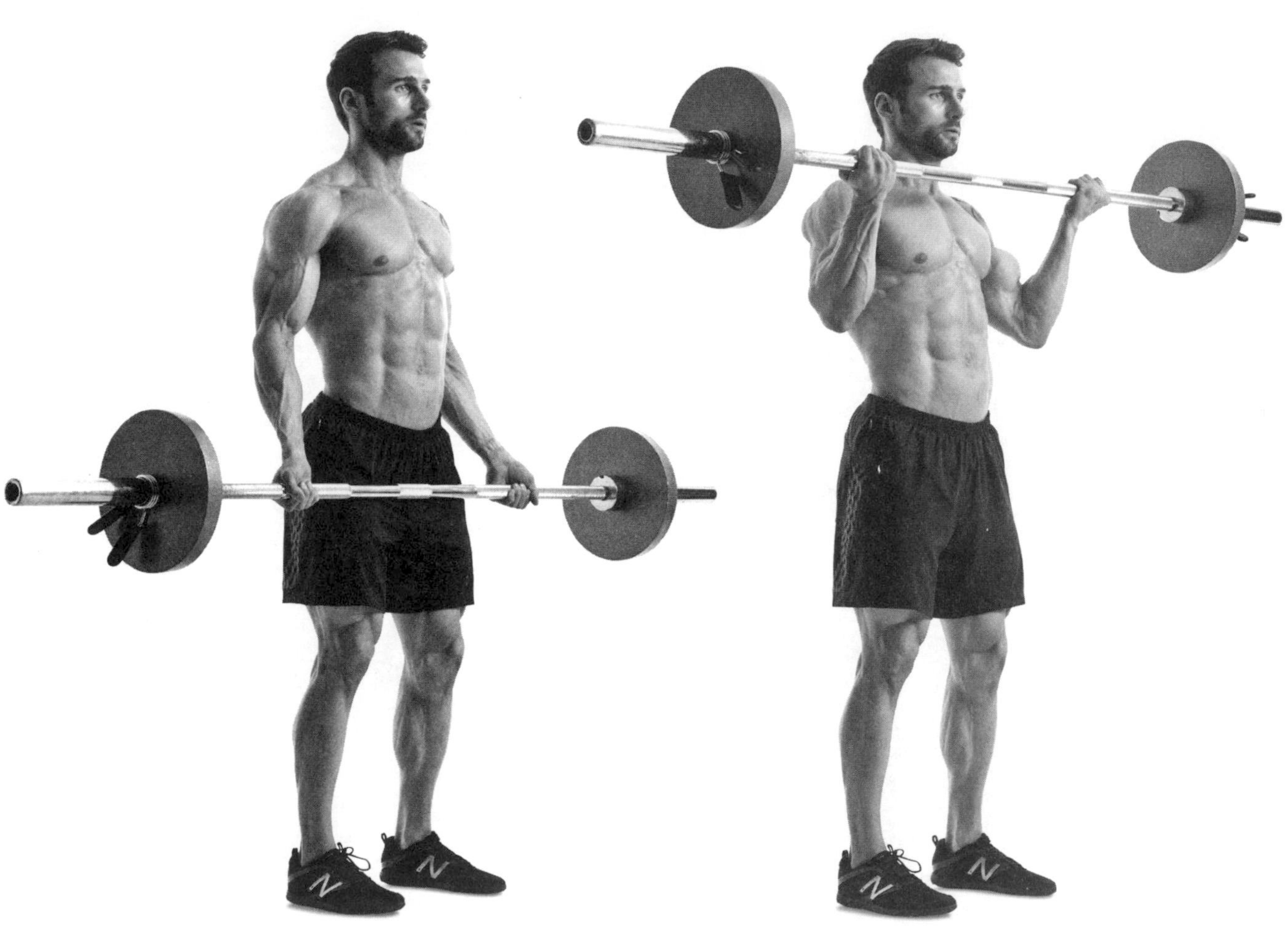

WIDE-GRIP CURL

PURPOSE
Target your biceps.

START
Grab a barbell with an underhand grip that is one and half times the width of your shoulders and allow the bar to hang at arm's length in front of your hips.

MOVEMENT
Do not move your upper arms as you bend your elbows and curl the bar as high as you can.

FINISH
Pause briefly, then lower the weight back to the starting position.

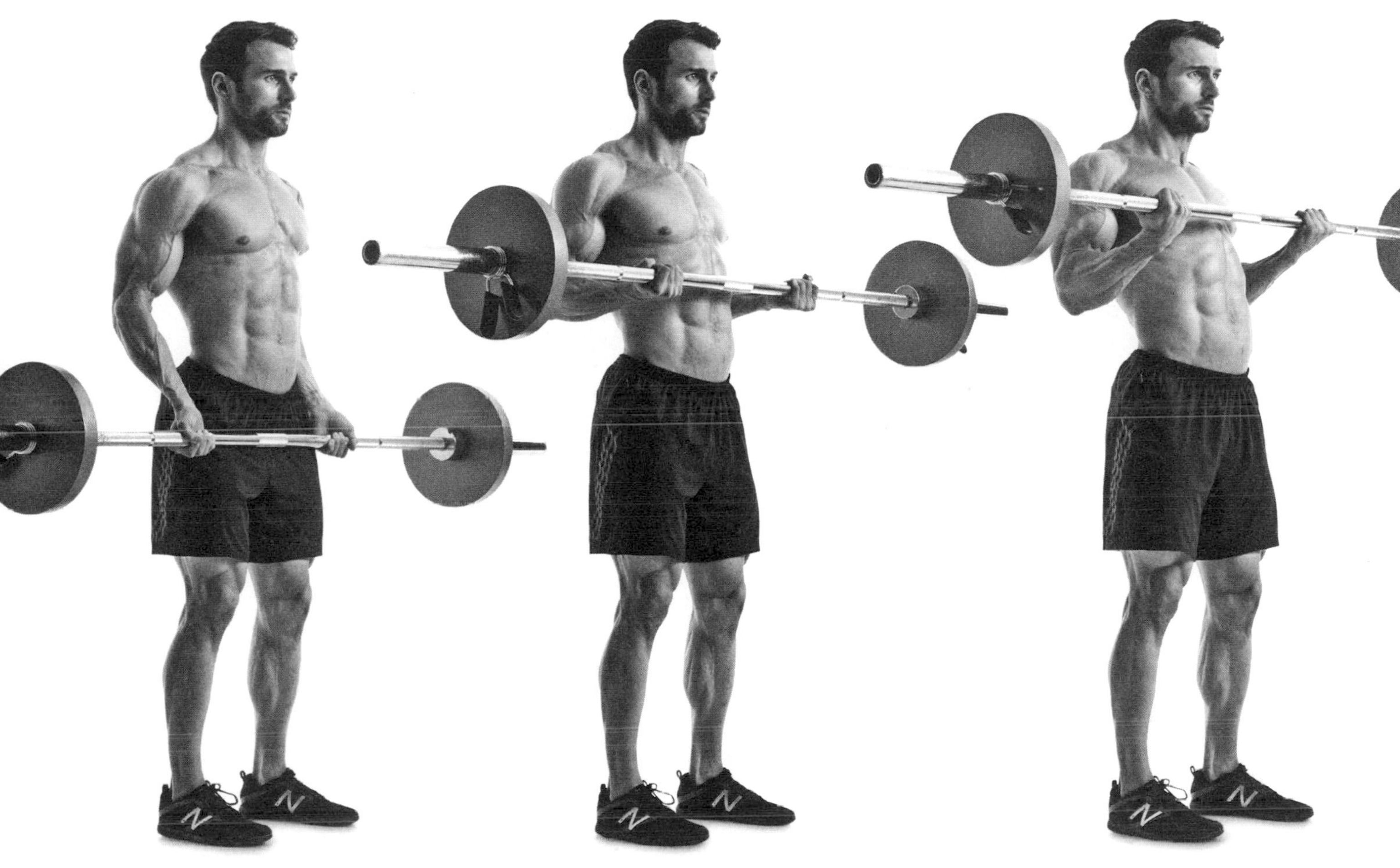

DRAG CURL

PURPOSE
Target your biceps.

START
Grab a barbell with an underhand grip that is shoulder width apart and allow the bar to hang at arm's length in front of your hips.

MOVEMENT
Instead of curling the bar, move your elbows up and back (but not out), allowing the bar to "drag" up the front of your body without ever quite touching your torso.

FINISH
Pause when your elbows are as high as they can go, then lower the weight back to the starting position.

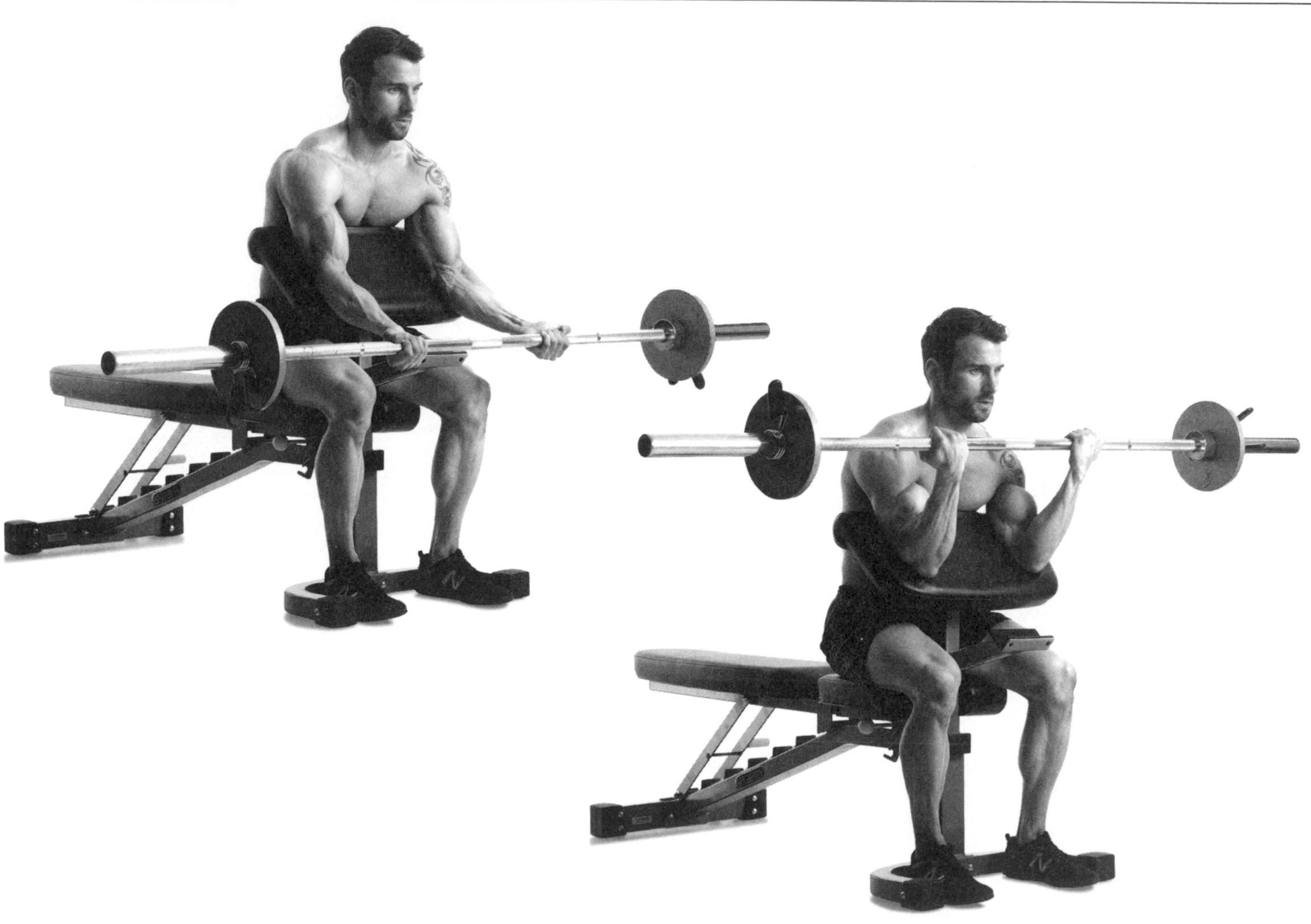

PREACHER CURL

PURPOSE
Target your biceps.

START
Grab a barbell with an underhand grip that is shoulder width apart and sit on a preacher bench so the top of the pad almost touches your armpits.

MOVEMENT
Do not move your upper arms as you bend your elbows and curl the bar just short of perpendicular to the floor (higher is just too easy to do and reduces the workload).

FINISH
Pause briefly, then lower the weight back to the starting position.

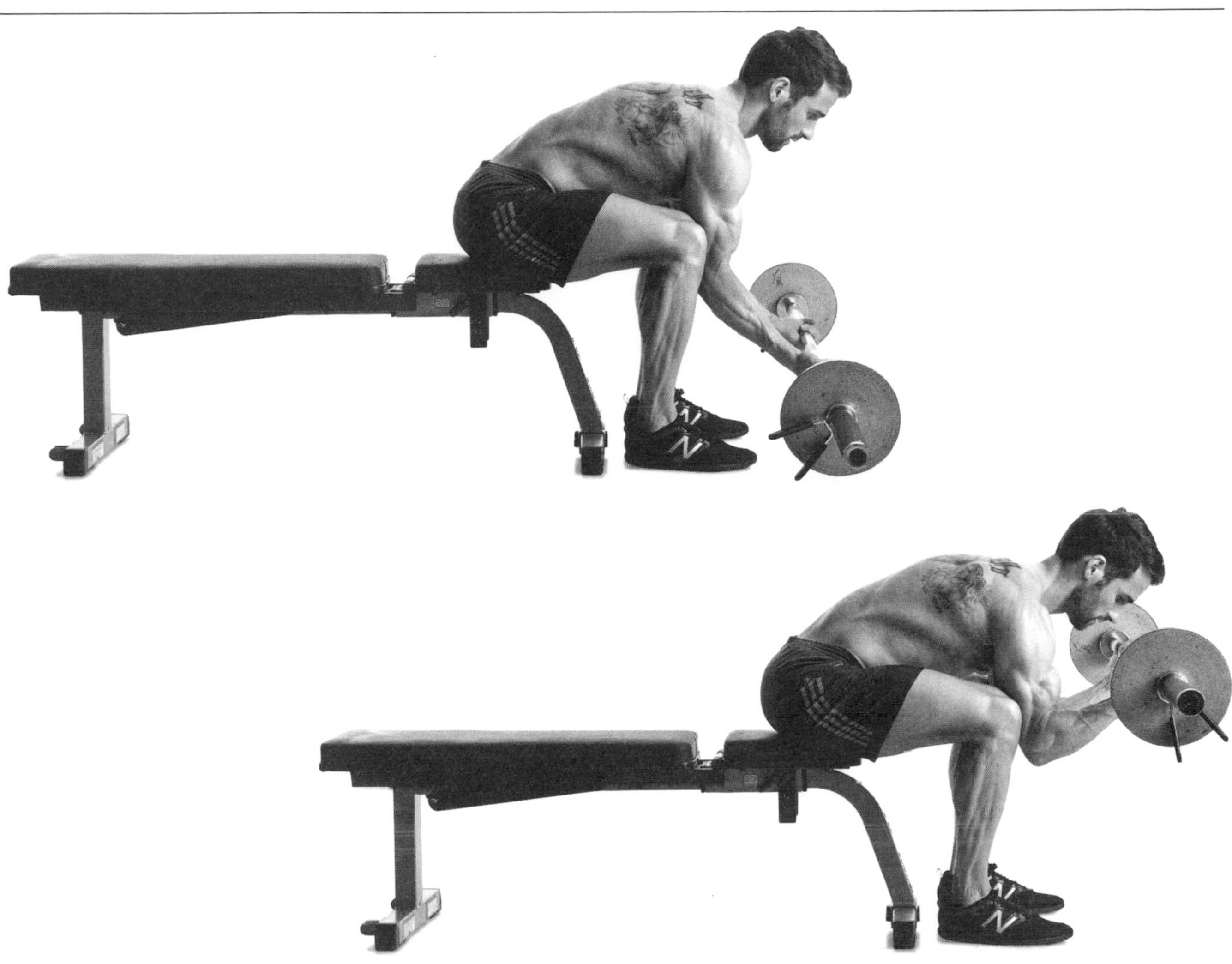

SEATED CLOSE-GRIP CONCEN-TRATION CURL

PURPOSE
Target your biceps.

START
Grab a barbell with an underhand grip that is shoulder width apart. Sit on the edge of a bench and allow the bar to hang at arm's length in front of your hips.

MOVEMENT
Do not move your upper arms as you bend your elbows and curl the bar as high as you can.

FINISH
Pause briefly, then lower the weight back to the starting position.

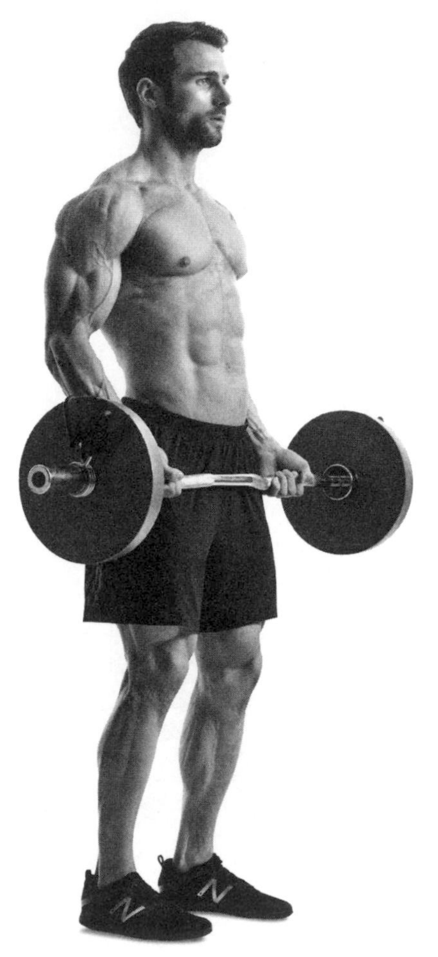

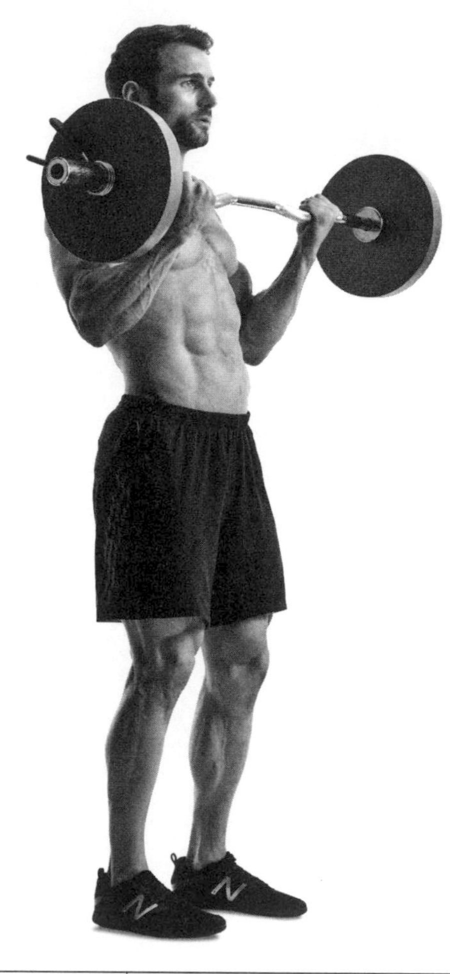

STANDING CURL

PURPOSE
Target your biceps.

START
Grab an EZ bar with an underhand grip that is shoulder width apart and allow the bar to hang at arm's length in front of your hips.

MOVEMENT
Do not move your upper arms as you bend your elbows and curl the bar as high as you can.

FINISH
Pause briefly, then lower the weight back to the starting position.

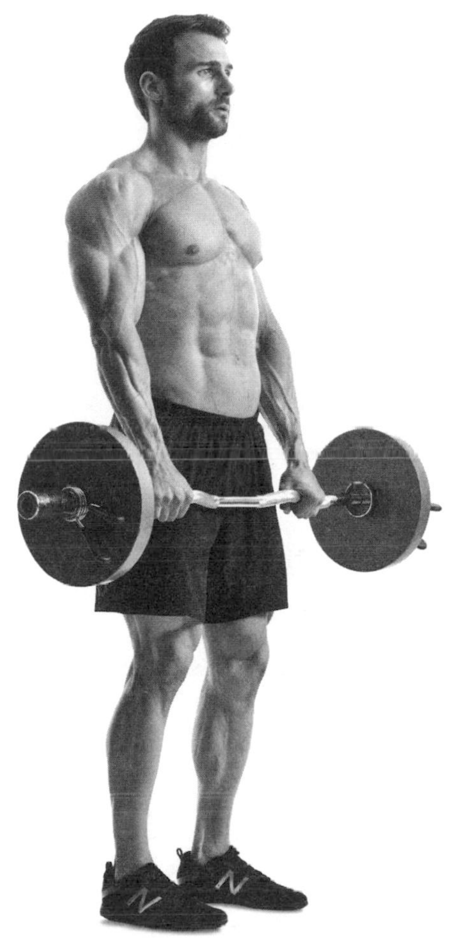

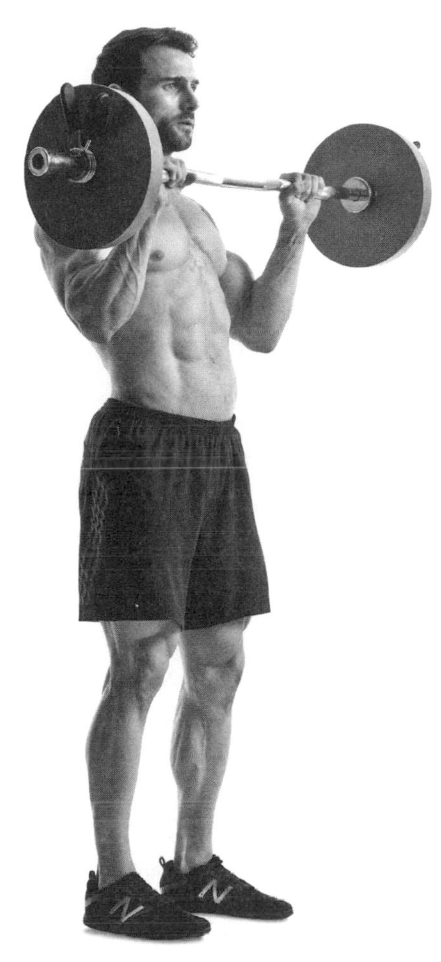

REVERSE-GRIP CURL

PURPOSE
Target your biceps.

START
Grab an EZ bar with an overhand grip that is shoulder width apart and allow the bar to hang at arm's length in front of your hips.

MOVEMENT
Do not move your upper arms as you bend your elbows and curl the bar as high as you can.

FINISH
Pause briefly, then lower the weight back to the starting position.

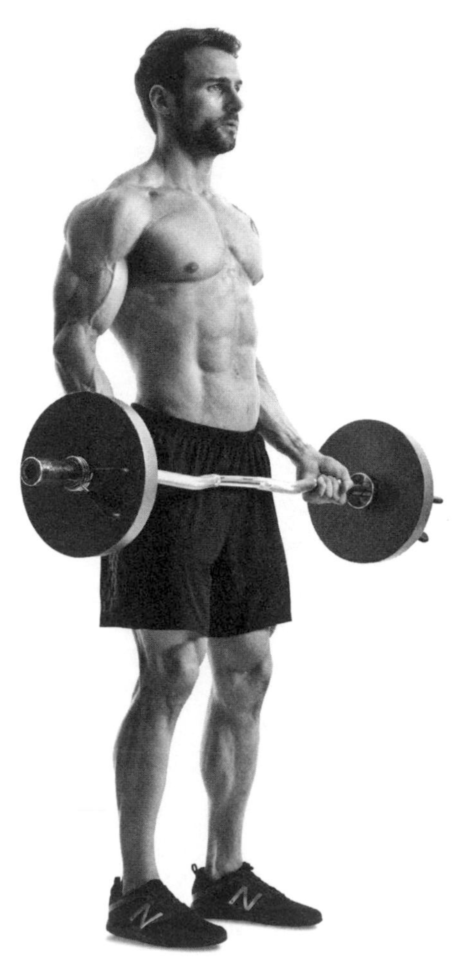

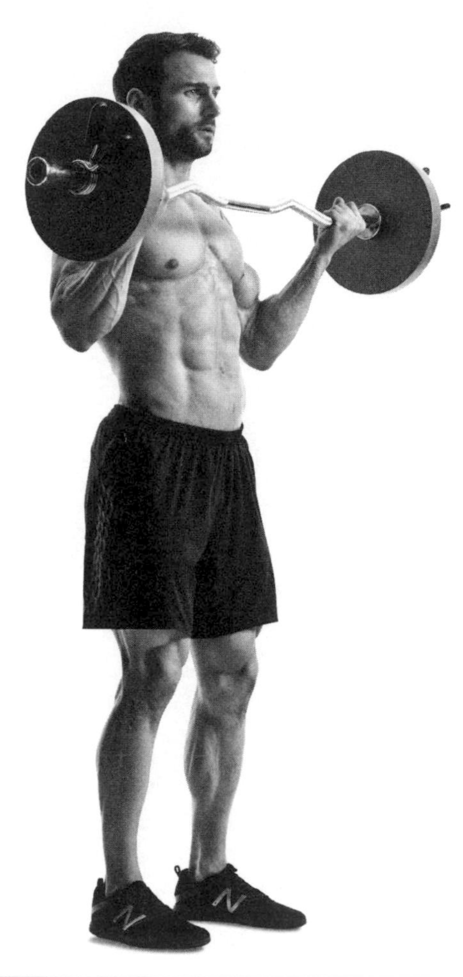

WIDE-GRIP CURL

PURPOSE
Target your biceps.

START
Grab an EZ bar with an underhand grip that is one and a half times the width of your shoulders and allow the bar to hang at arm's length in front of your hips.

MOVEMENT
Do not move your upper arms as you bend your elbows and curl the bar as high as you can.

FINISH
Pause briefly, then lower the weight back to the starting position.

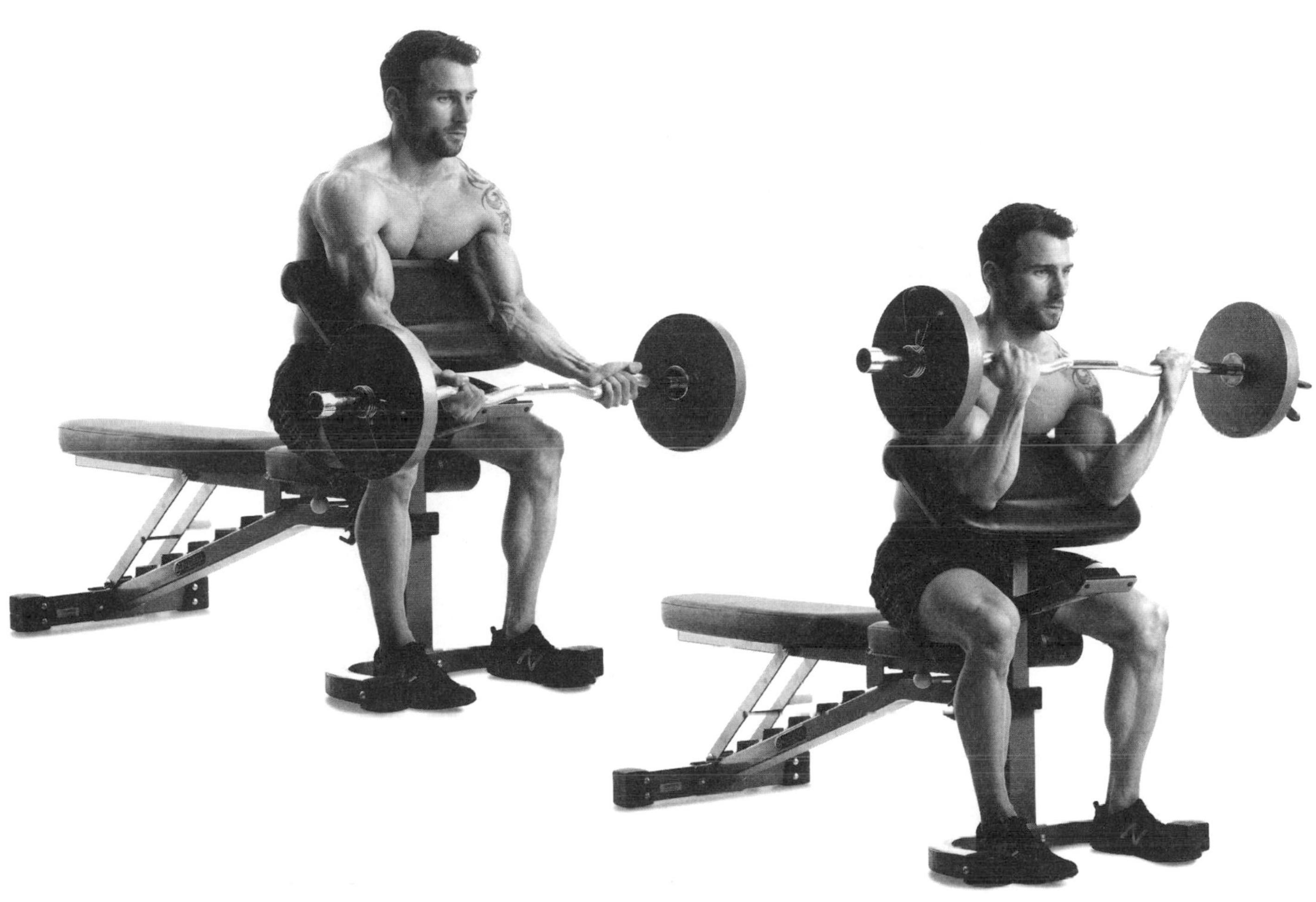

PREACHER CURL

PURPOSE

Target your biceps.

START

Grab an EZ bar with an underhand grip that is shoulder width apart and sit on a preacher bench so the top of the pad almost touches your armpits.

MOVEMENT

Do not move your upper arms as you bend your elbows and curl the bar just short of perpendicular to the floor (higher is just too easy to do and reduces the workload).

FINISH

Pause briefly, then lower the weight back to the starting position.

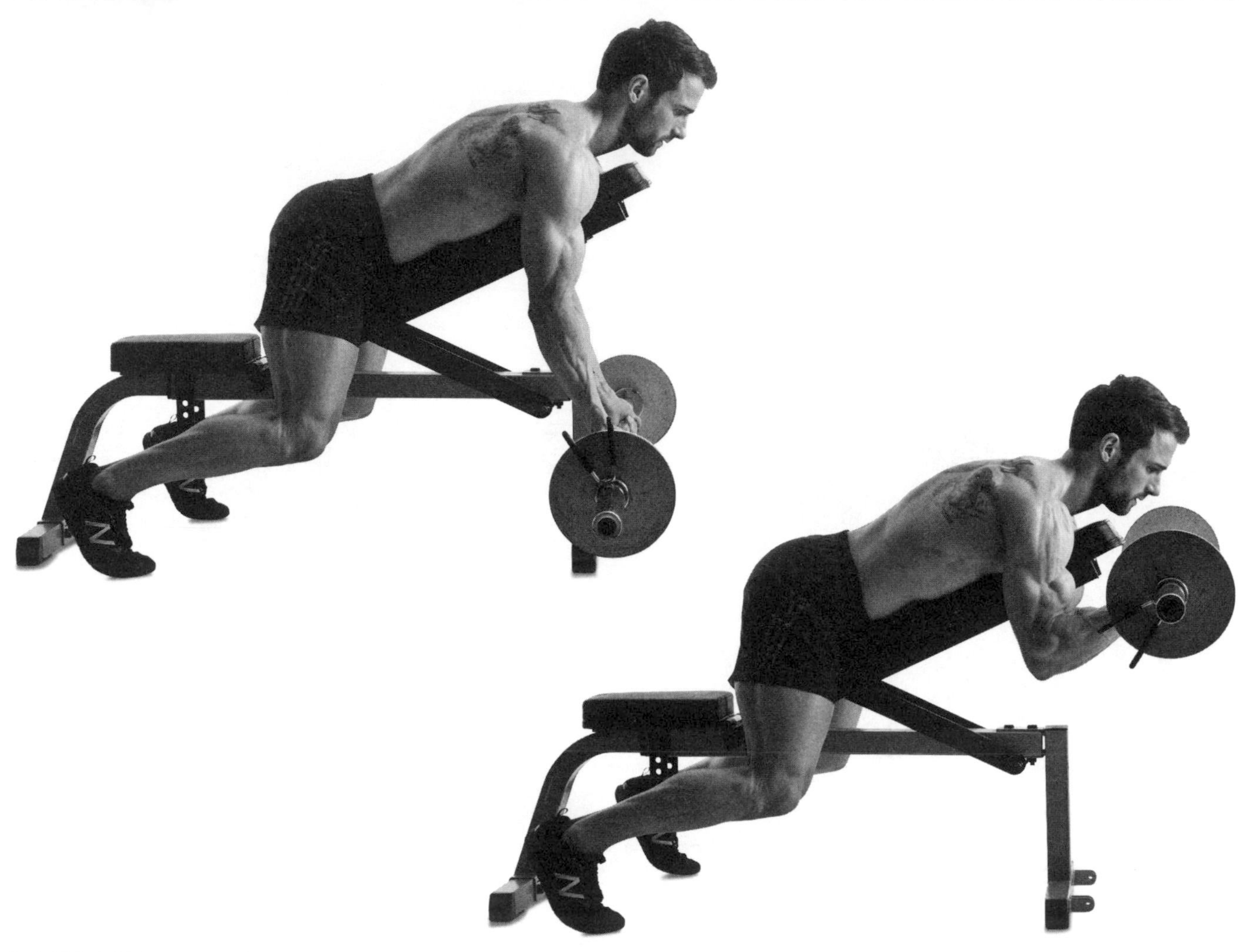

CHEST-SUPPORTED SPIDER CURL

PURPOSE
Target your biceps.

START
Lie with your chest against an incline bench set to 10 to 30 degrees. Keep the balls of your feet on the ground. Grab an EZ bar with an underhand grip that is shoulder width apart and allow the bar to hang out in front of your chest.

MOVEMENT
Do not move your upper arms as you bend your elbows and curl the bar as high as you can.

FINISH
Pause briefly, then lower the weight back to the starting position.

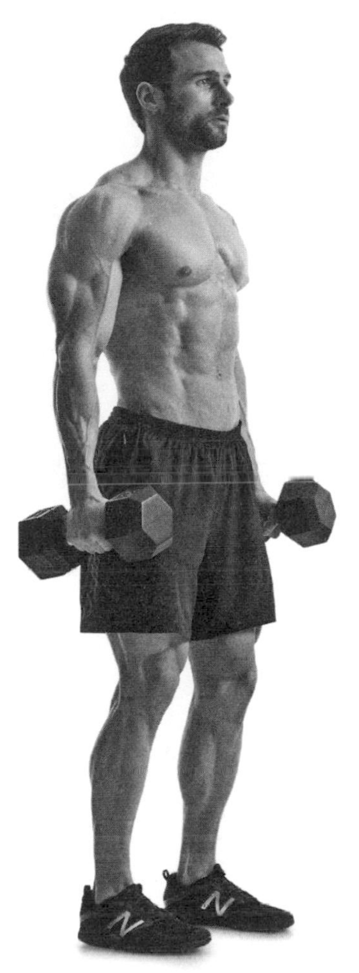

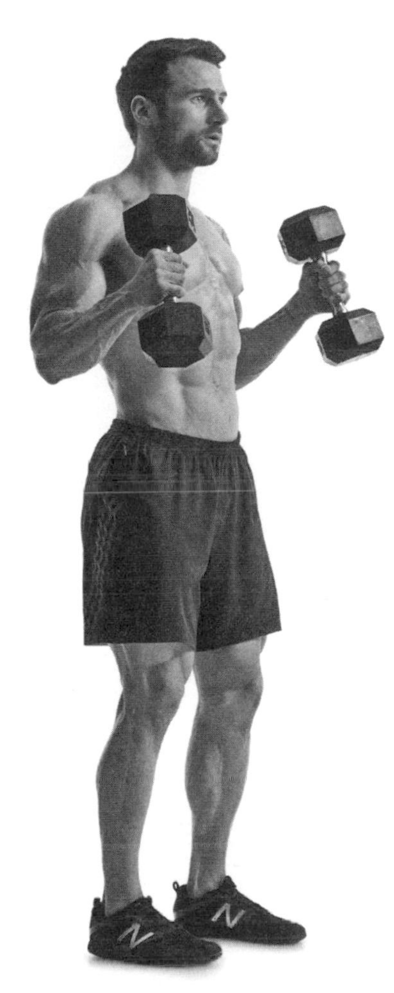

STANDING HAMMER CURL

PURPOSE
Target your biceps.

START
Grab a pair of dumbbells with a neutral grip. Allow the dumbbells to hang at arm's length at your sides, your palms facing each other.

MOVEMENT
Do not move your upper arms as you bend your elbows and curl the dumbbells as high as you can.

FINISH
Pause briefly, then lower the weight back to the starting position.

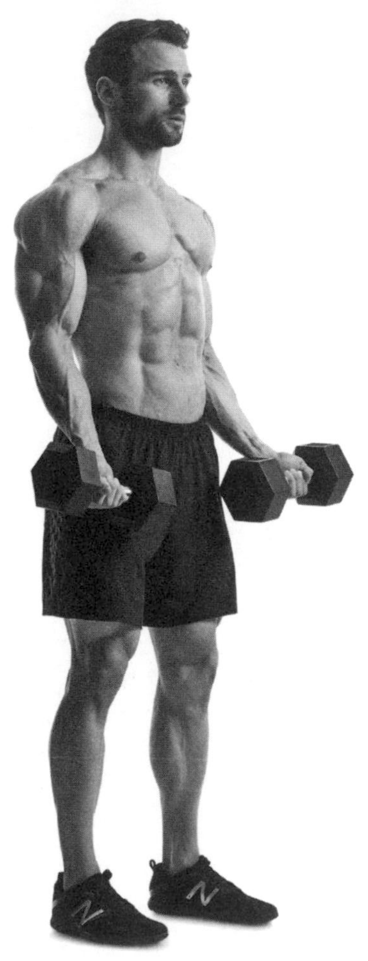

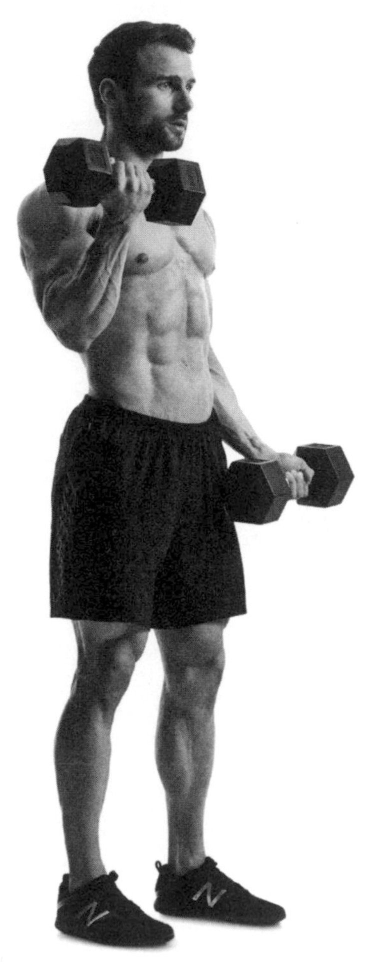

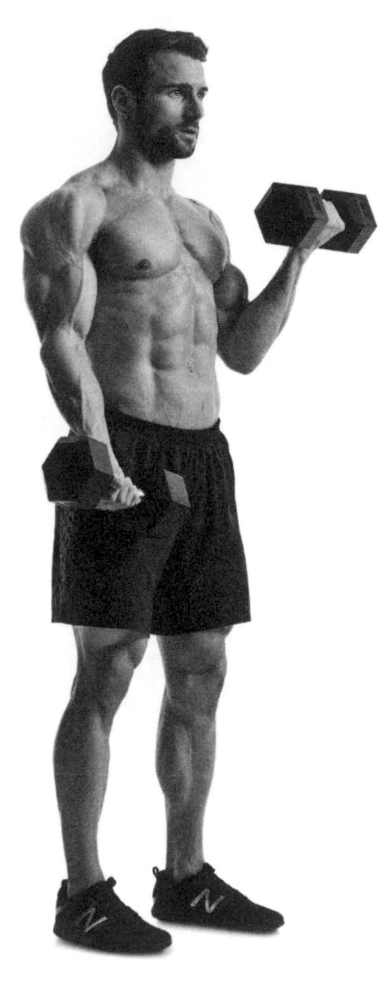

STANDING ALTERNATE BICEPS CURL

PURPOSE

Target your biceps.

START

Grab a pair of dumbbells with an underhand grip that is shoulder width apart. Allow the dumbbells to hang at arm's length at your sides.

MOVEMENT

Do not move your upper arm as you bend your elbow and curl one dumbbell as high as you can.

FINISH

Pause briefly, then lower the dumbbell and alternate sides continuously.

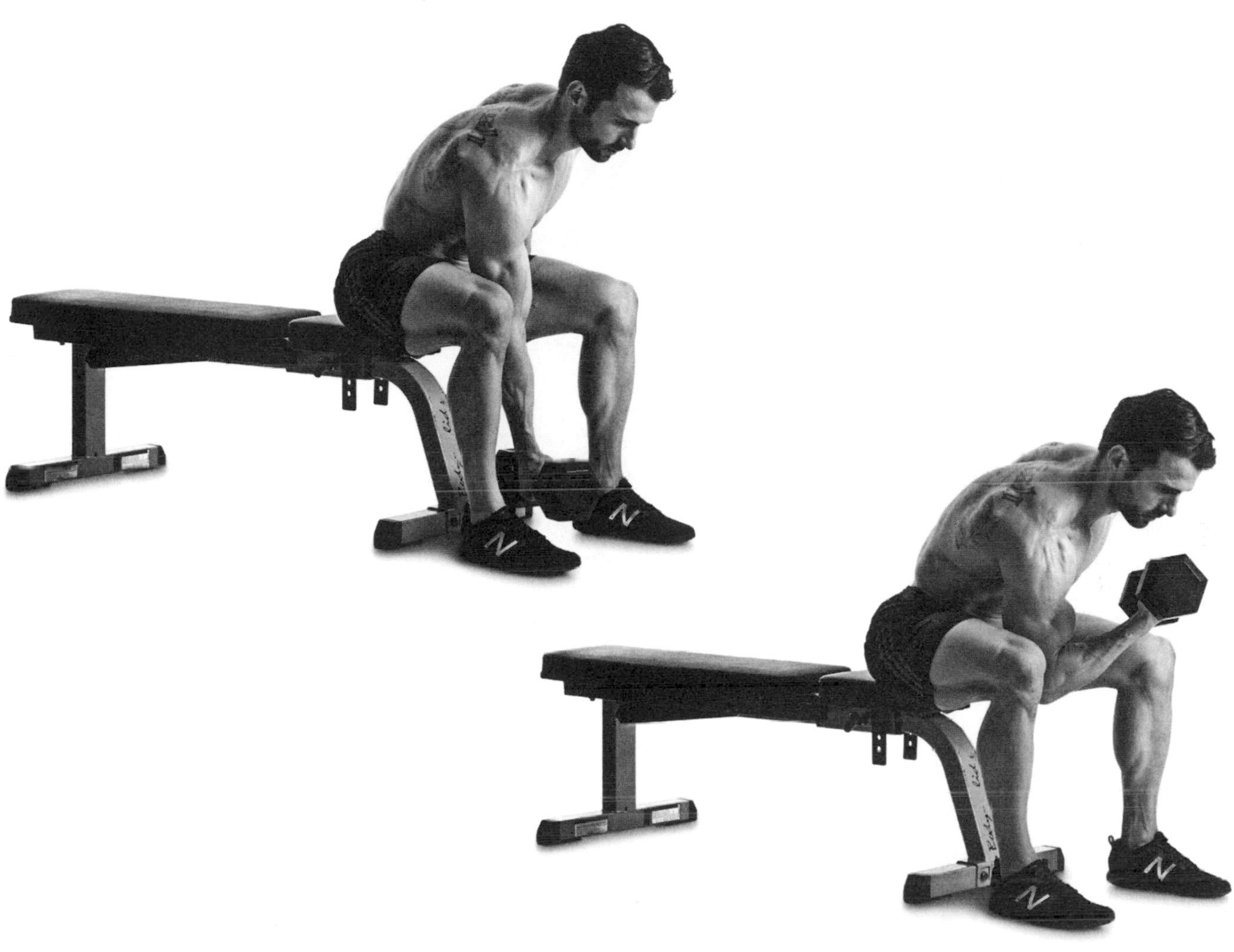

CONCEN-TRATION CURL

PURPOSE

Target the biceps.

START

Grab a single dumbbell with your right hand, sit at the end of a bench and support that arm by resting your right elbow on your quad. Allow your arm to hang at arm's length between your legs.

MOVEMENT

Do not curl the dumbbell straight up to your chest, but instead focus on angling the weight toward your body. Bending over at your hips with your arm fully extended, curl the weight toward your shoulder and flex your biceps at the top. Once at the top pause for 2 seconds.

FINISH

Slowly lower the weight back to the starting position.

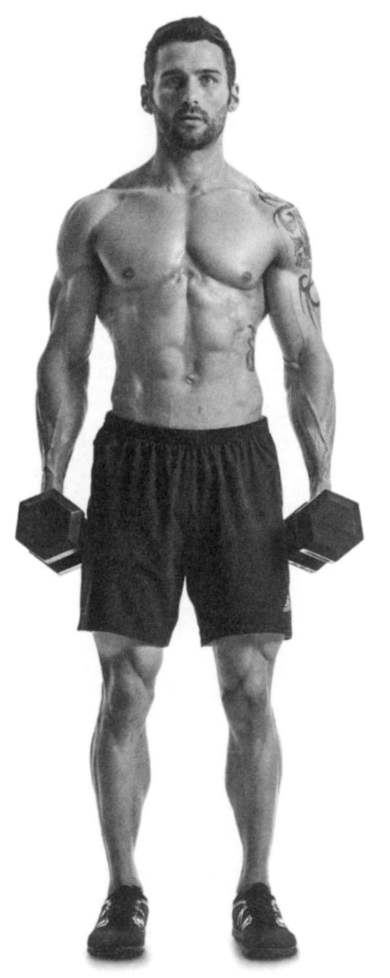
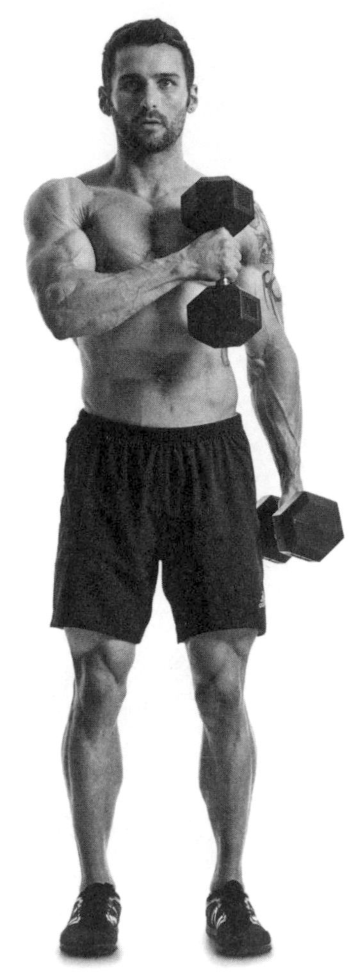
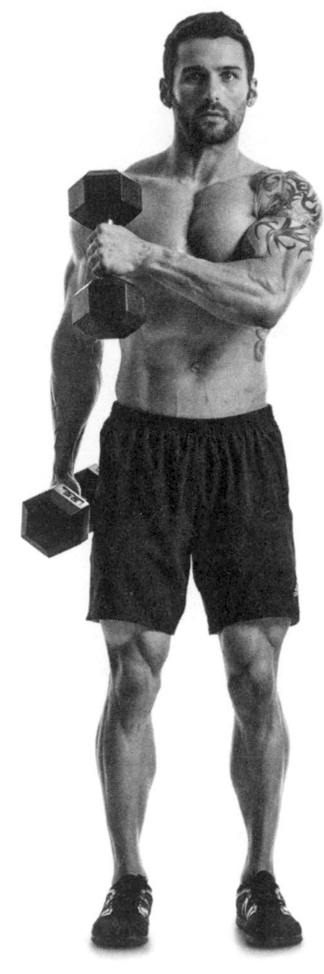

CROSS-BODY HAMMER CURL

PURPOSE
Target your biceps.

START
Grab a pair of dumbbells with a neutral grip. Allow the dumbbells to hang at arm's length at your sides.

MOVEMENT
Do not move your upper arm as you bend your elbow and curl one dumbbell across the front of your torso toward the opposing shoulder, as high as you can.

FINISH
Pause briefly, then lower the dumbbell and alternate sides continuously.

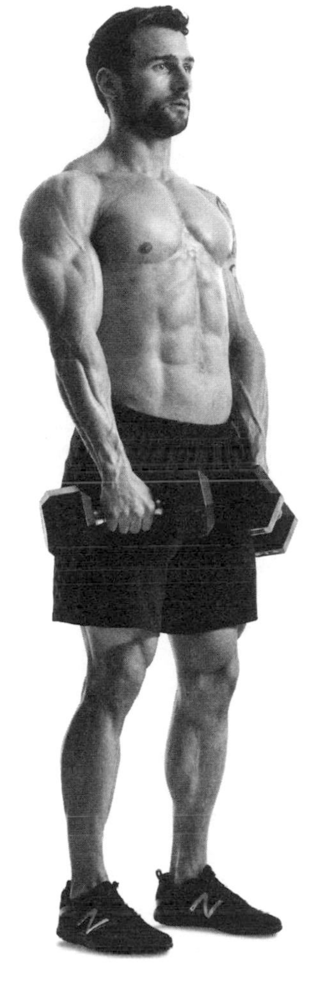

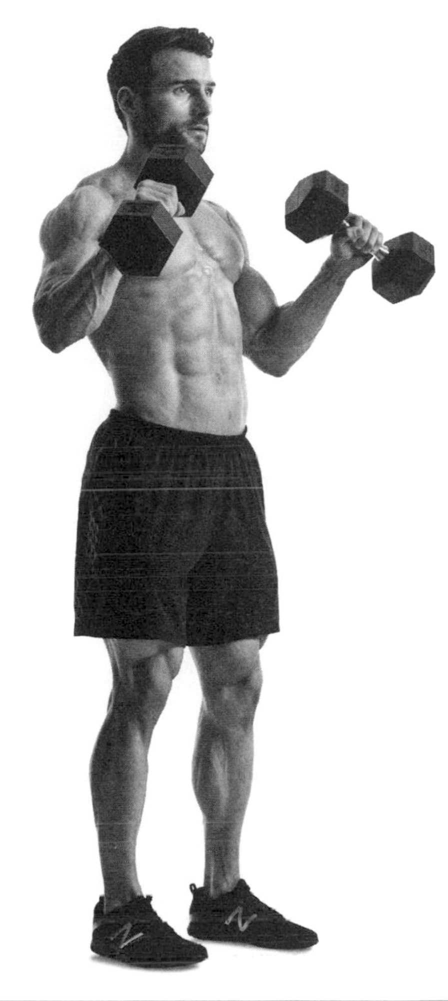

STANDING REVERSE CURL

PURPOSE

Target your biceps.

START

Grab a pair of dumbbells with an overhand grip and allow the dumbbells to hang at arm's length at your sides.

MOVEMENT

Do not move your upper arms as you bend your elbows and curl the dumbbells up as high as possible, keeping your palms facing away from you, using the overhand grip, throughout the movement.

FINISH

Pause briefly, then lower the weight back to the starting position.

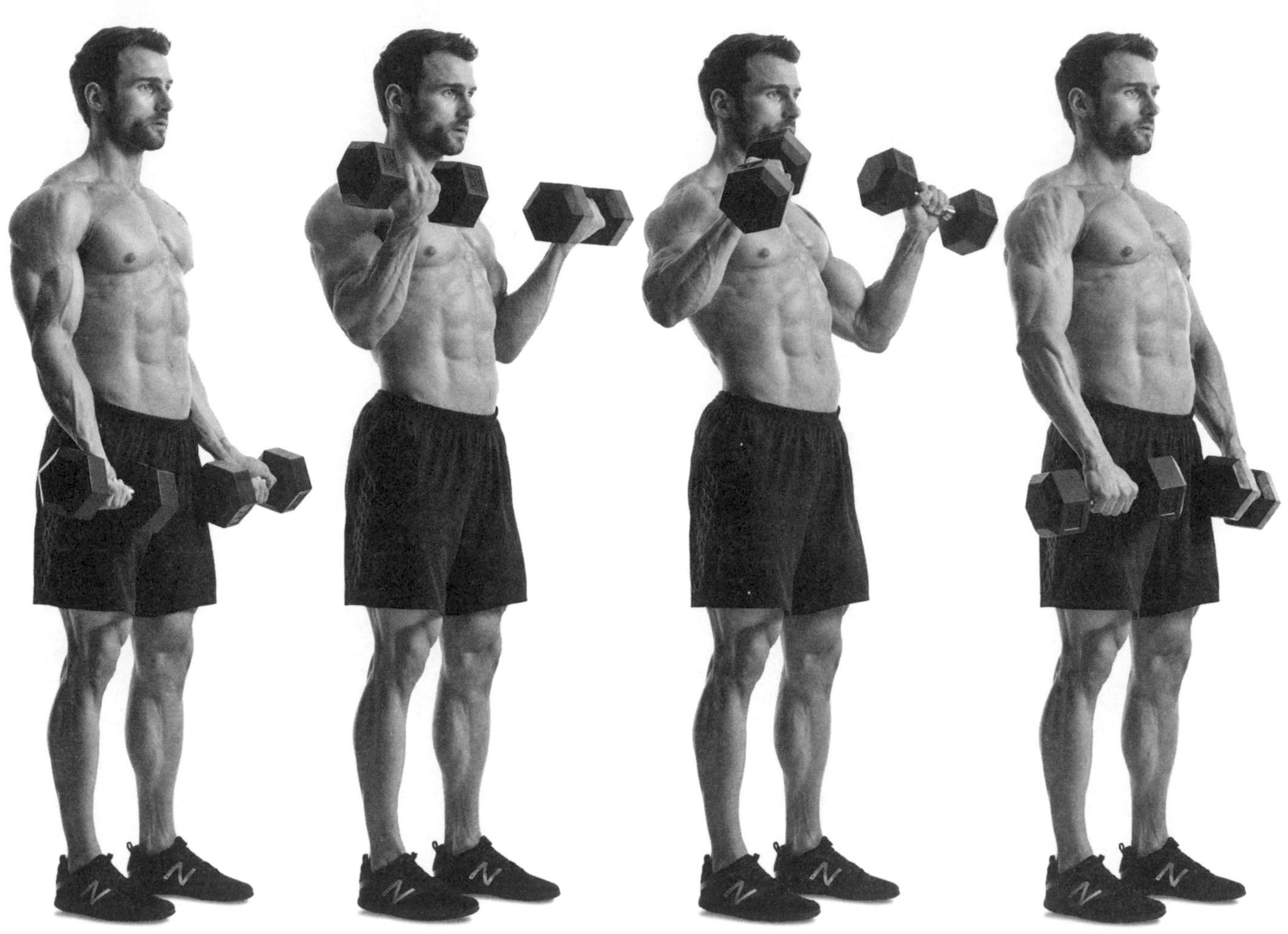

STANDING ZOTTMAN CURL

PURPOSE
Target your biceps.

START
Grab a pair of dumbbells and allow them to hang at arm's length at your sides. Your palms should face forward.

MOVEMENT
Without moving your upper arms, bend your elbows to curl the weights toward your shoulders. At the top of the curl, when your palms are facing your shoulders, rotate your wrists outward so your palms face forward. Now slowly lower the weights while keeping your hands in that position.

FINISH
When your arms are extended straight down at your sides, rotate your wrists and dumbbells back to the palms-forward starting position and repeat.

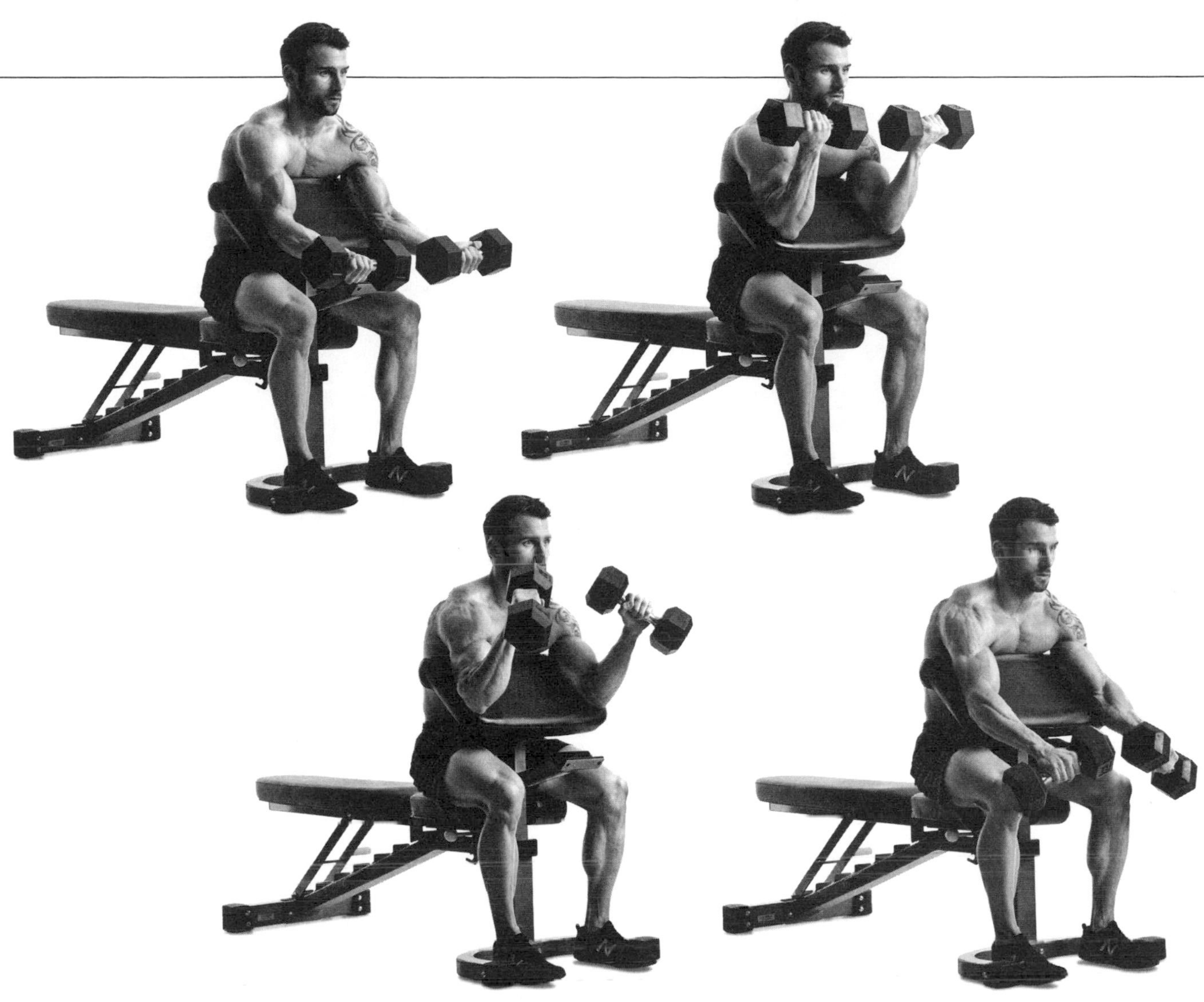

ZOTTMAN PREACHER CURL

PURPOSE
Target your biceps.

START
Grab a pair of dumbbells with an underhand grip and sit on a preacher bench so the top of the pad almost touches your armpits.

MOVEMENT
Without moving your upper arms, curl the weights toward your shoulders just short of perpendicular to the floor (higher is just too easy to do and reduces the workload). At the top of the curl, rotate your wrists outward so your palms face forward. Slowly lower the weights in that position.

FINISH
When your weights are down, rotate your wrists and dumbbells to the palms-up starting position and repeat.

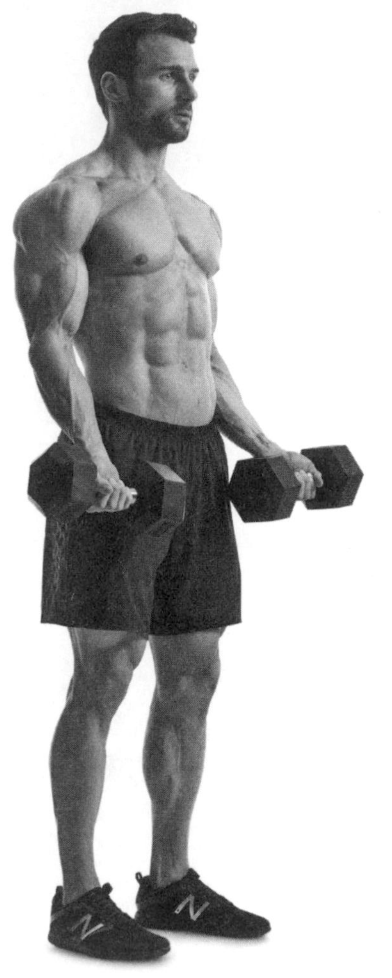

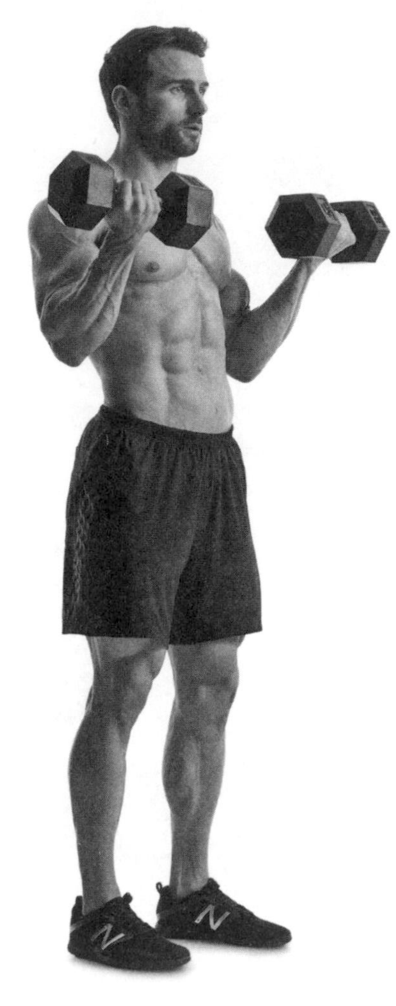

STANDING BICEPS CURL

PURPOSE

Target your biceps.

START

Grab a pair of dumbbells with an underhand grip. Allow the dumbbells to hang at arm's length at your sides.

MOVEMENT

Do not move your upper arms as you bend your elbows and curl the dumbbells as high as you can.

FINISH

Pause briefly, then lower the weight back to the starting position.

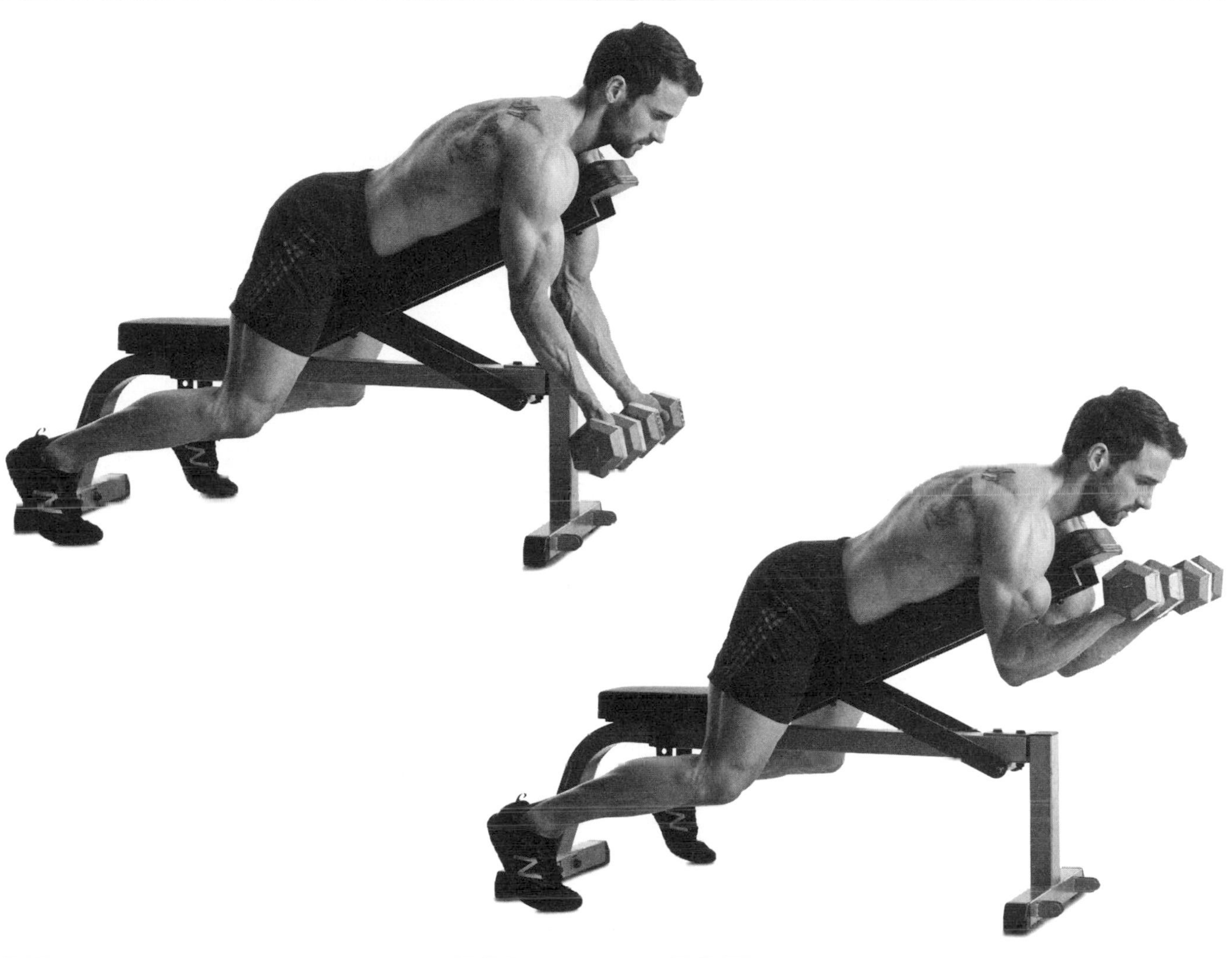

CHEST-SUPPORTED SPIDER CURL

PURPOSE

Target your biceps.

START

Lie with your chest against an incline bench set to 10 to 30 degrees. Keep the balls of your feet on the ground. Grab a pair of dumbbells with an underhand grip and allow the dumbbells to hang out in front of your chest.

MOVEMENT

Do not move your upper arms as you bend your elbows and curl the dumbbells as high as you can.

FINISH

Pause briefly, then lower the weight back to the starting position.

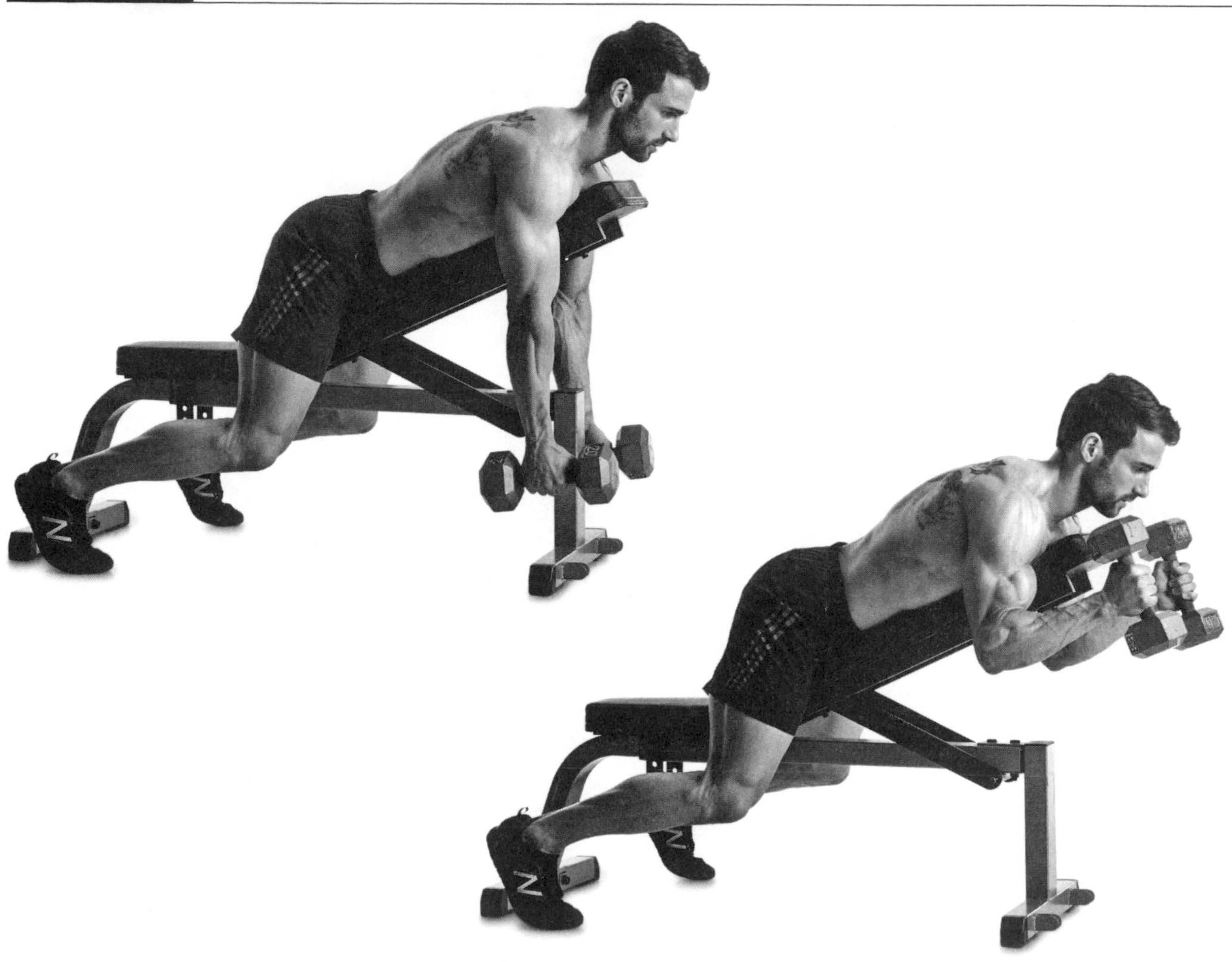

HAMMER-GRIP SPIDER CURL

PURPOSE
Target your biceps.

START
Lie with your chest against an incline bench set to 10 to 30 degrees. Keep the balls of your feet on the ground. Grab a pair of dumbbells with a neutral grip and allow the dumbbells to hang out in front of your chest.

MOVEMENT
Do not move your upper arms as you bend your elbows and curl the dumbbells as high as you can, keeping your palms facing each other.

FINISH
Pause briefly, then lower the weight back to the starting position.

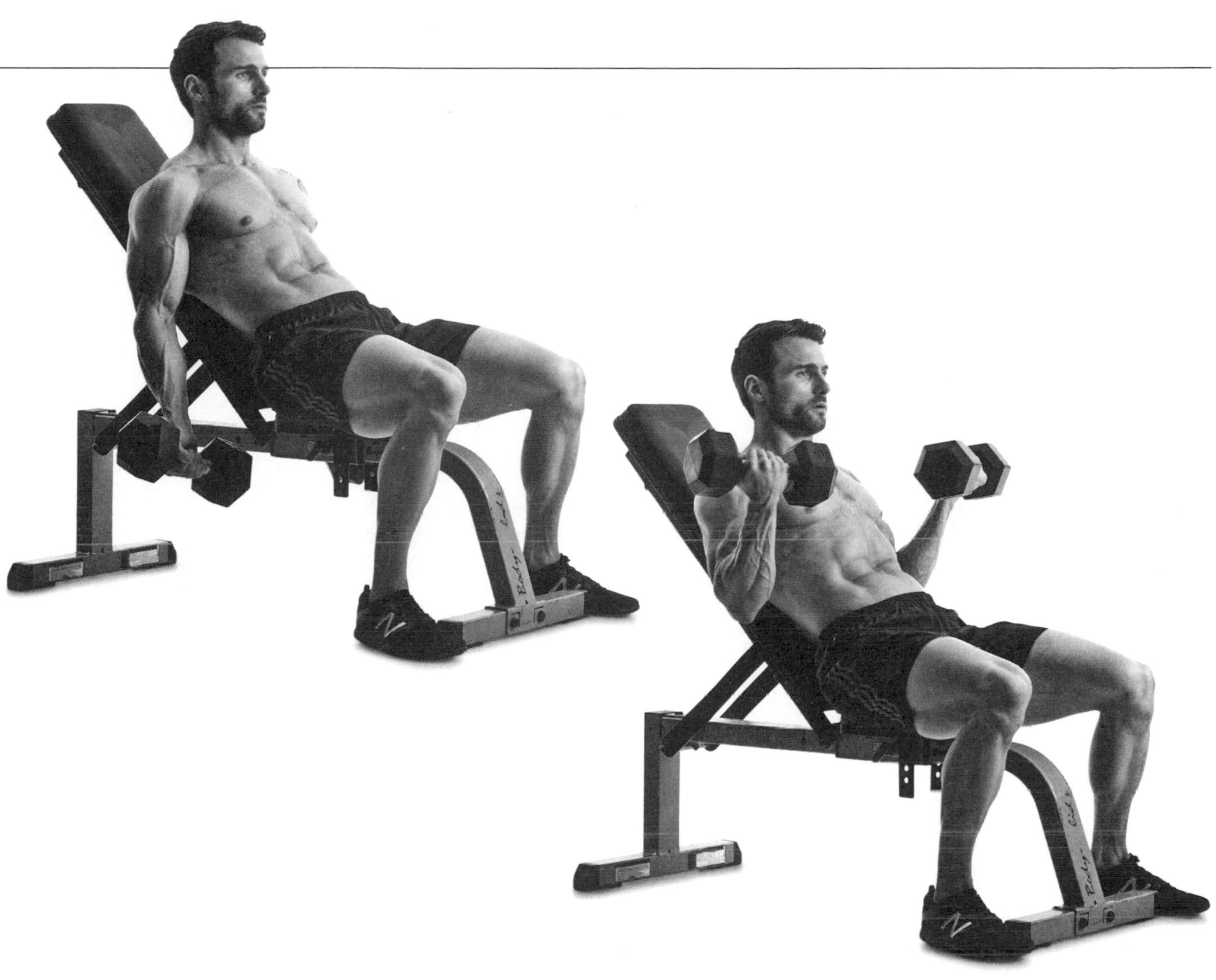

INCLINE CURL

PURPOSE

Target your biceps.

START

Sit on an incline bench set to 30 to 45 degrees. Grab a pair of dumbbells with an underhand grip. Allow your arms to rest at your sides.

MOVEMENT

Do not move your upper arms as you bend your elbows and curl the dumbbells as high as possible.

FINISH

Pause briefly, then lower the weight back to the starting position.

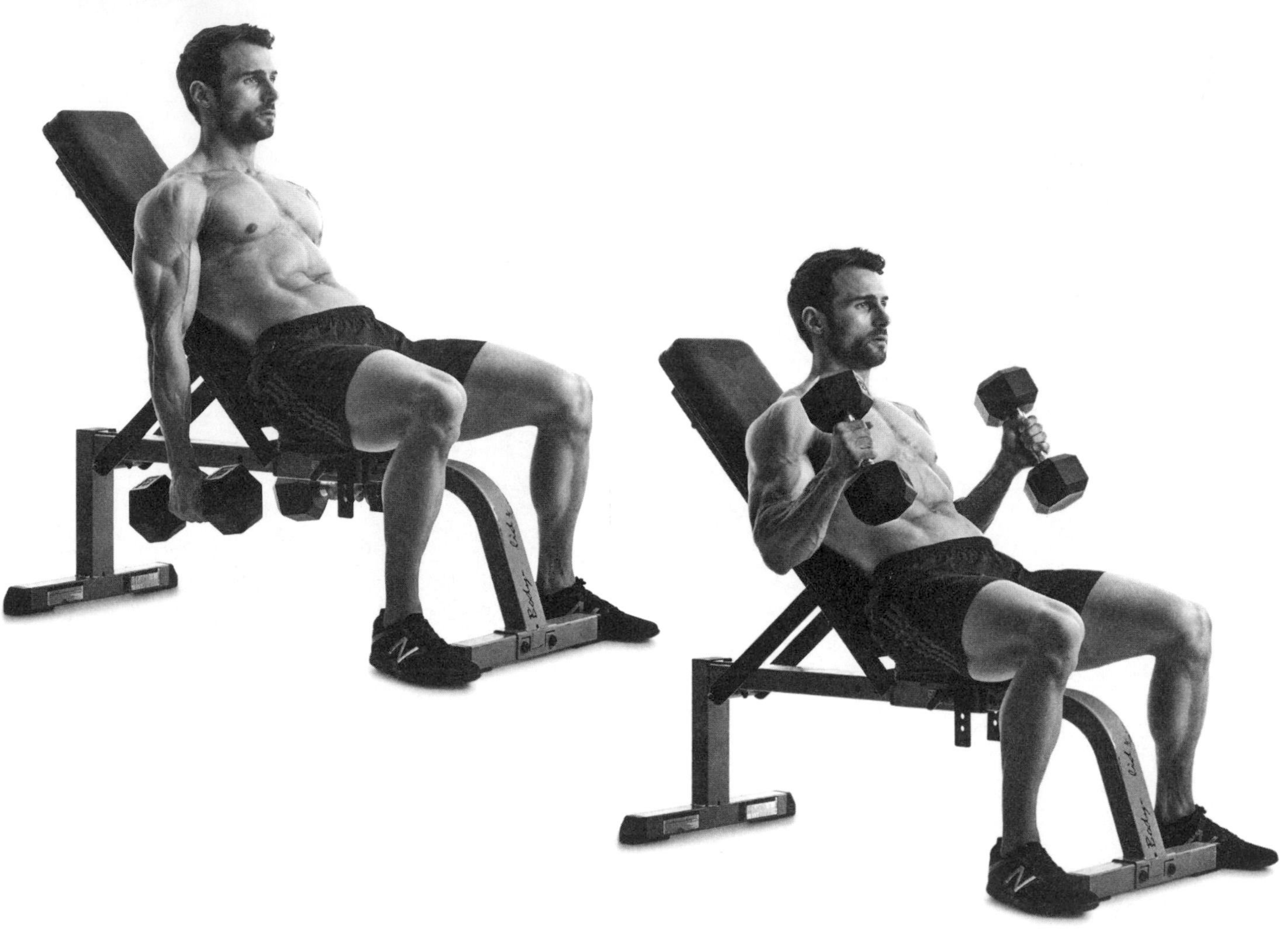

INCLINE HAMMER CURL

PURPOSE

Target your biceps.

START

Sit on an incline bench set to 30 to 45 degrees. Grab a pair of dumbbells with a neutral grip and allow your arms to rest at your sides.

MOVEMENT

Do not move your upper arms as you bend your elbows and curl the dumbbells as high as possible while keeping your palms facing each other.

FINISH

Pause briefly, then lower the weight back to the starting position.

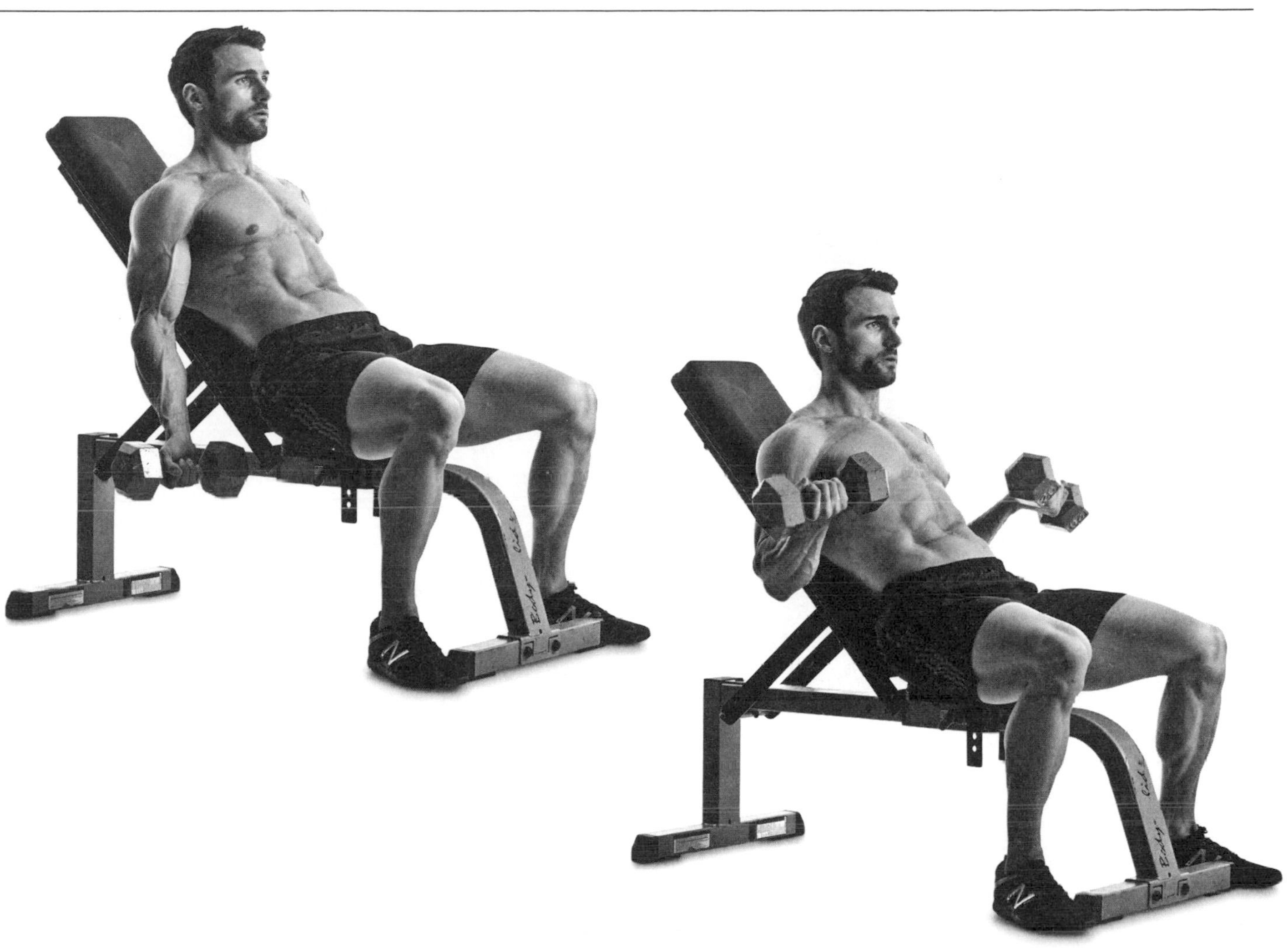

FLEXOR INCLINE CURL

PURPOSE

Target your biceps.

START

Sit on an incline bench set to 45 degrees. Grab a pair of dumbbells with an underhand grip. Allow your arms to rest at your sides.

MOVEMENT

Do not move your upper arms as you bend your elbows and curl the dumbbells as high as possible while keeping your palms forward and thumbs pointing away from you (maintain this position throughout with no rotation of the dumbbell).

FINISH

Pause briefly, then lower the weight back to the starting position.

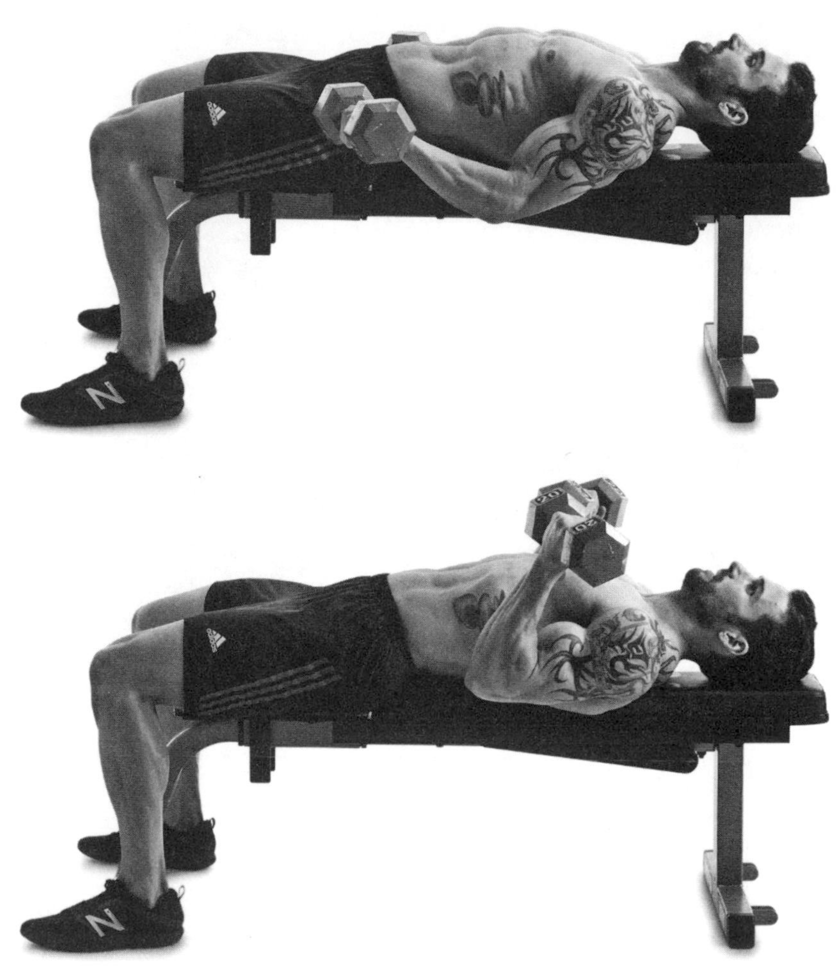

SUPINE FLAT-BENCH CURL

PURPOSE
Target your biceps.

START
Lie on your back on a flat bench. Grab a pair of dumbbells with an underhand grip. Your arms should be fully extended at your sides so the dumbbells rest at your hips with your palms facing the ceiling.

MOVEMENT
Do not move your upper arms as you bend your elbows and curl the dumbbells as high as possible toward your shoulders.

FINISH
Pause briefly, then lower the weight back to the starting position.

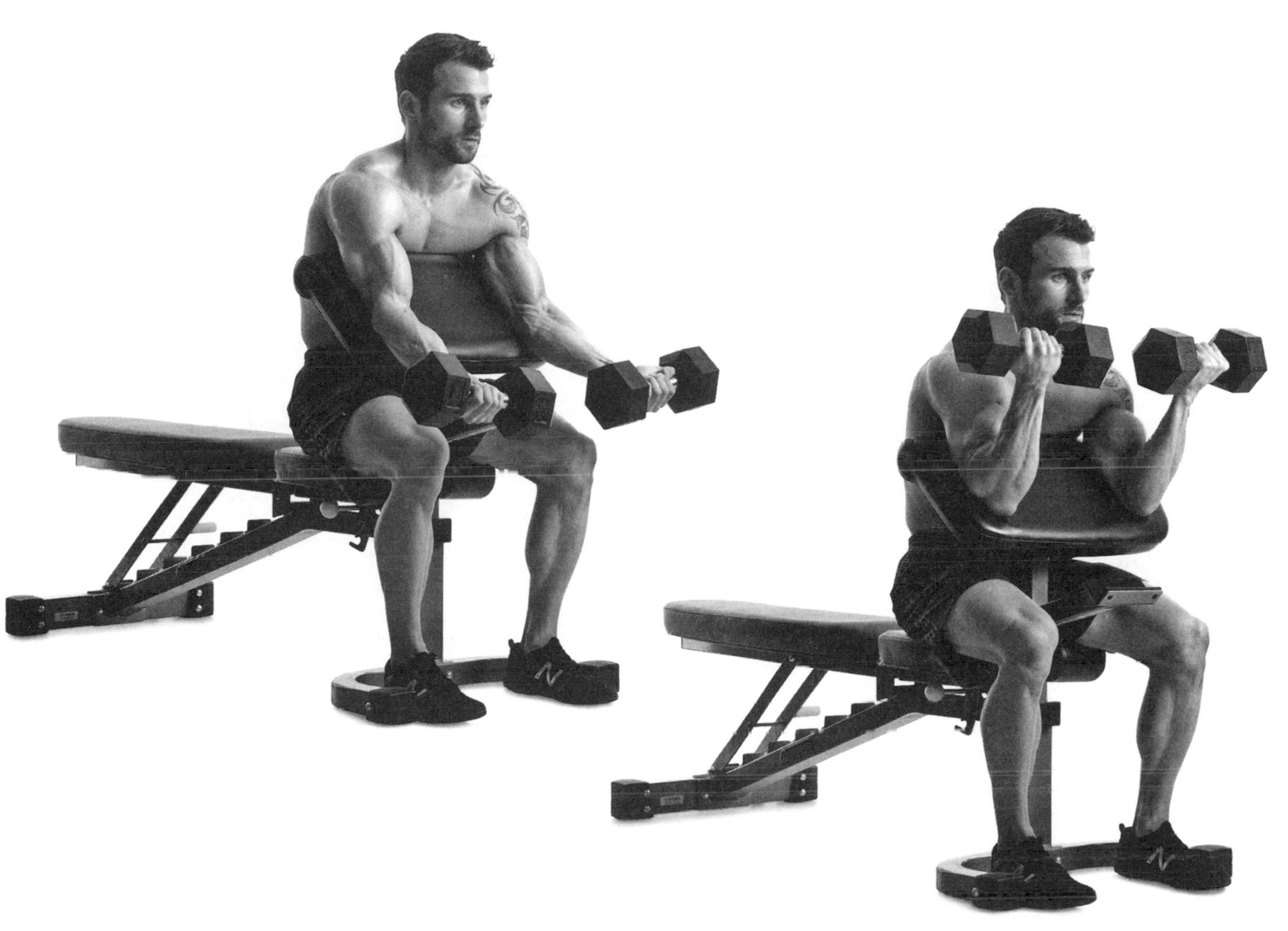

PREACHER CURL

PURPOSE
Target your biceps.

START
Grab a pair of dumbbells with an underhand grip and sit on a preacher bench so the top of the pad almost touches your armpits.

MOVEMENT
Do not move your upper arms as you bend your elbows and curl the dumbbells just short of perpendicular to the floor (higher is just too easy to do and reduces the workload).

FINISH
Pause briefly, then lower the weight back to the starting position.

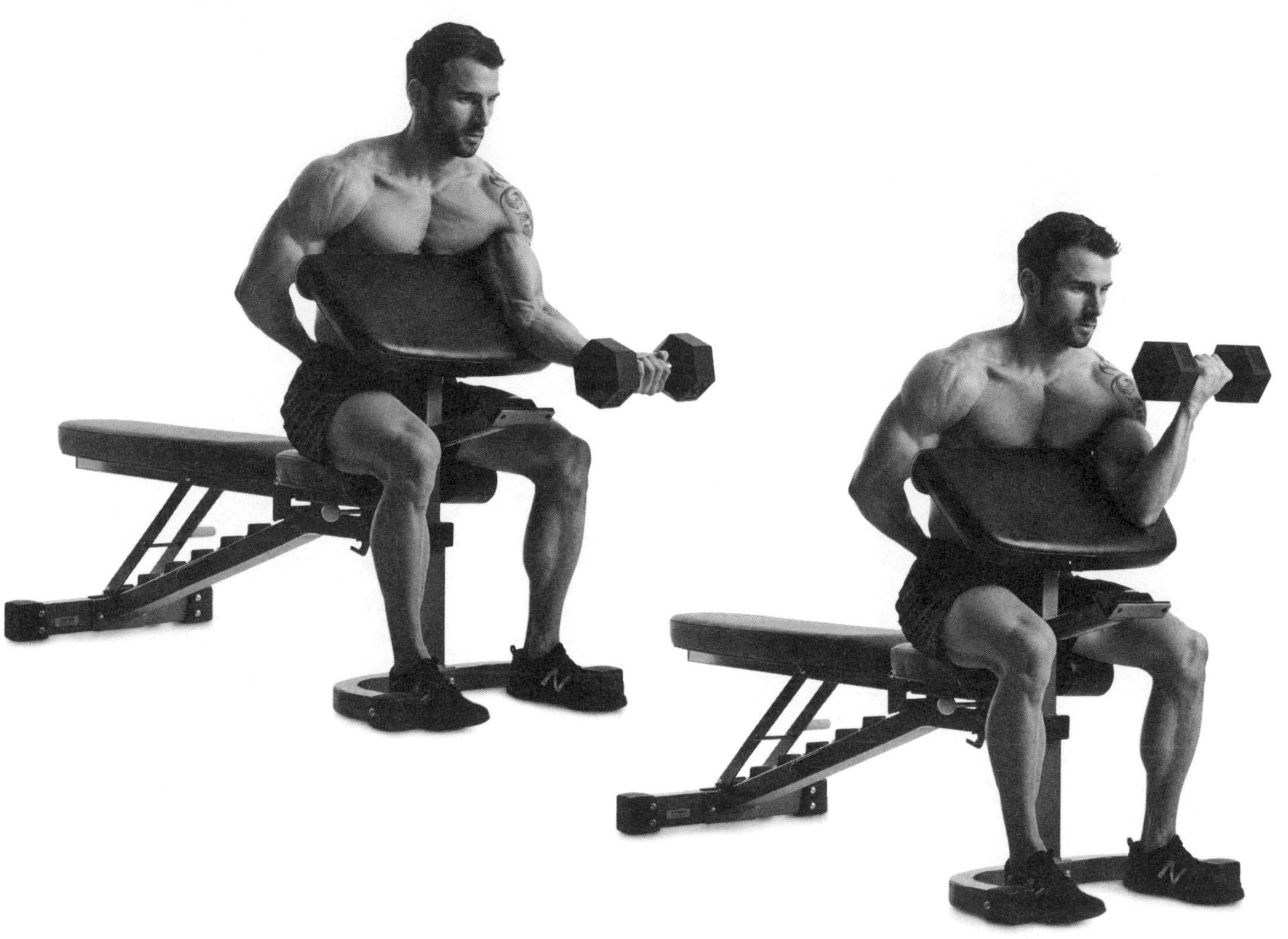

ONE-ARM PREACHER CURL

PURPOSE

Target your biceps.

START

Grab one dumbbell with an underhand grip and sit on a preacher bench so the top of the pad almost touches your armpits.

MOVEMENT

Do not move your upper arm as you bend your elbow and curl the dumbbell just short of perpendicular to the floor (higher is just too easy to do and reduces the workload).

FINISH

Pause briefly, then lower the weight back to the starting position.

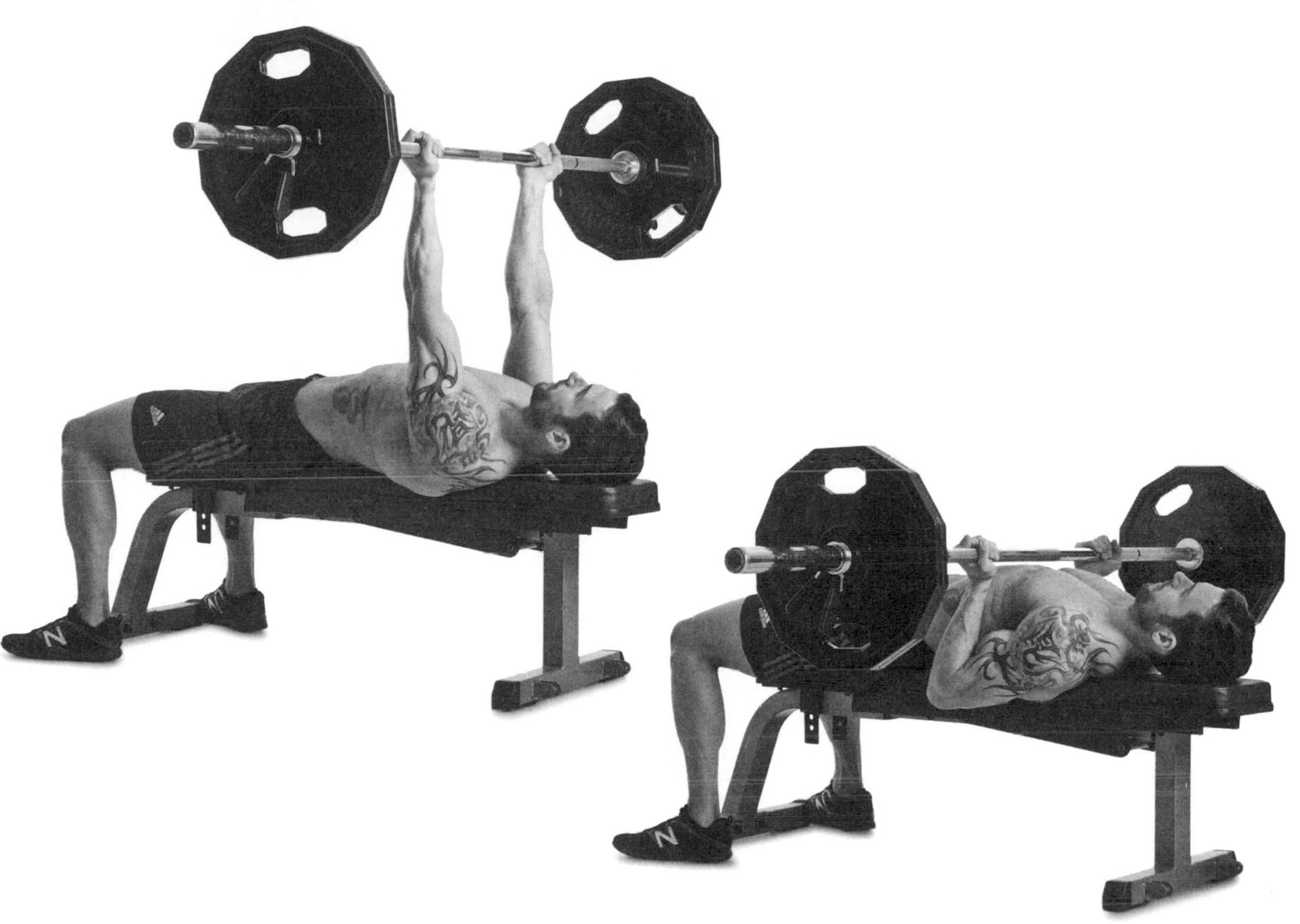

REVERSE-GRIP BENCH PRESS

Note: For safety, always use a spotter when performing this exercise.

PURPOSE

For overall chest and triceps development.

START

Lie on a bench with your head, torso, and hips pressed against the bench and your feet flat on the floor. Using an underhand grip, place your hands less than shoulder width apart (around 8 inches) on a barbell. Remove the bar from the uprights and with straight arms hold it over nipple line.

MOVEMENT

Keeping your shoulder blades together and your elbows tight to your sides, lower the bar in a slow and controlled manner to your mid chest (just above your nipples).

FINISH

Pause briefly, then press the bar back to finish just over your collarbone. (Stop just short of locking your elbows.)

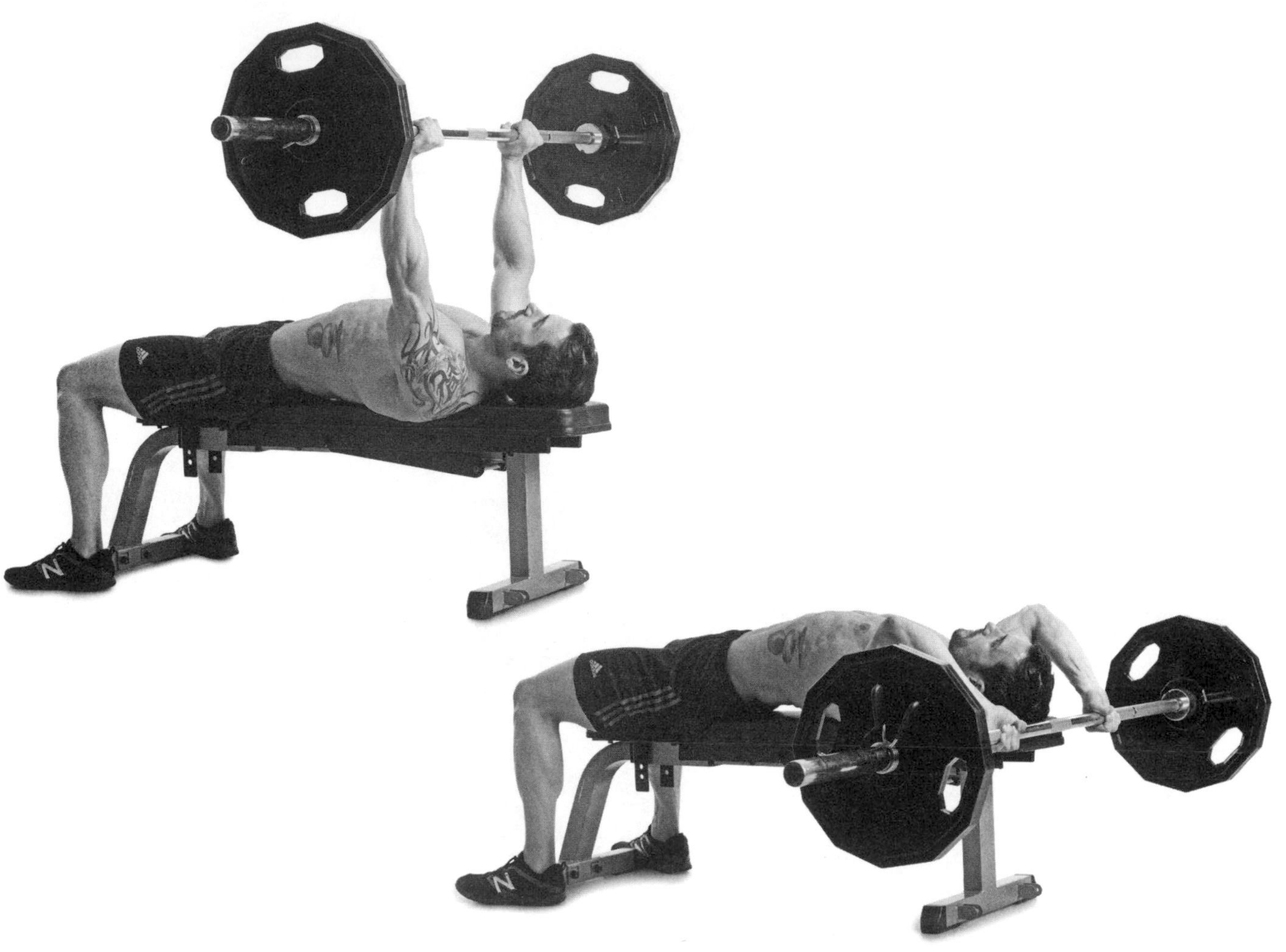

LYING TRICEPS EXTENSION

PURPOSE

For triceps development.

START

Grab a barbell with an overhand grip, your hands a little less than shoulder width apart. Lie on a bench with your head, torso, and hips pressed against the bench, keeping your feet flat on the ground. Hold the bar with your arms straight over your forehead, so your arms are at an angle.

MOVEMENT

Without moving your upper arms, bend at the elbows to allow the bar to lower until your forearms are past parallel.

FINISH

Pause briefly, then lift the weight back to the starting position.

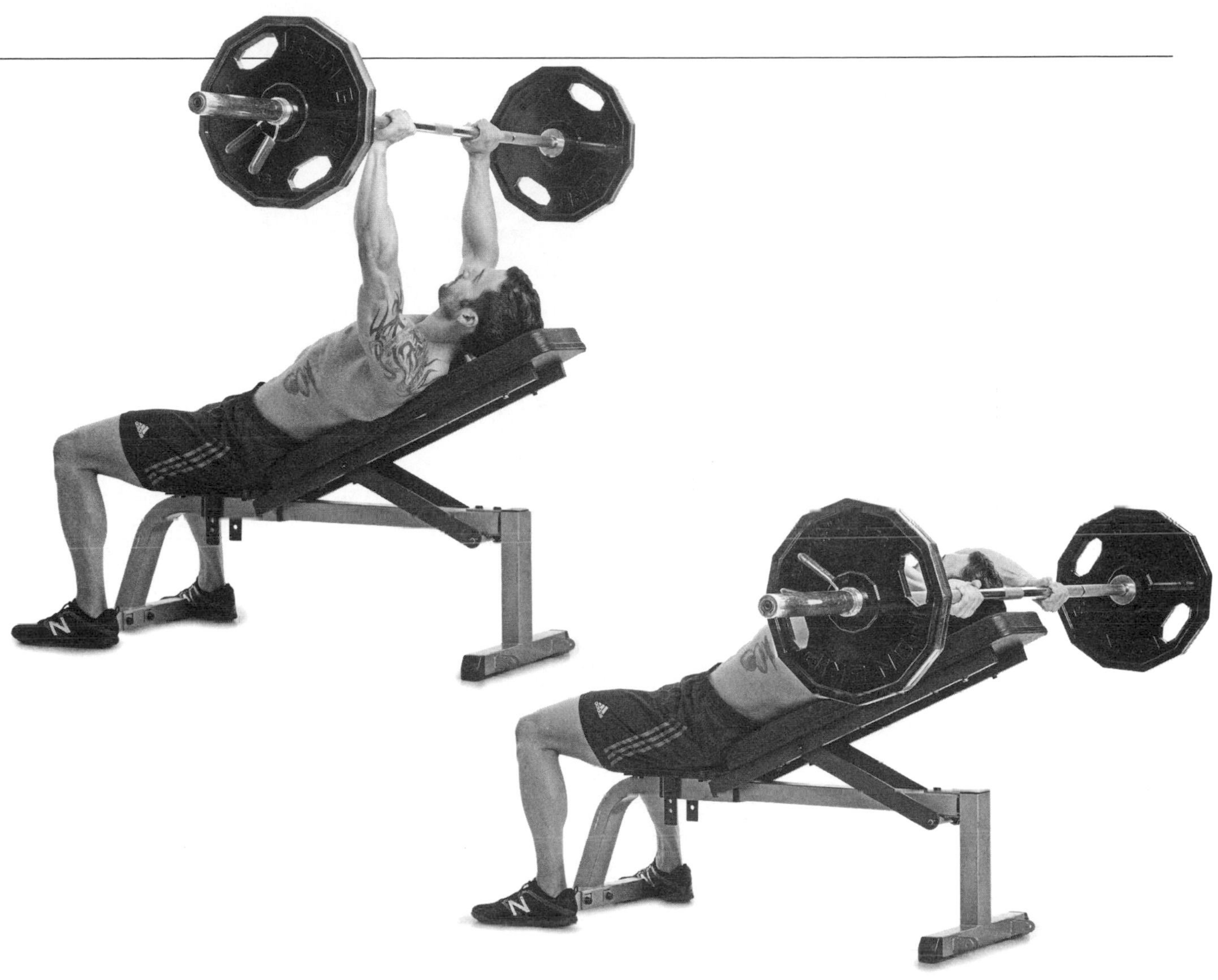

INCLINE TRICEPS EXTENSION

PURPOSE

For triceps development.

START

Grab a barbell with an overhand grip, your hands a little less than shoulder width apart. Lie on an incline bench set to 10 to 30 degrees with your head, torso, and hips pressed against the bench and keeping your feet flat on the ground. Hold the bar with your arms straight over your forehead, so your arms are at an angle.

MOVEMENT

Without moving your upper arms, bend at the elbows to allow the bar to lower until your forearms are past parallel.

FINISH

Pause briefly, then lift the weight back to the starting position.

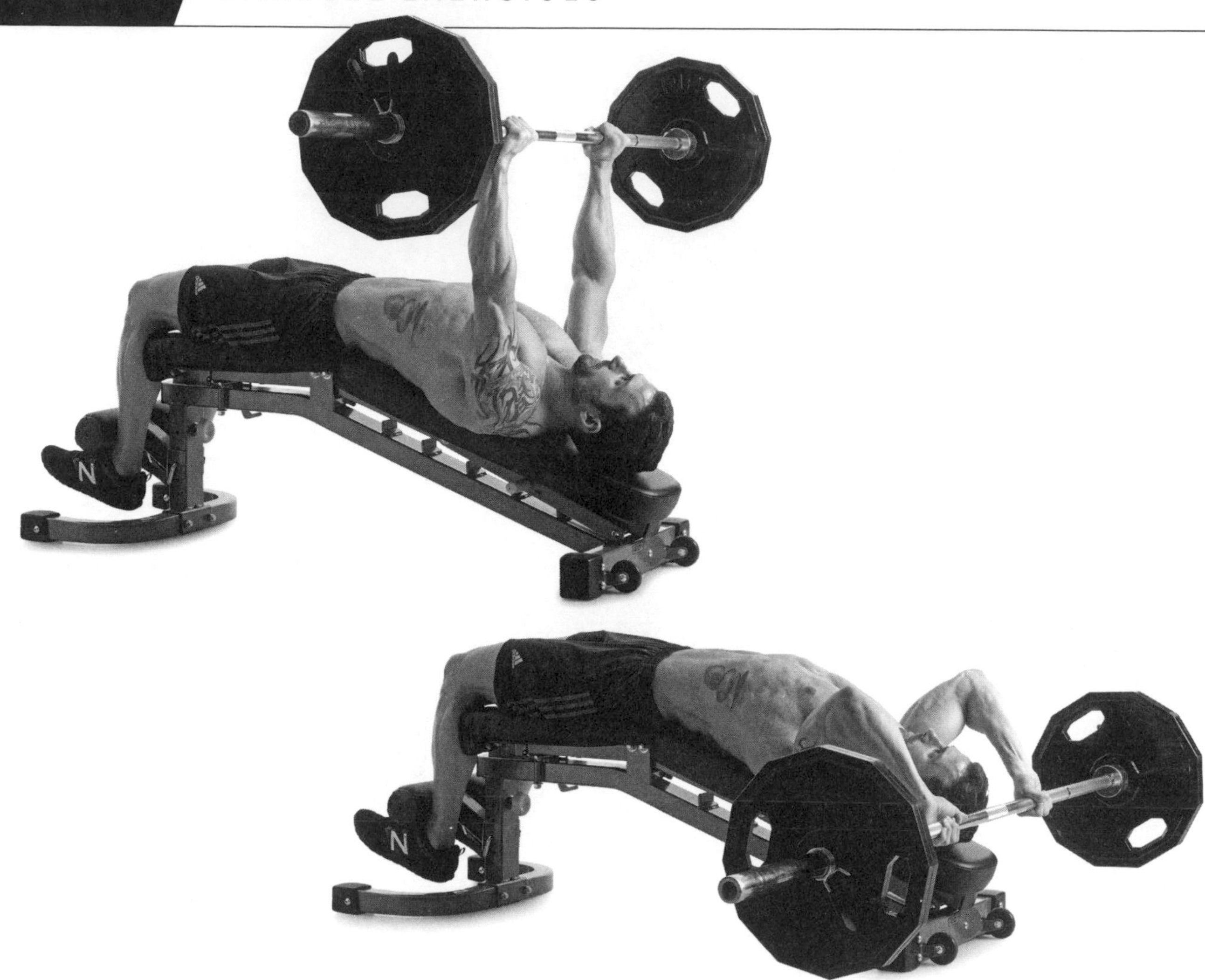

DECLINE CLOSE-GRIP SKULL CRUSHER

PURPOSE

For triceps development.

START

Grab a barbell with an overhand grip, your hands a little less than shoulder width apart. Lie on a decline bench with your head, torso, and hips press against the bench and keep your feet in the ankle supports. Hold the bar with your arms straight over your forehead, so your arms are at an angle.

MOVEMENT

Without moving your upper arms, bend at the elbows to allow the bar to lower until your forearms are past parallel.

FINISH

Pause briefly, then lift the weight back to the starting position.

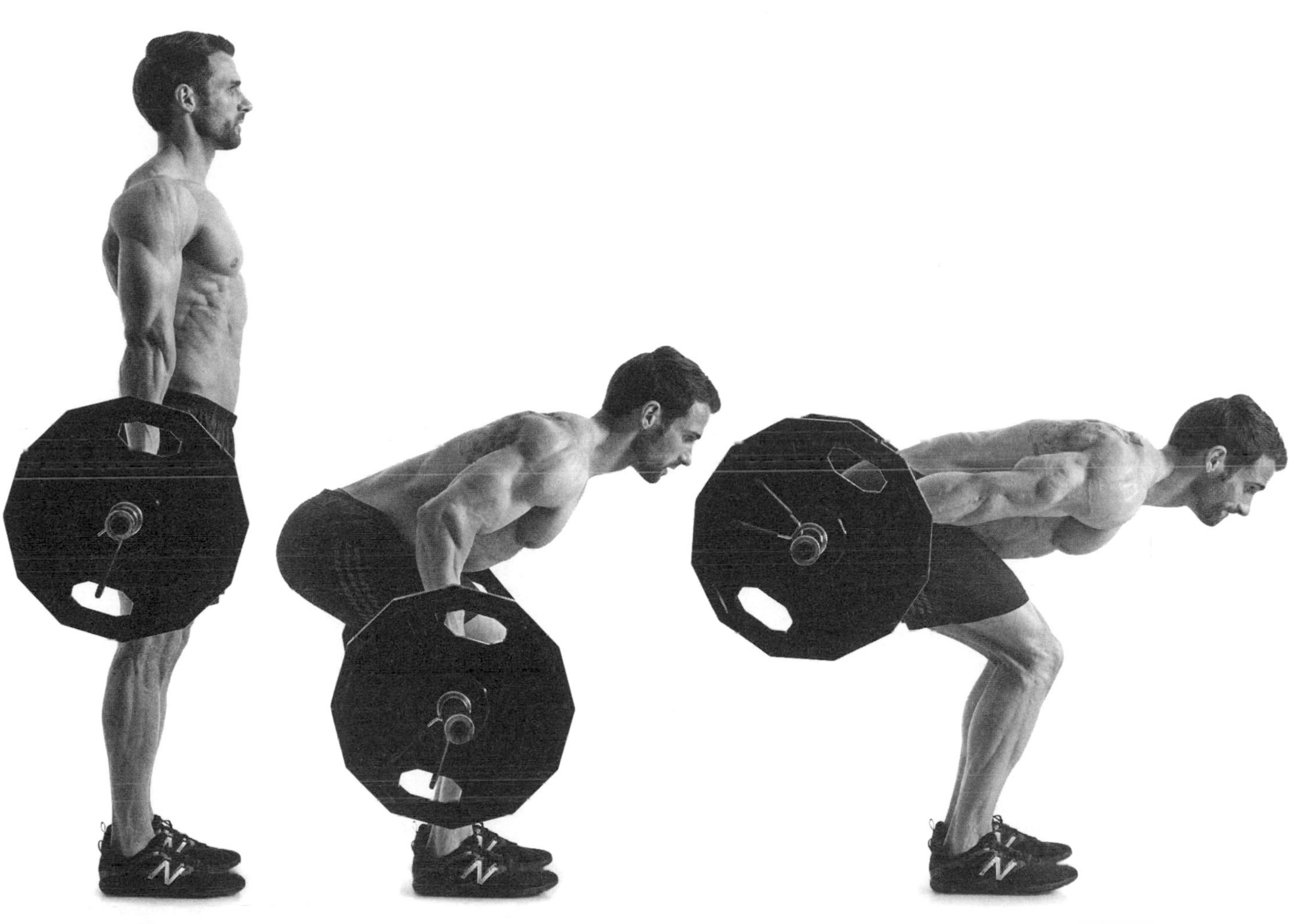

BEHIND-THE-LEG TRICEPS KICKBACK

PURPOSE

For triceps development.

START

Grab a barbell behind your back with an overhand grip, your hands a little less than shoulder width apart. Bend your knees, hinge at your hips, and bring your torso toward the floor, keeping the natural arch to your back.

MOVEMENT

Without moving your upper arms, bend at the elbows and allow the bar to stay above your knees. Push the bar back to extend your arms behind your back.

FINISH

Pause briefly, then lower the weight back to the starting position.

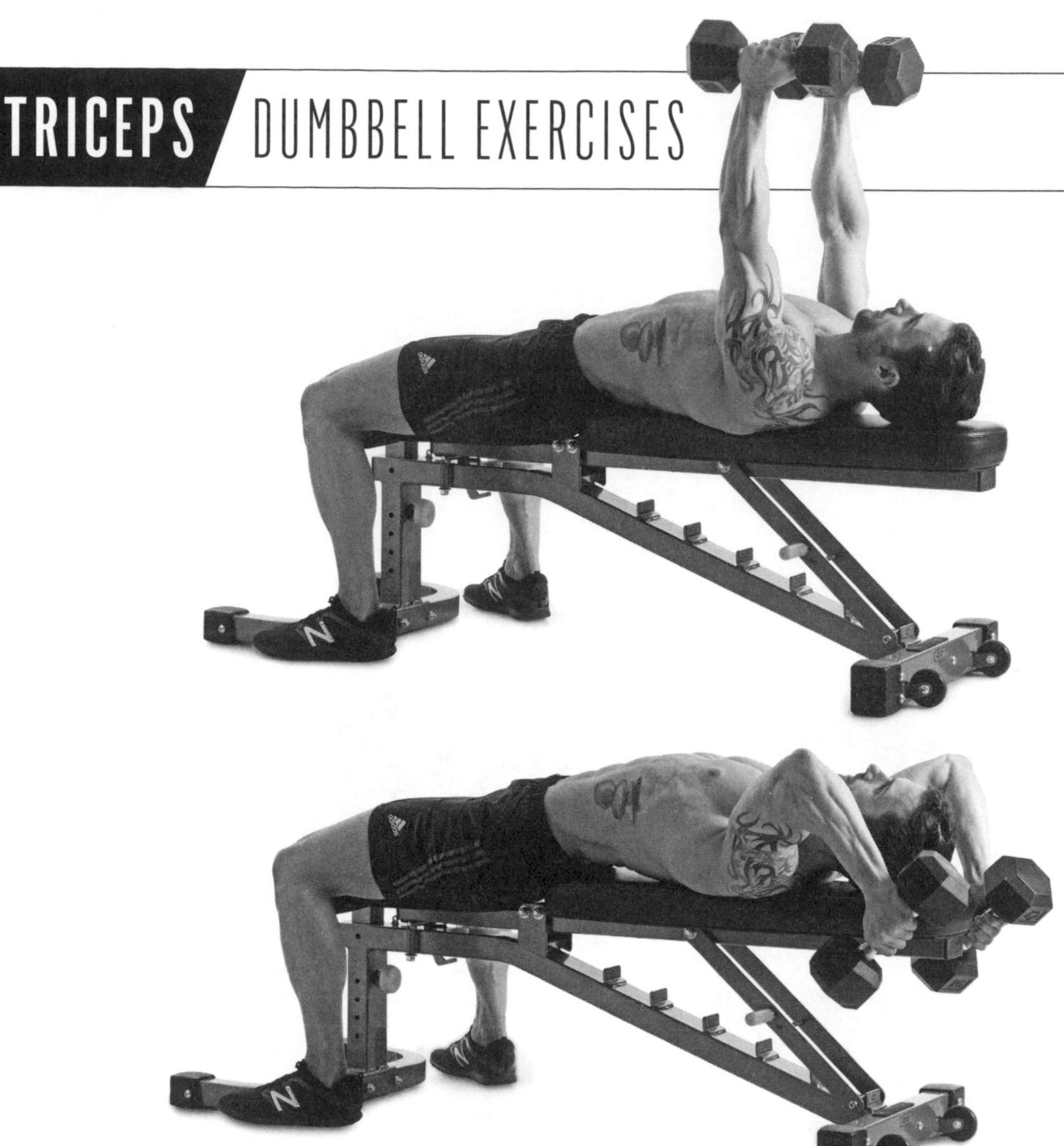

SKULL CRUSHER

PURPOSE
For triceps development.

START
Grab a pair of dumbbells with a neutral grip. Lie on a bench with your head, torso, and hips pressed against the bench and keep your feet flat on the ground. Hold the dumbbells with your arms straight over your forehead, so your arms are at an angle.

MOVEMENT
Without moving your upper arms, bend at the elbows to allow the dumbbells to lower until your forearms are lower than parallel to the floor.

FINISH
Pause briefly, then lift the weight back to the starting position.

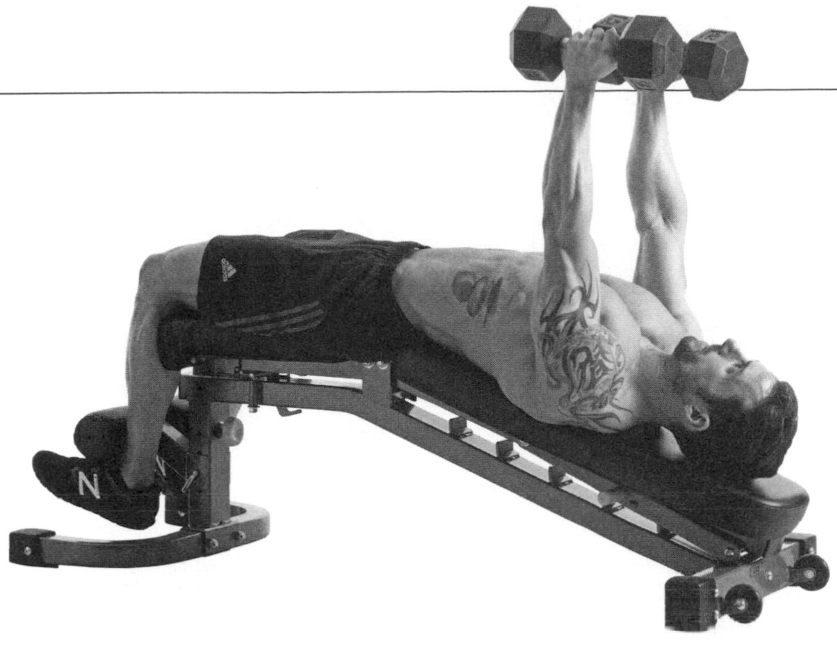

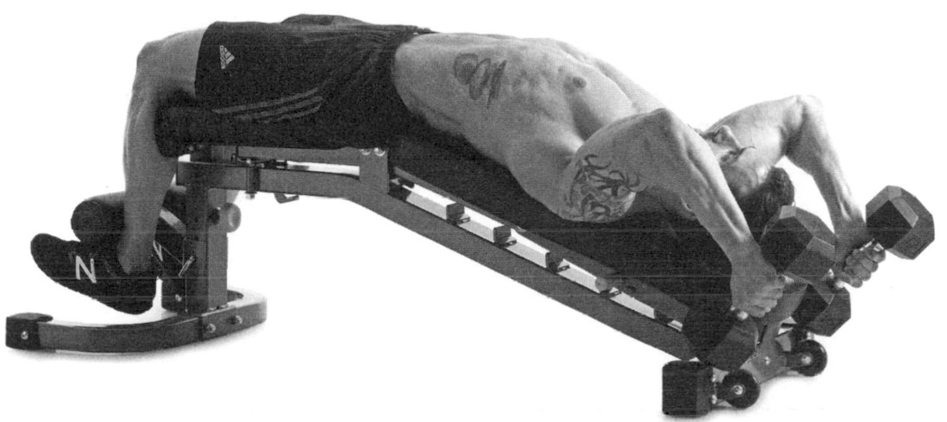

DECLINE SKULL CRUSHER

PURPOSE

For triceps development.

START

Grab a pair of dumbbells with a neutral grip. Lie on a decline bench with your head, torso, and hips pressed against the bench and keep your ankles in the supports. Hold the dumbbells with your arms straight over your forehead, so your arms are at an angle.

MOVEMENT

Without moving your upper arms, bend at the elbows to allow the dumbbells to lower until your forearms are past parallel.

FINISH

Pause briefly, then lift the weight back to the starting position.

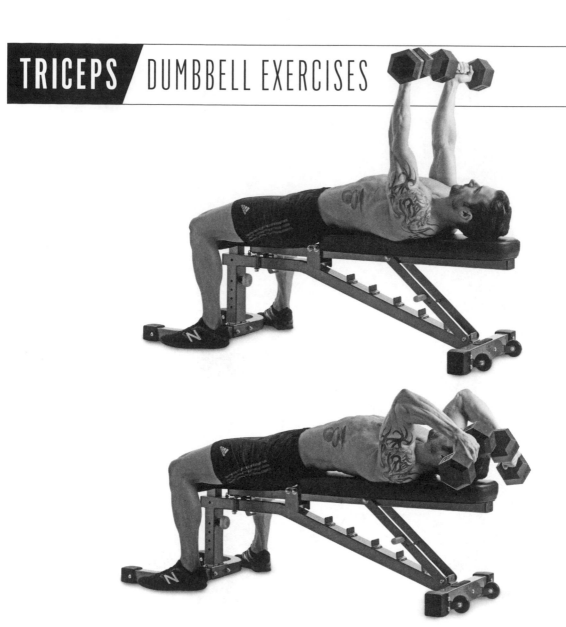

LYING PRONATED TRICEPS EXTENSION

PURPOSE
For triceps development.

START
Grab a pair of dumbbells with an underhand grip. Lie on a bench with your head, torso, and hips pressed against the bench and keep your feet flat on the ground. Hold the dumbbells with your arms straight over your forehead.

MOVEMENT
Without moving your upper arms, bend at the elbows to allow the dumbbells to lower until your forearms are past parallel. (Keep the dumbbells and palms pronated.)

FINISH
Pause briefly, then lift the weight back to the starting position.

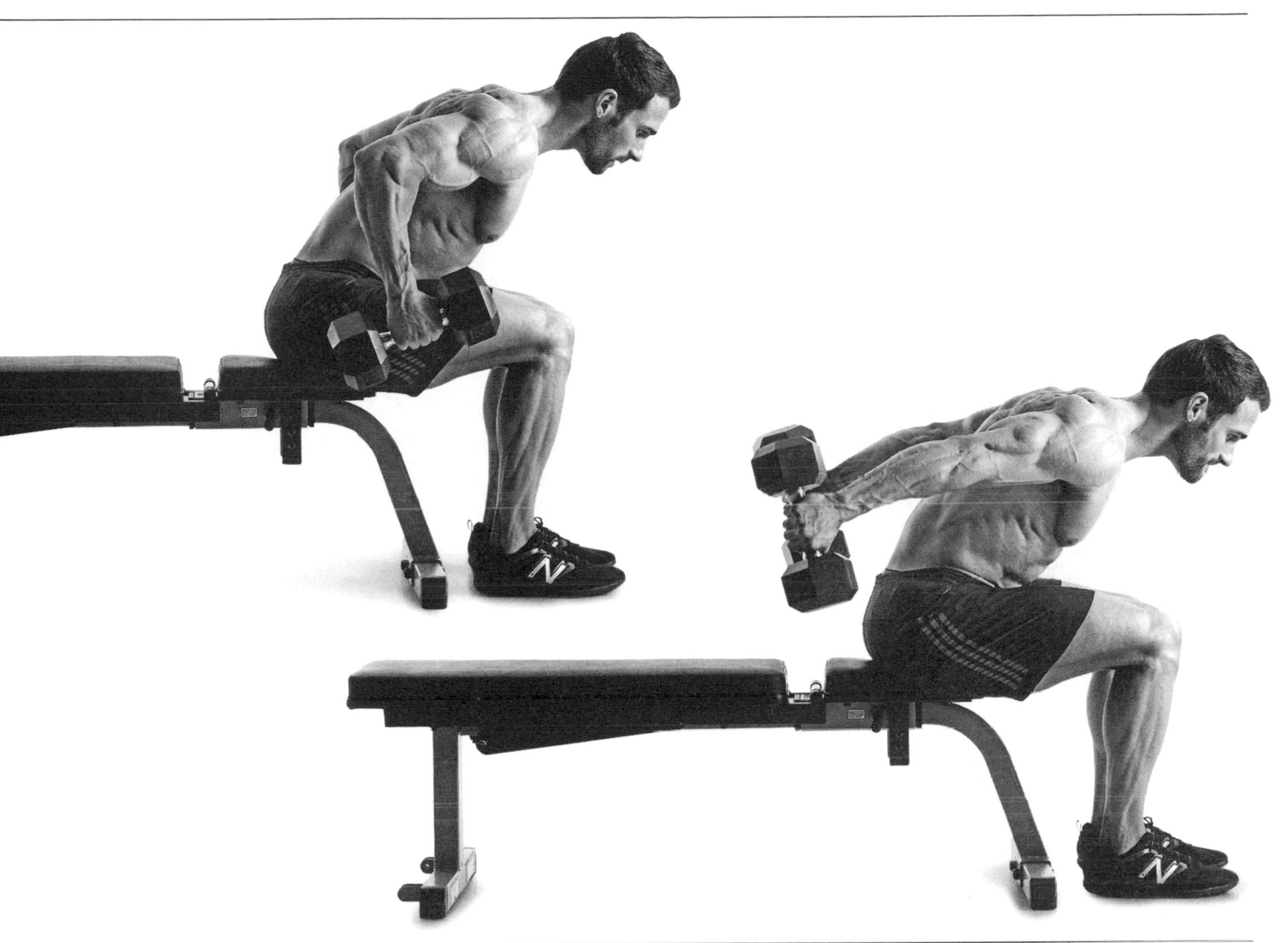

SEATED TRICEPS KICKBACK

PURPOSE

For triceps development.

START

Grab a pair of dumbbells with a neutral grip. Sit on the end of a bench, keeping your feet flat on the ground. Lean your torso forward while simultaneously keeping your elbows back at your sides and slightly bent.

MOVEMENT

Without moving your upper arms, straighten your elbows to allow the dumbbells to extend toward your hips.

FINISH

Pause briefly, then bend your arms back to the starting position.

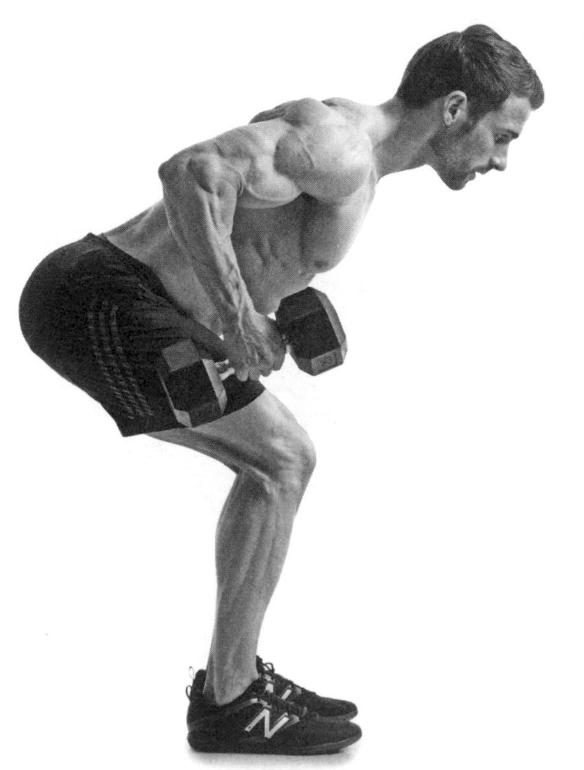

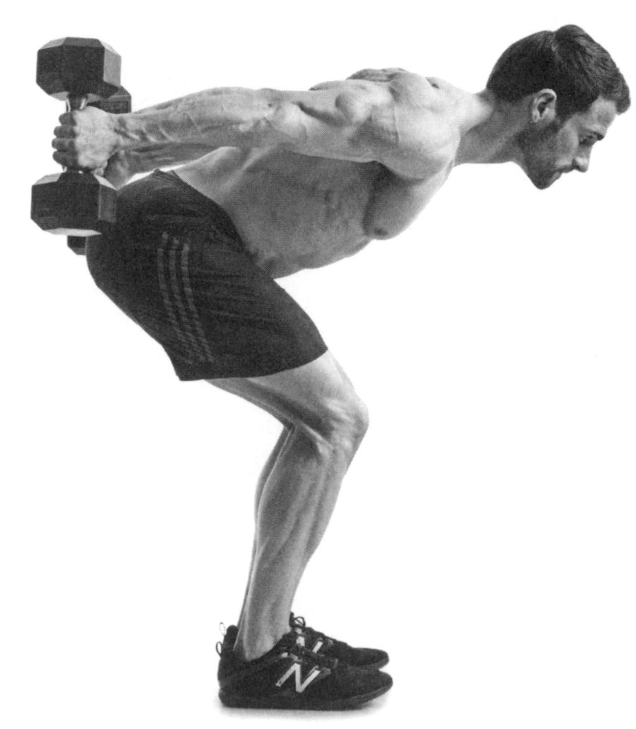

STANDING TRICEPS KICKBACK

PURPOSE

For triceps development.

START

Grab a pair of dumbbells with a neutral grip, then bend your knees and hinge at your hips to bring your torso toward the floor. Allow the dumbbells to hang out in front of your shoulders. Bend your elbows and pull them back.

MOVEMENT

Without moving your upper arms, raise your fore-arms until your arms are com-pletely straight behind you.

FINISH

Pause briefly, then lower the weights back to the starting position.

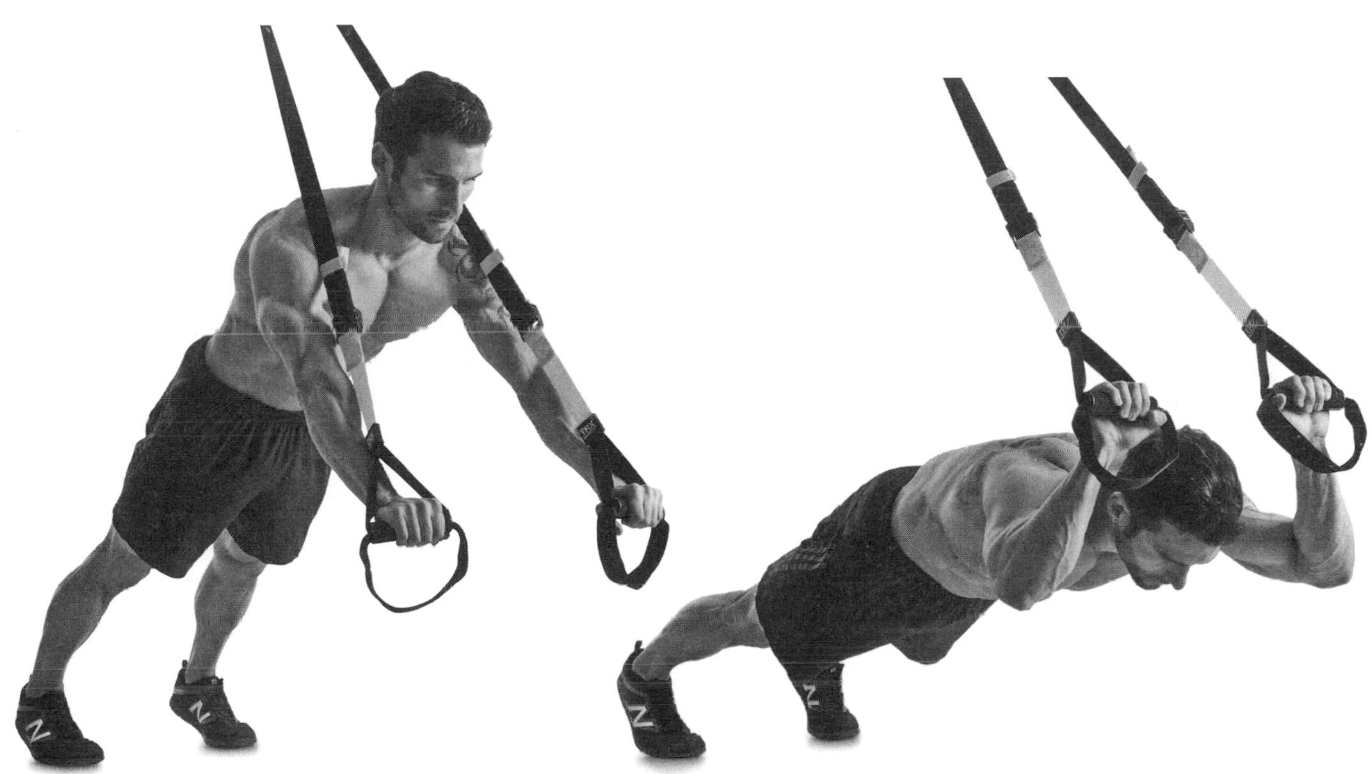

SUSPENDED PRONE TRICEPS EXTENSION (WITH TRX STRAPS)

PURPOSE
To develop the triceps.

START
Grab the handles with an overhand grip and your arms extended forward just overhead. Keep your torso straight and your body in a prone position. Your arms are holding your weight and your feet are shoulder width apart. Keep your elbows in.

MOVEMENT
Without moving your upper arms, bend at the elbows to allow your forearms to travel past parallel while lowering your body until your forehead passes beyond your hands.

FINISH
Pause, then push your body back to the starting position.

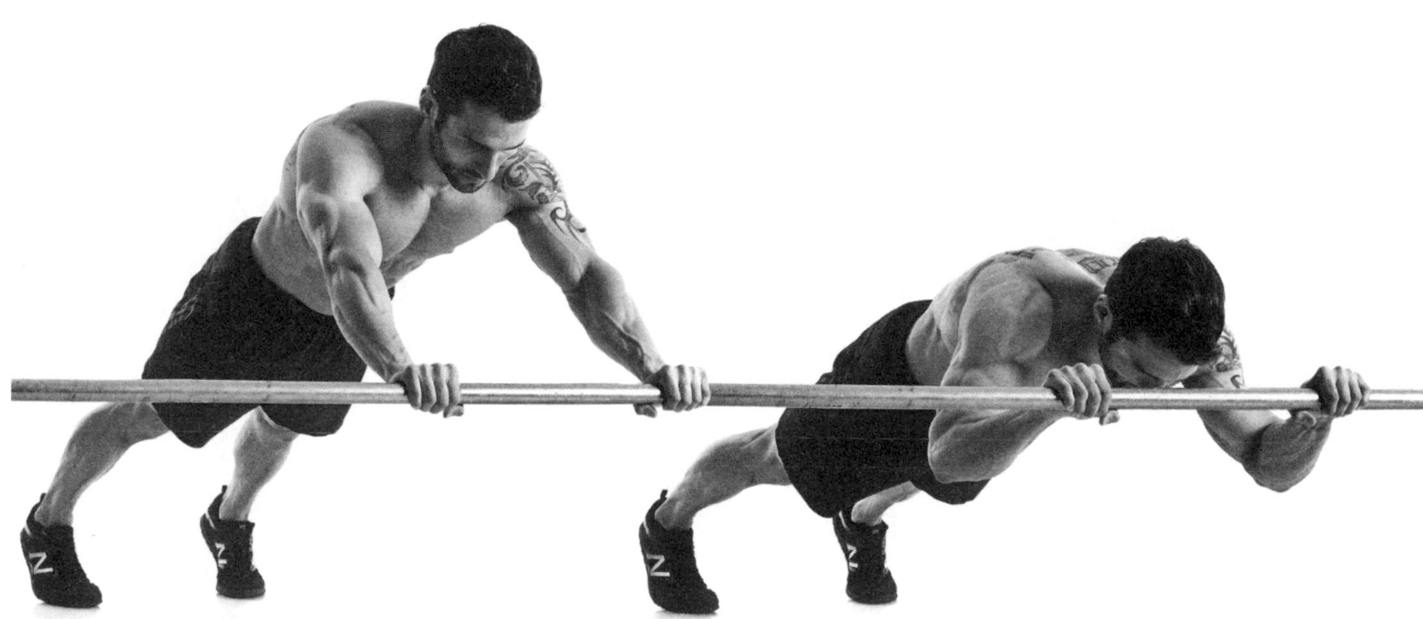

PRONE TRICEPS EXTENSION

PURPOSE

To develop the triceps.

START

Grab the barbell with an overhand grip and your arms extended forward overhead. Keep your torso straight and your body in a prone position. Your arms are holding your weight and your feet are shoulder width apart. Keep your elbows in.

MOVEMENT

Without moving your upper arms, bend at the elbows to allow your forearms to travel past parallel while lowering your body until your forehead touches the bar.

FINISH

Pause and push your body back to the starting position.

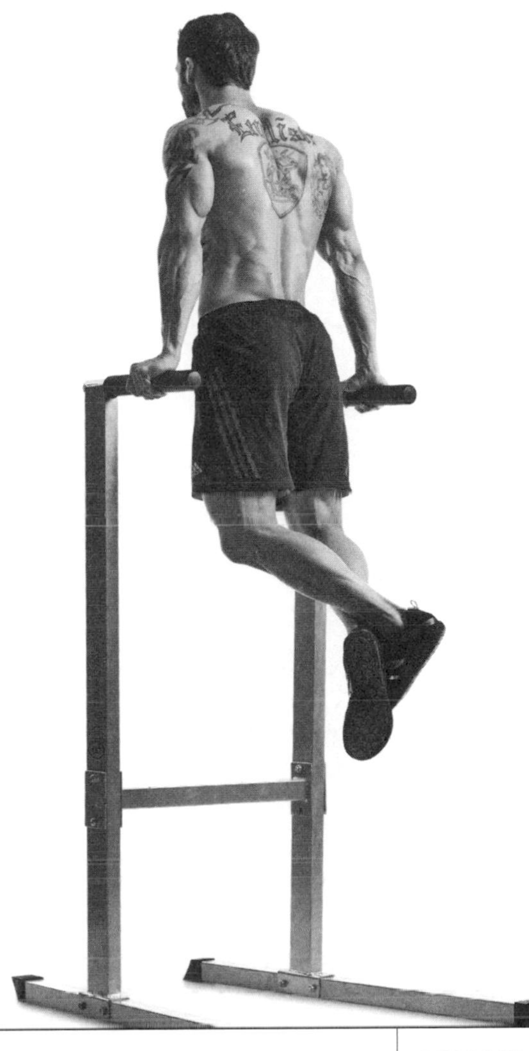

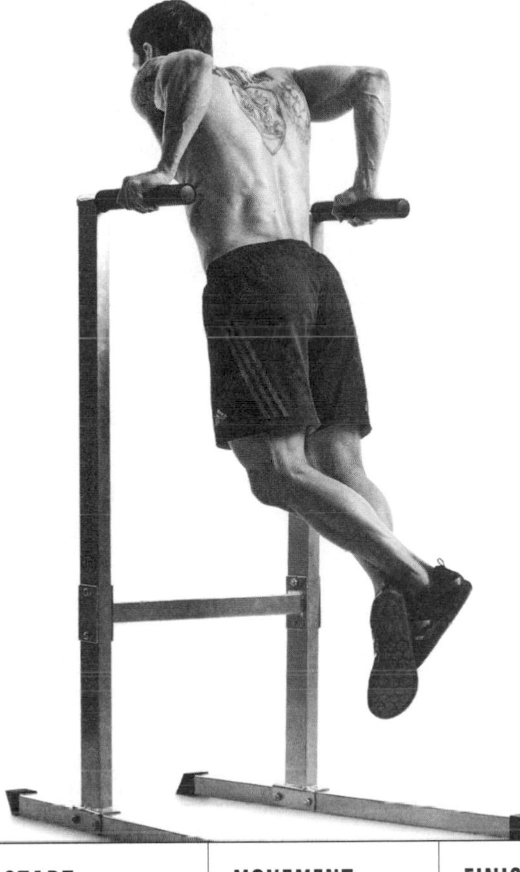

PARALLEL DIP

PURPOSE

To develop the chest and triceps.

START

Place your hands on the parallel bars of a dip station and press your body up so your arms are straight, elbows locked, and your feet are off the ground. Bend your legs behind you and cross one foot over the other.

MOVEMENT

Bend your elbows to slowly lower yourself, keeping your head facing forward. Your chest and shoulders should remain upright and straight. Keep your upper arms close to your body as you lower yourself to isolate the triceps.

FINISH

Press your body upward, finishing in the lockout position.

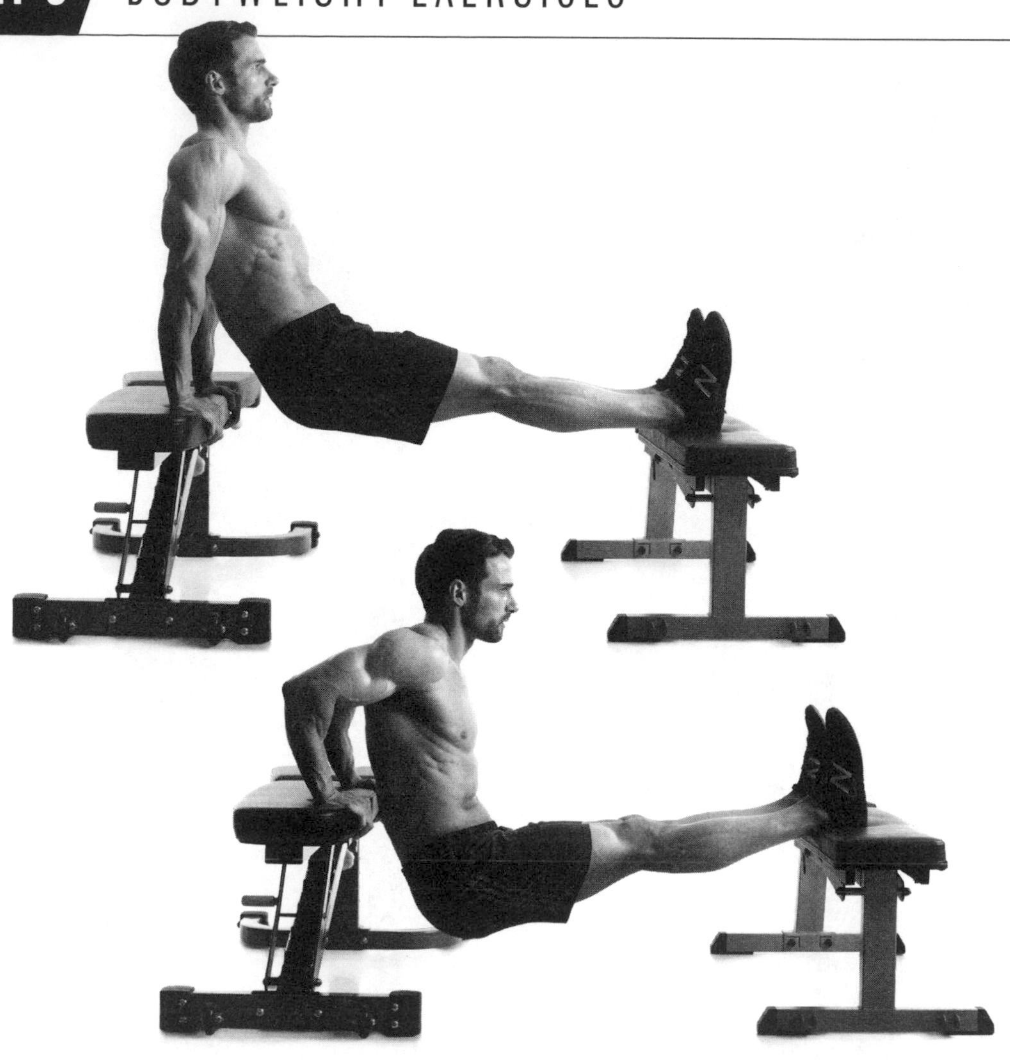

BENCH DIP

PURPOSE
To develop the triceps.

START
Place two flat benches parallel to each other. Sit between the two benches with your feet on one bench and your palms on the other. Your body should resemble an L.

MOVEMENT
Lower your body toward the floor in a slow controlled movement. Continue until your arms and forearms create a 90-degree angle.

FINISH
Push yourself back to the starting position at the top.

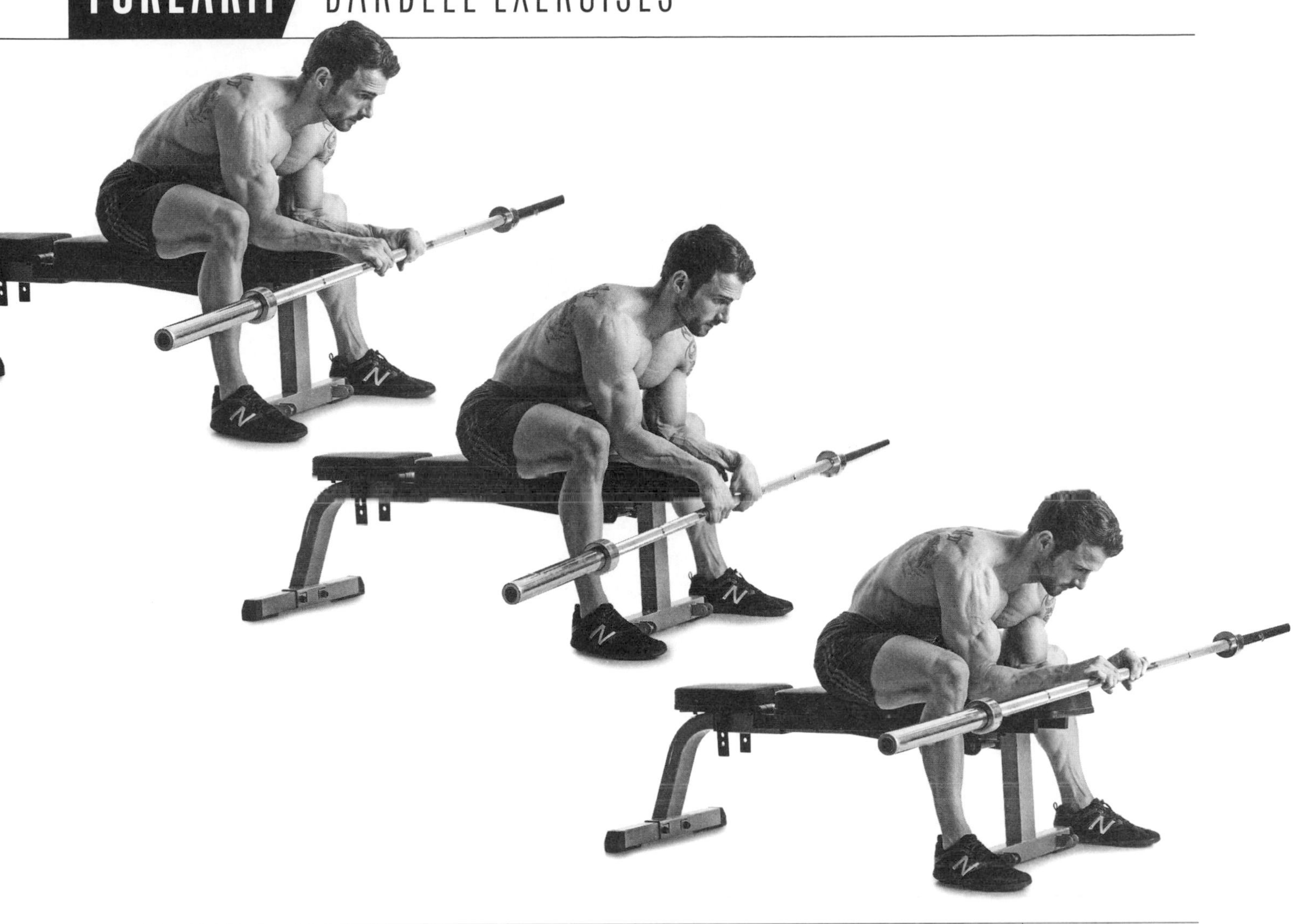

SEATED PALMS-DOWN WRIST CURL

PURPOSE

To isolate the forearms.

START

Grab a barbell with an overhand grip, hands about 2 inches apart. Sit on a bench. Place your forearms on the bench so that your palms are facing down and your hands are hanging off the bench. Allow your wrists to bend.

MOVEMENT

Reverse curl the barbell by raising the backs of your hands toward your body.

FINISH

Lower the bar to the starting position.

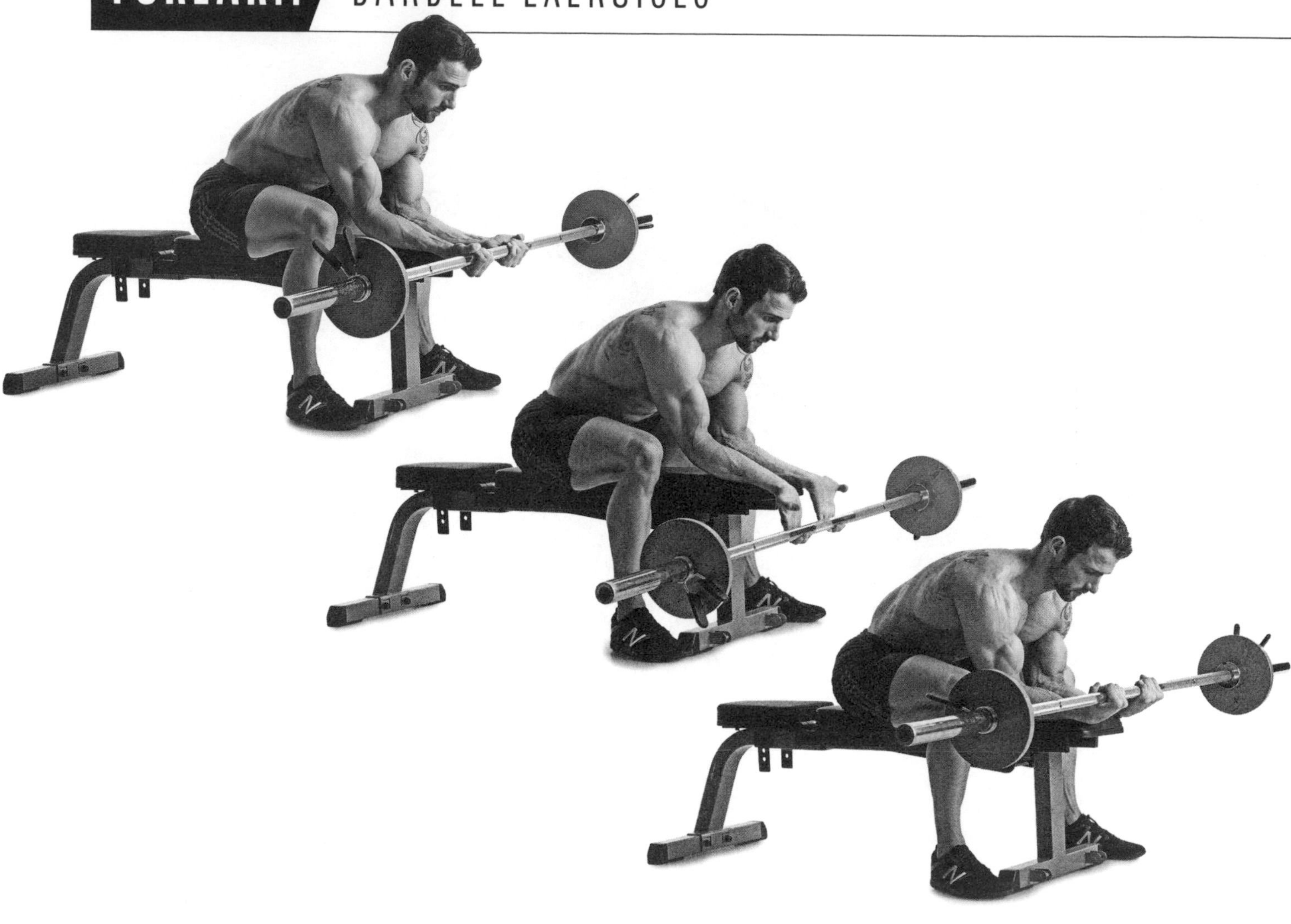

SEATED PALMS-UP WRIST CURL

PURPOSE
To isolate the forearms.

START
Grab a barbell with an underhand grip. Sit on a bench. Place your forearms so that your palms are facing up and your hands are hanging off the bench. Allow your wrists to bend from the weight of the bar.

MOVEMENT
Curl the barbell by raising your palms toward your body.

FINISH
Reverse the movement to return to the starting position.

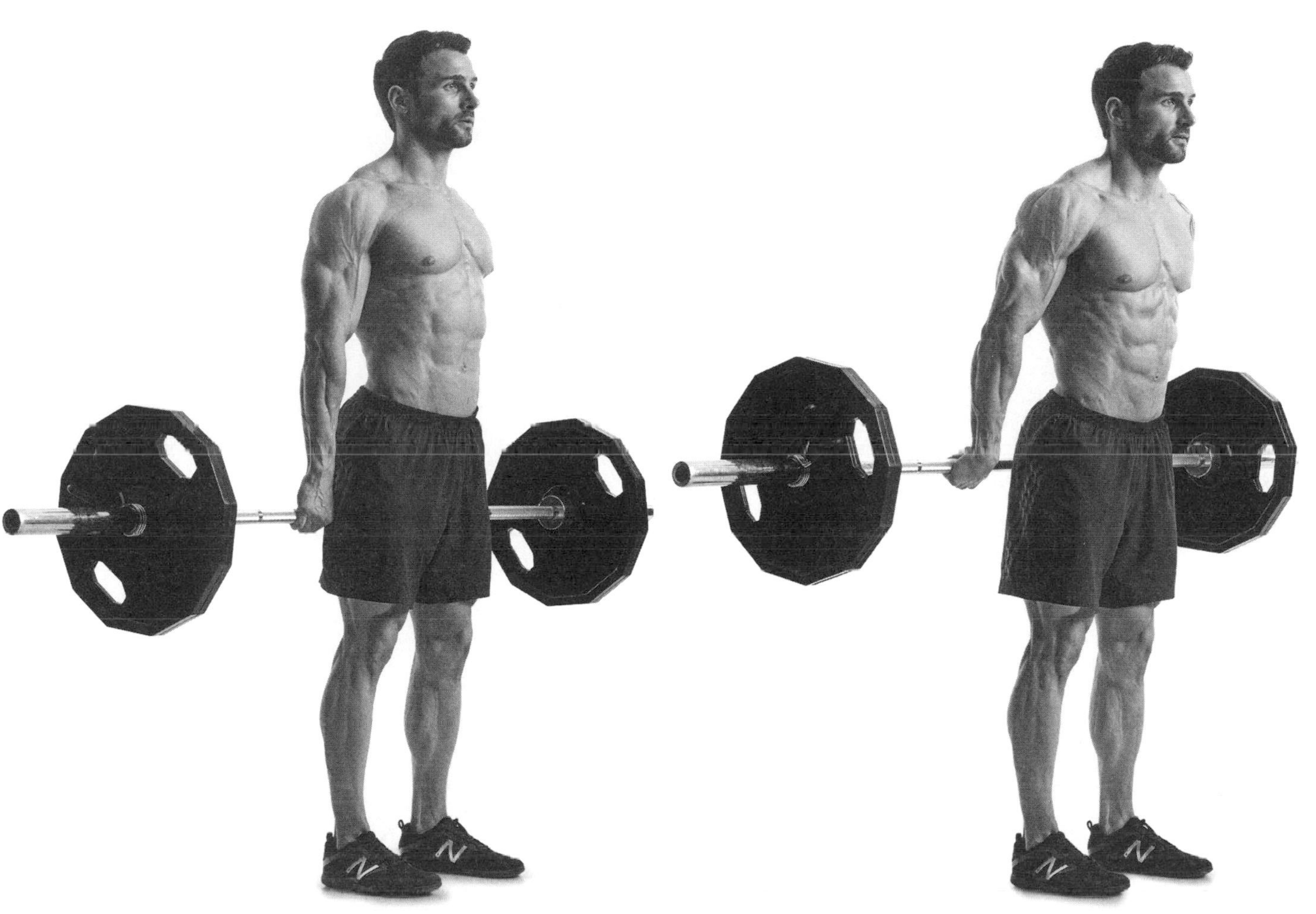

STANDING PALMS-UP BEHIND-THE-BACK WRIST CURL

PURPOSE
To develop the forearms.

START
Grab a barbell behind your back, with an overhand grip.

MOVEMENT
Curl your wrists with your palms up toward the ceiling.

FINISH
Allow the barbell to lower back to the starting position.

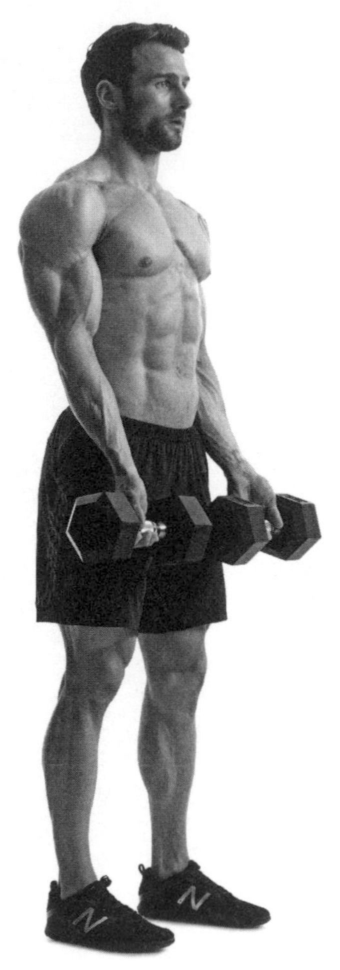

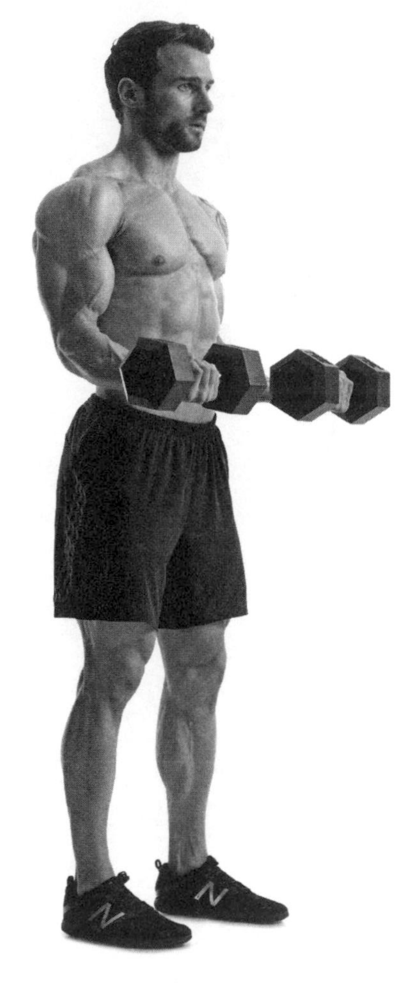

DUAL WRIST CURL

PURPOSE

To isolate the forearms.

START

Stand and grab a pair of dumbbells with an underhand grip and allow the dumbbells to hang in front of your thighs. With palms facing forward, allow your wrists to bend from the weight of the dumbbells.

MOVEMENT

Bend your elbows slightly and using only your wrists, curl the dumbbells up by raising your palms toward your body.

FINISH

Reverse the movement to return to the starting position.

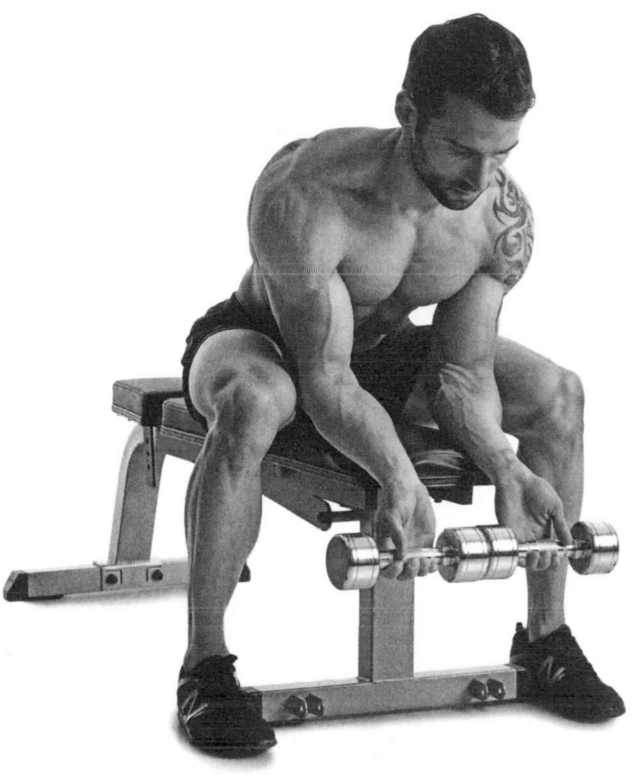

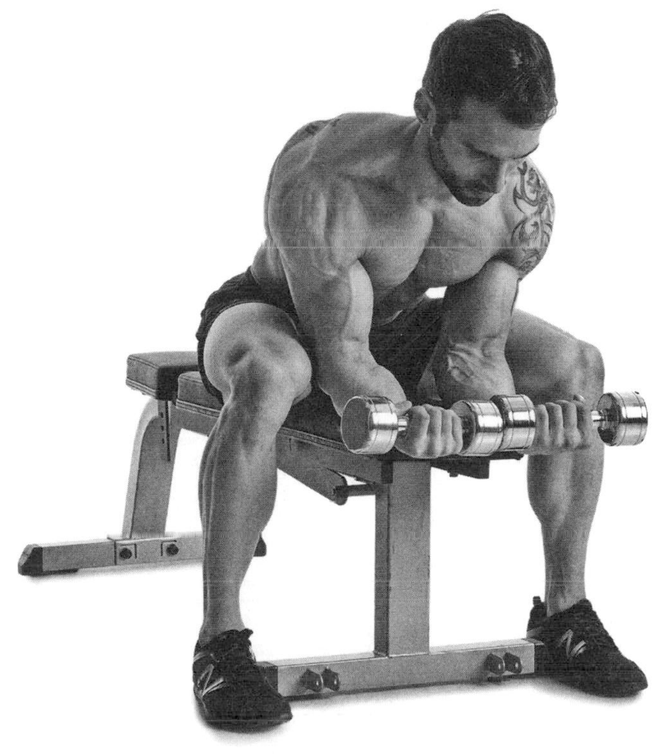

SEATED PALMS-UP WRIST CURL

PURPOSE

To isolate the forearms.

START

Grab a pair of dumbbells with an underhand grip. Sit on the front of a bench. Rest your forearms on the bench so that your palms-up hands hang off the bench. Allow your wrists to bend.

MOVEMENT

Curl the dumbbells by raising your palms toward your body.

FINISH

Reverse the movement to return to the starting position.

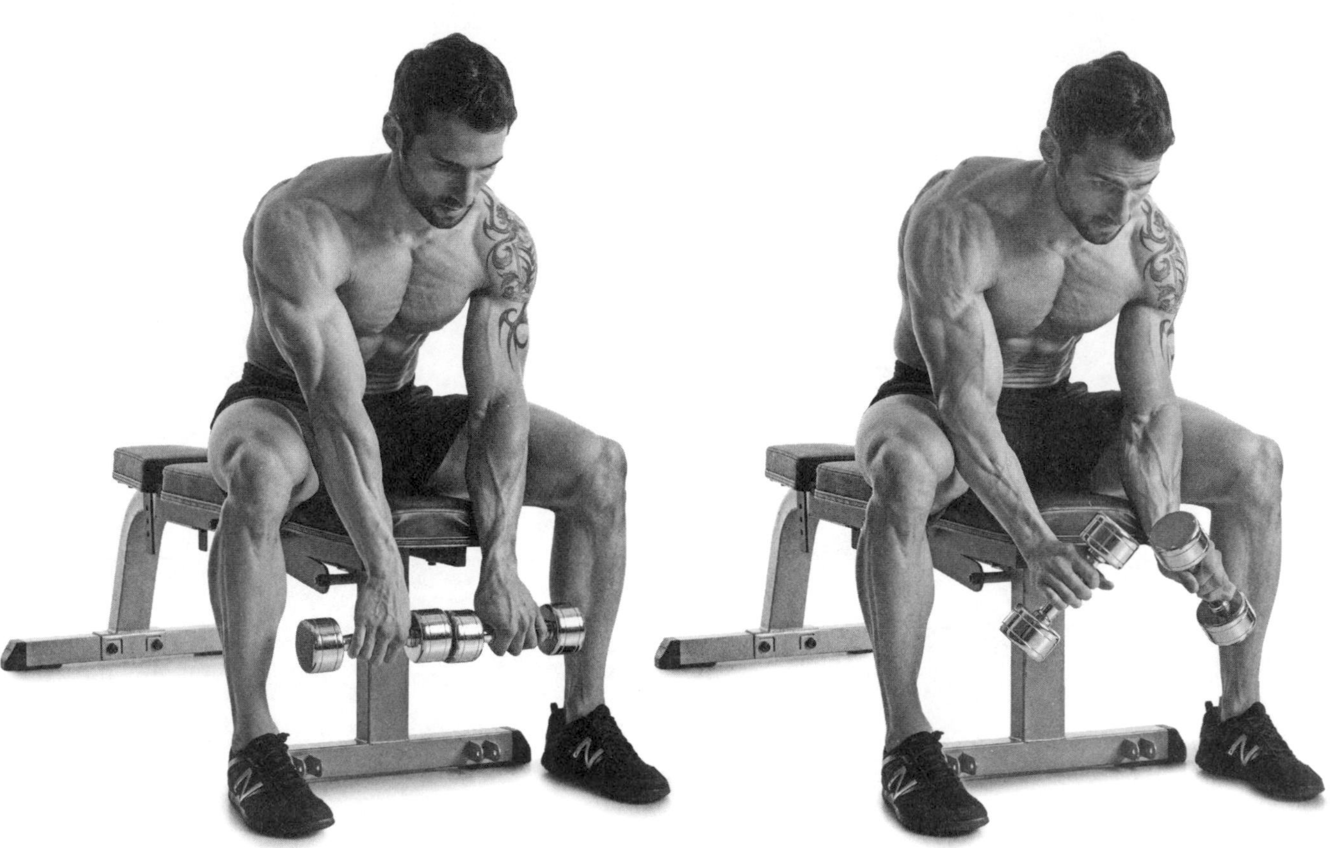

SEATED PALMS-DOWN WRIST CURL

PURPOSE

To isolate the forearms.

START

Grab a pair of dumbbells with an overhand grip. Sit on the front of a bench. Rest your forearms on the edge of the bench and allow your palms-down hands to hang. Allow your wrists to bend.

MOVEMENT

Reverse curl the dumbbells by raising the backs of your hands toward your body.

FINISH

Slowly lower the weights to the starting position.

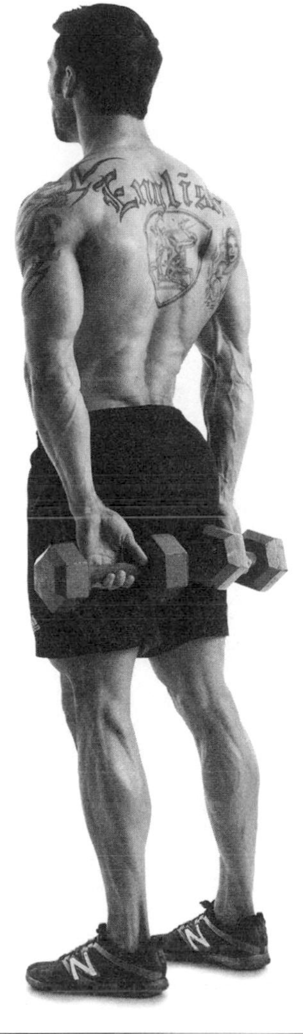

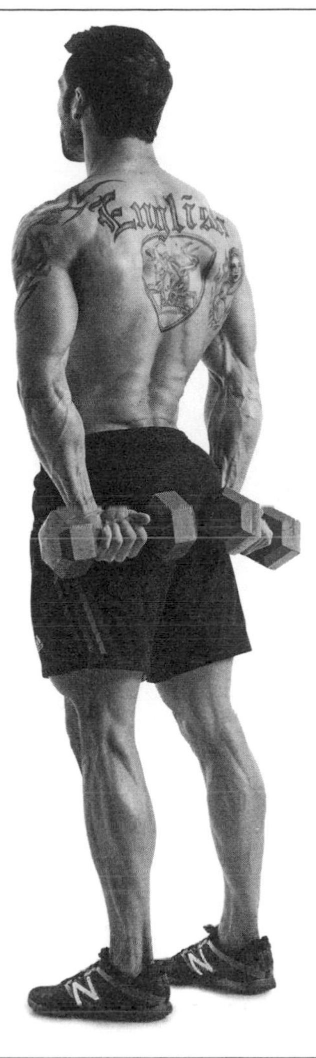

STANDING PALMS-UP BEHIND-THE-BACK WRIST CURL

PURPOSE

To isolate the forearms.

START

Stand and grab a pair of dumbbells with an overhand grip. Move the weights behind your glutes.

MOVEMENT

With your palms facing behind you, keep your arms still and perform a wrist curl by raising your palms up toward the ceiling.

FINISH

Allow the dumbbells to extend and return to the starting position.

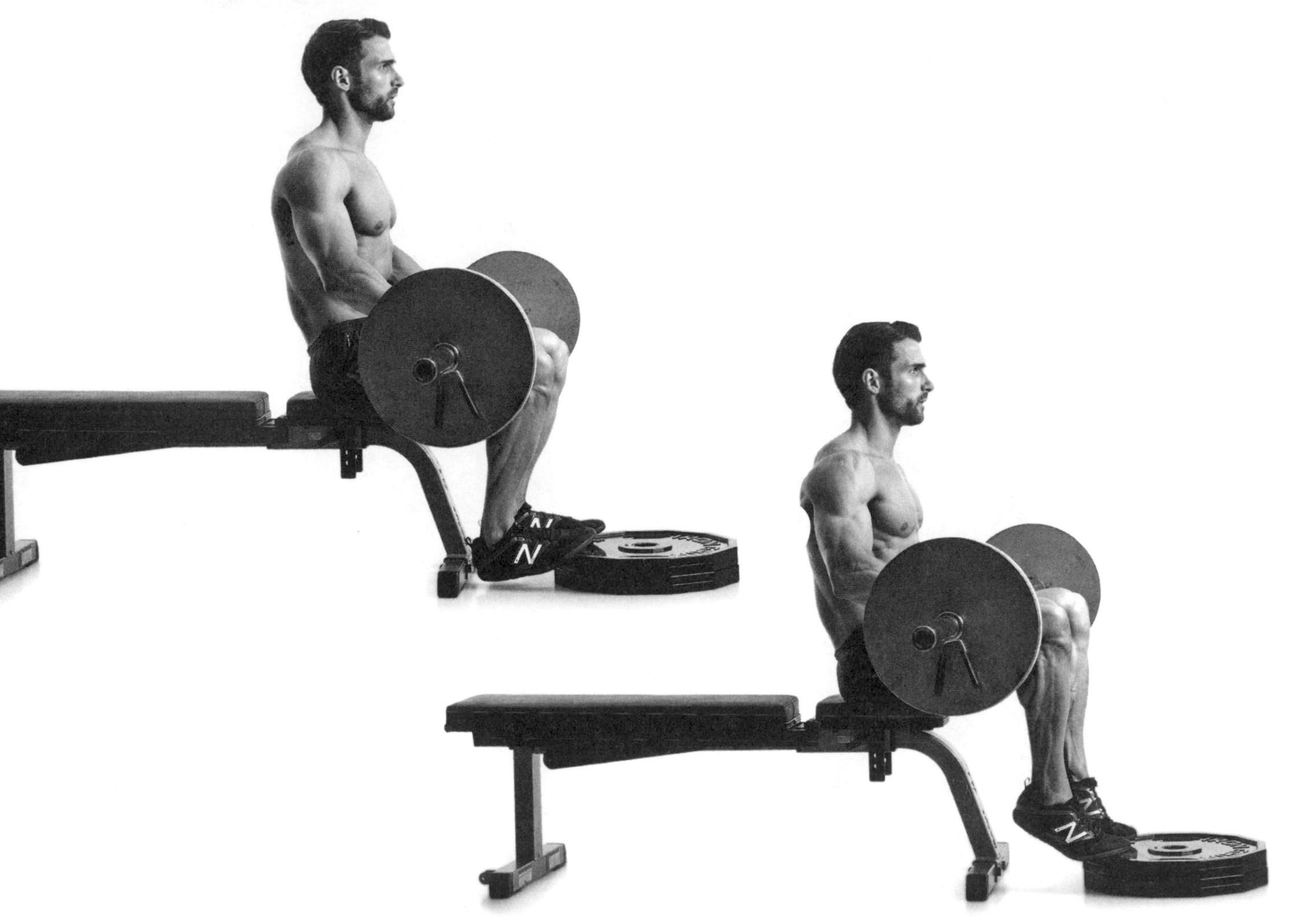

SEATED CALF RAISE

PURPOSE

Target the calves.

START

Grab a barbell and rest it on your thighs while sitting on the edge of a bench. Place the balls of your feet on two stacked 25-pound weight plates. Keep your torso tight and sit tall.

MOVEMENT

Rise up on your toes as high as you can.

FINISH

Pause, then slowly lower to the starting position.

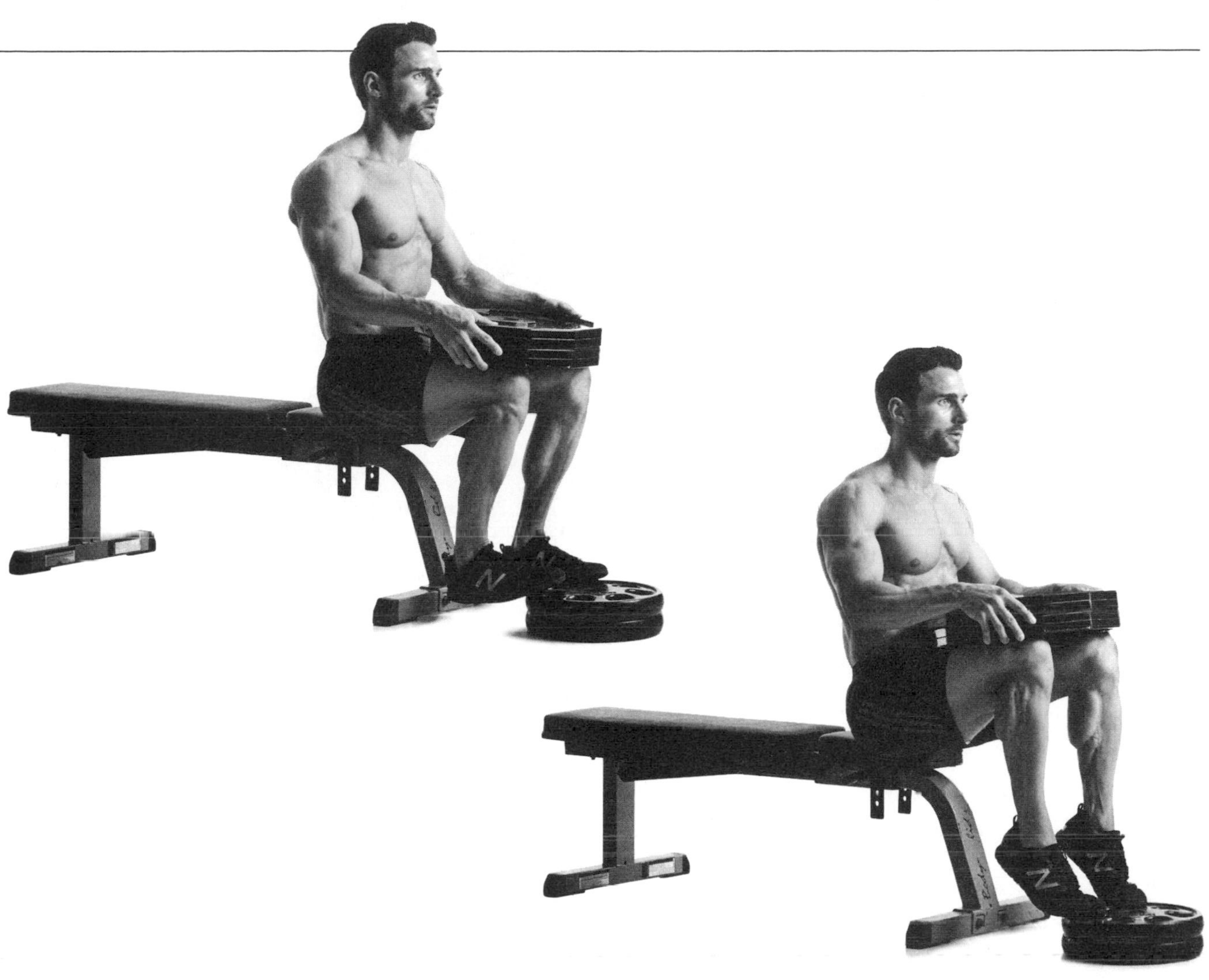

SEATED PLATE CALF RAISE

PURPOSE
Target the calves.

START
Grab two weight plates and rest them on top of your thighs while sitting on the edge of a bench. Place your feet on two stacked 25-pound weight plates. Keep your torso tight and sit tall.

MOVEMENT
Rise up on your toes as high as you can.

FINISH
Pause, then slowly lower to the starting position.

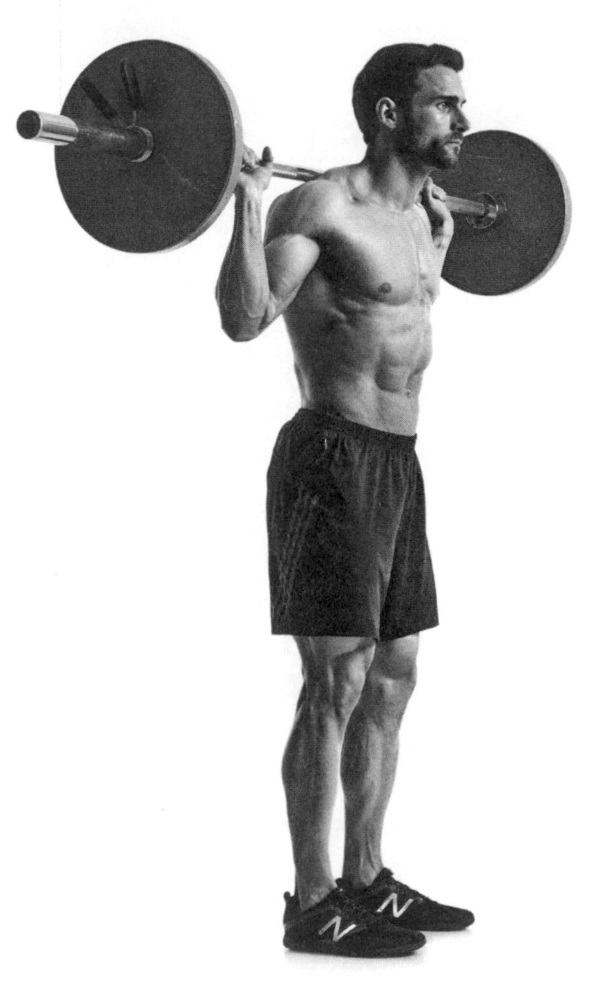

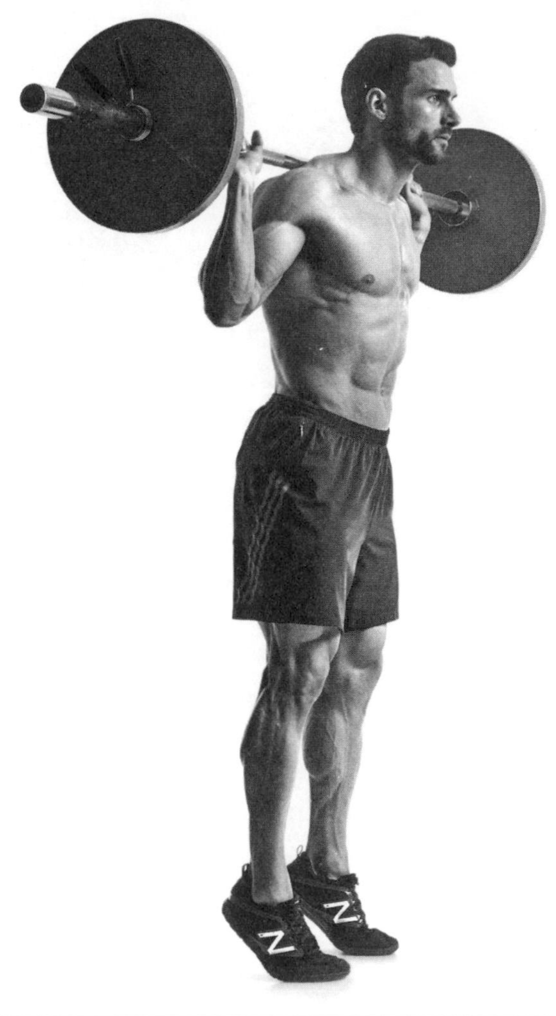

STANDING CALF RAISE

PURPOSE
Target the calves.

START
Grab a barbell with an overhand grip and place it so that it rests on your upper back. Keep your torso tight and stand tall.

MOVEMENT
Rise up on your toes as high as you can.

FINISH
Pause, then slowly lower to the starting position.

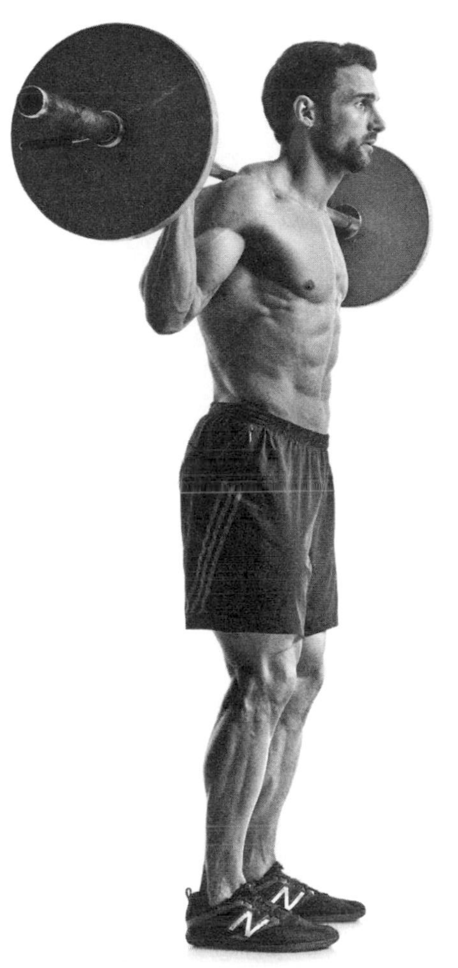

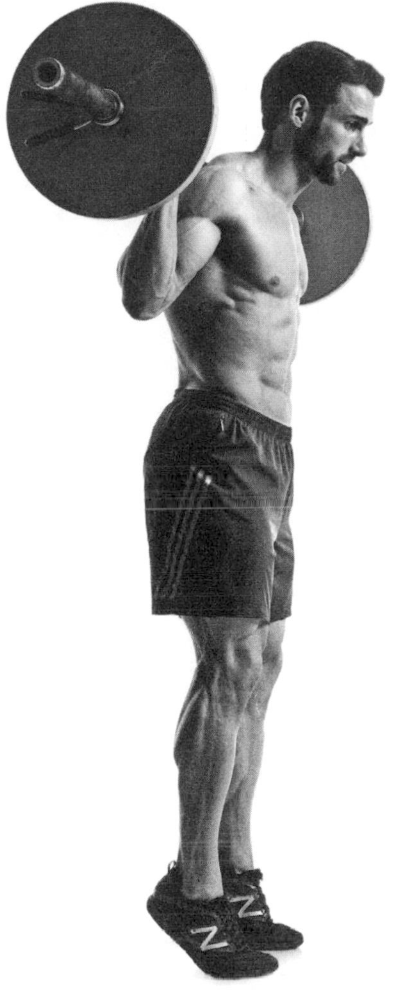

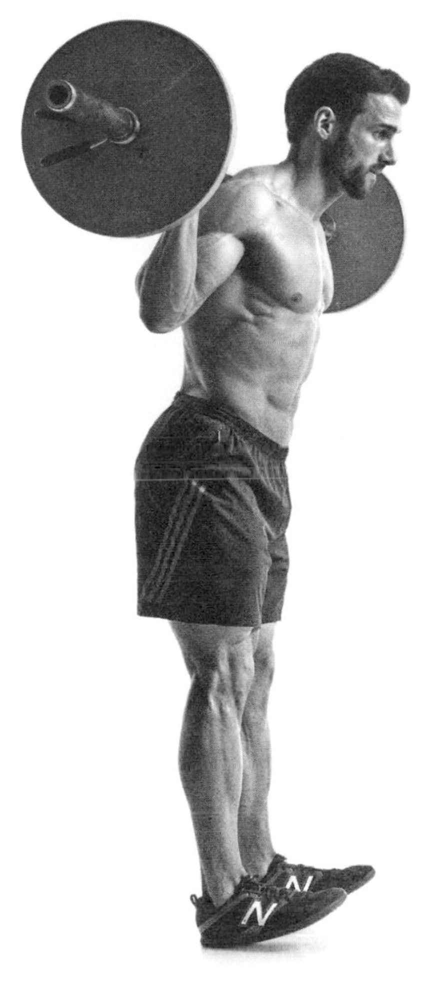

ROCKING STANDING CALF RAISE

PURPOSE

Target the calves.

START

Grab a barbell with an overhand grip and place it so that it rests on your upper back. Keep your torso tight and stand tall.

MOVEMENT

Rise up on your toes as high as you can, then rock back on your heels, keeping constant tension in your calves. That's one rep.

FINISH

Continue to rock back and forth for the allotted number of reps.

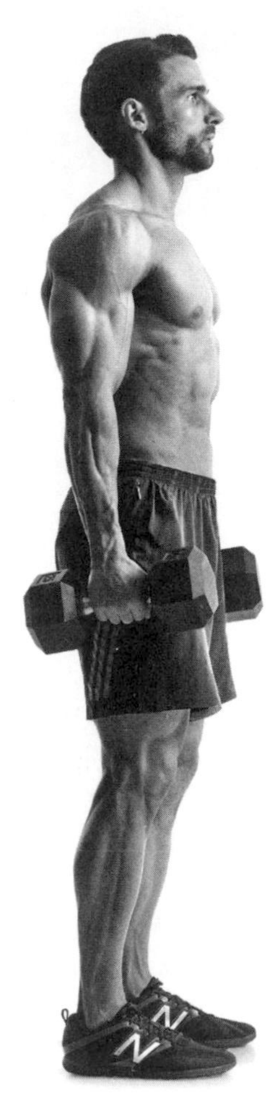

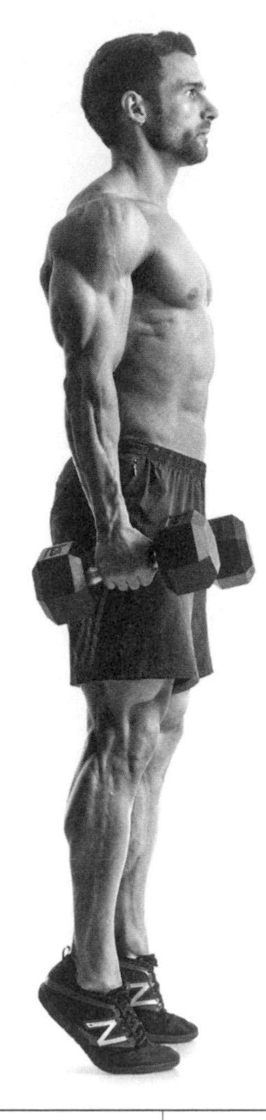

STANDING CALF RAISE

PURPOSE
Target the calves.

START
Grab a pair of dumbbells with a neutral grip and allow them to hang at arm's length at your sides. Keep your torso tight and stand tall.

MOVEMENT
Rise up on your toes as high as you can.

FINISH
Pause, then slowly lower to the starting position.

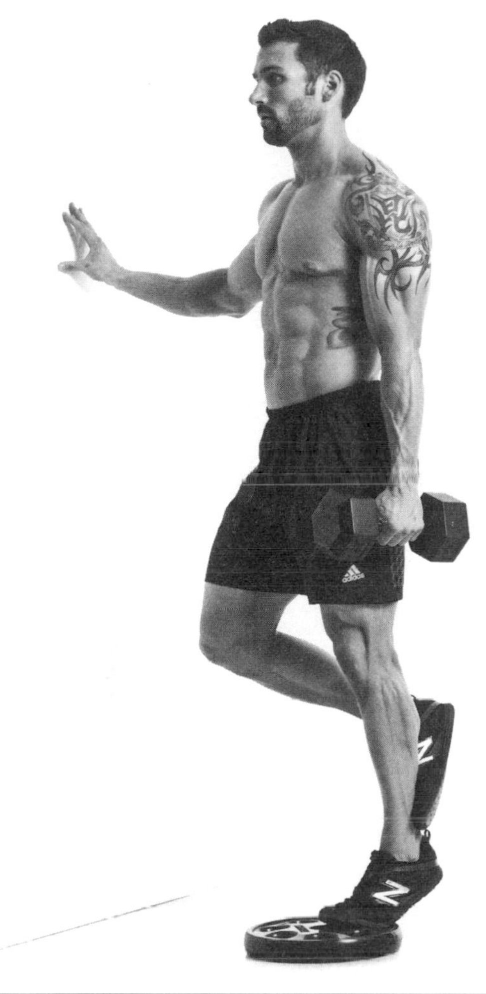

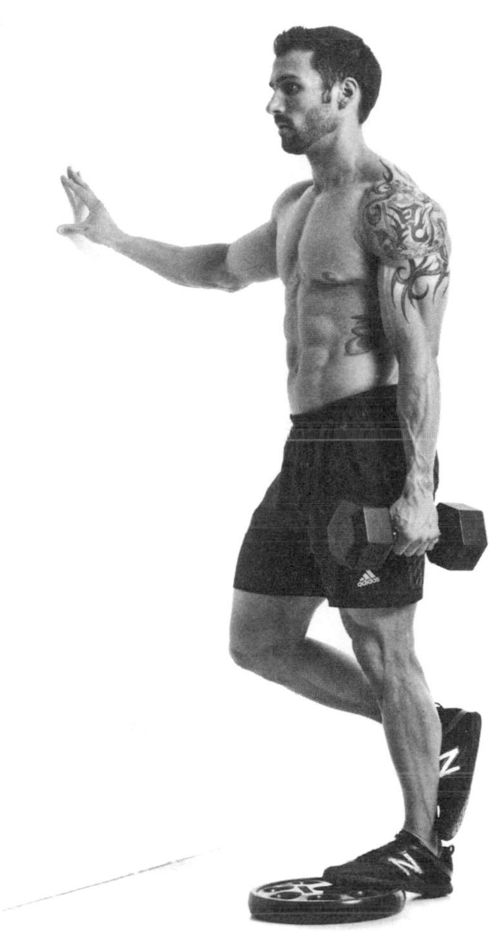

STANDING BENT-KNEE ONE-LEGGED CALF RAISE

PURPOSE

Target the soleus.

START

Grab a dumbbell and hold on to a wall or rack with the other hand. Place one foot on a 25-pound weight plate. Lift the opposing foot off the ground and wrap it around the back of your straight leg. Keep your torso tight.

MOVEMENT

Rise up on your toes as high as you can.

FINISH

Pause, then slowly lower to the starting position, repeat on other side.

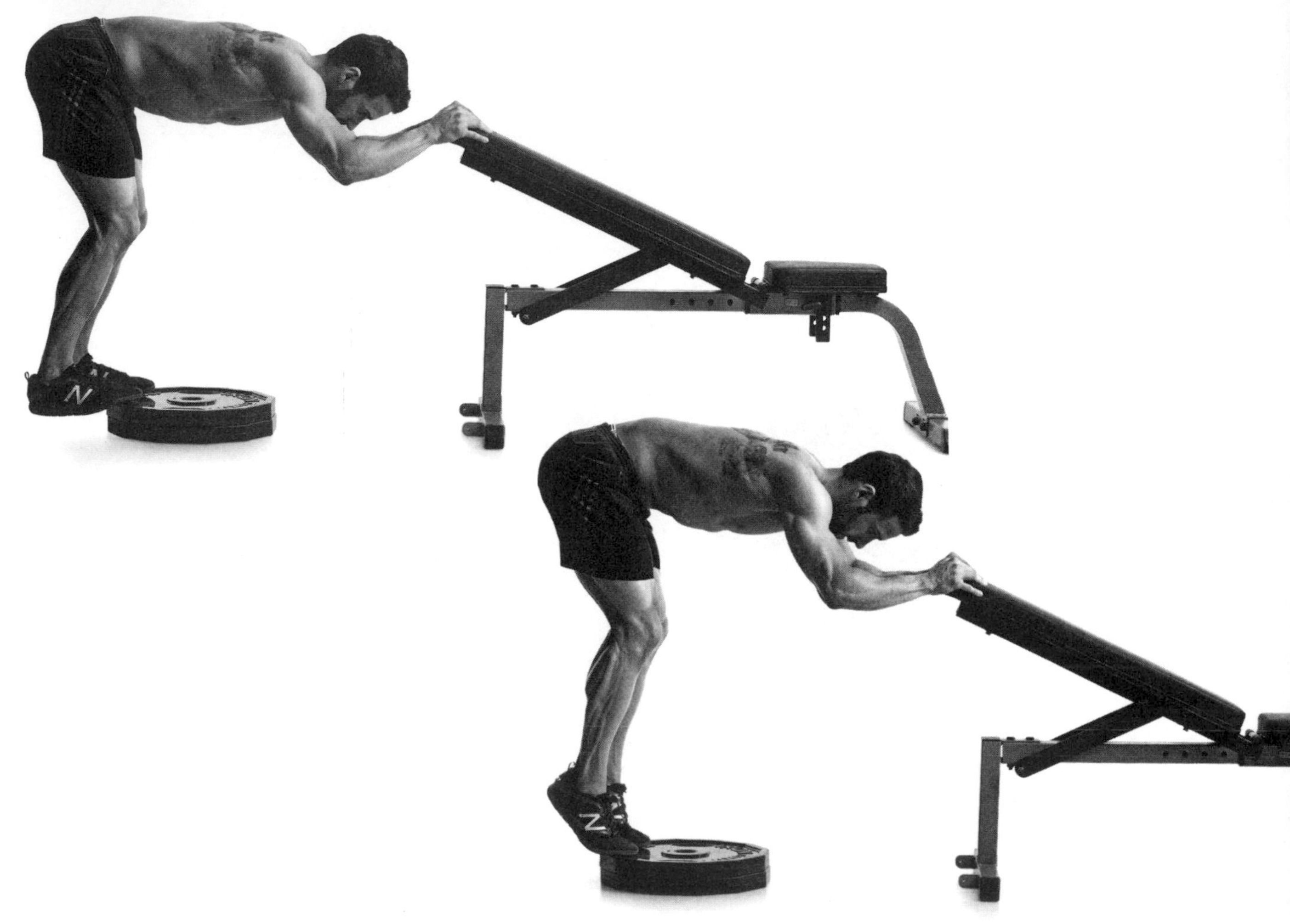

DONKEY CALF RAISE

PURPOSE
Target the calves.

START
Stand on the edge of two stacked weight plates. Keeping a natural arch to your back, bend at the hips and lower your torso until your upper body is parallel to the floor. Place your hands on a sturdy object like a squat rack or incline bench as shown.

MOVEMENT
Rise up on your toes as high as you can.

FINISH
Pause, then slowly lower to the starting position.

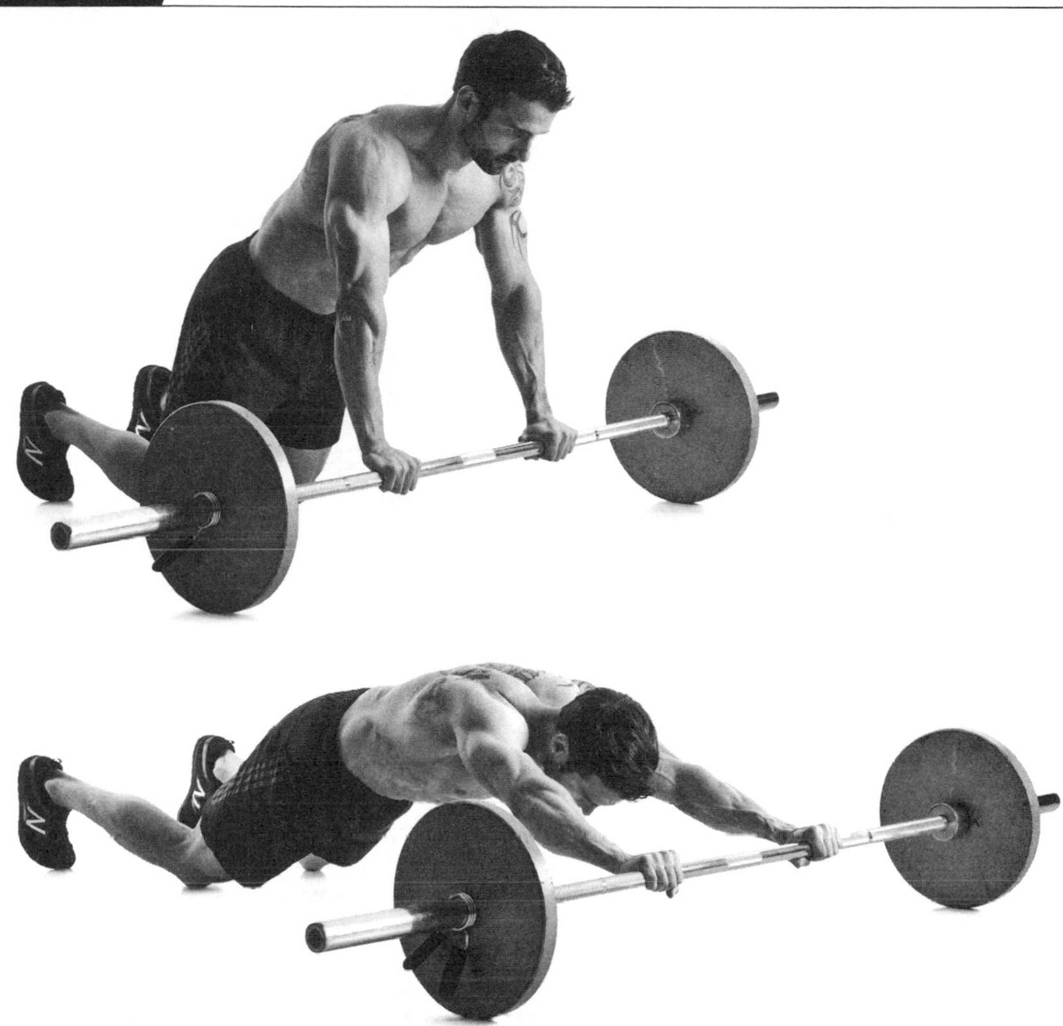

ROLLOUT

PURPOSE

Target your abdominals.

START

Load a barbell with a 10-pound weight plate on each side and use collars. Kneel on the floor and grab the bar with an overhand grip that is shoulder width apart. Start with your shoulders over the bar.

MOVEMENT

Slowly roll the bar forward, extending your body as far as you can without allowing your hips to fall. Brace your core and squeeze your glutes.

FINISH

Use your abdominals to pull the bar back toward your knees.

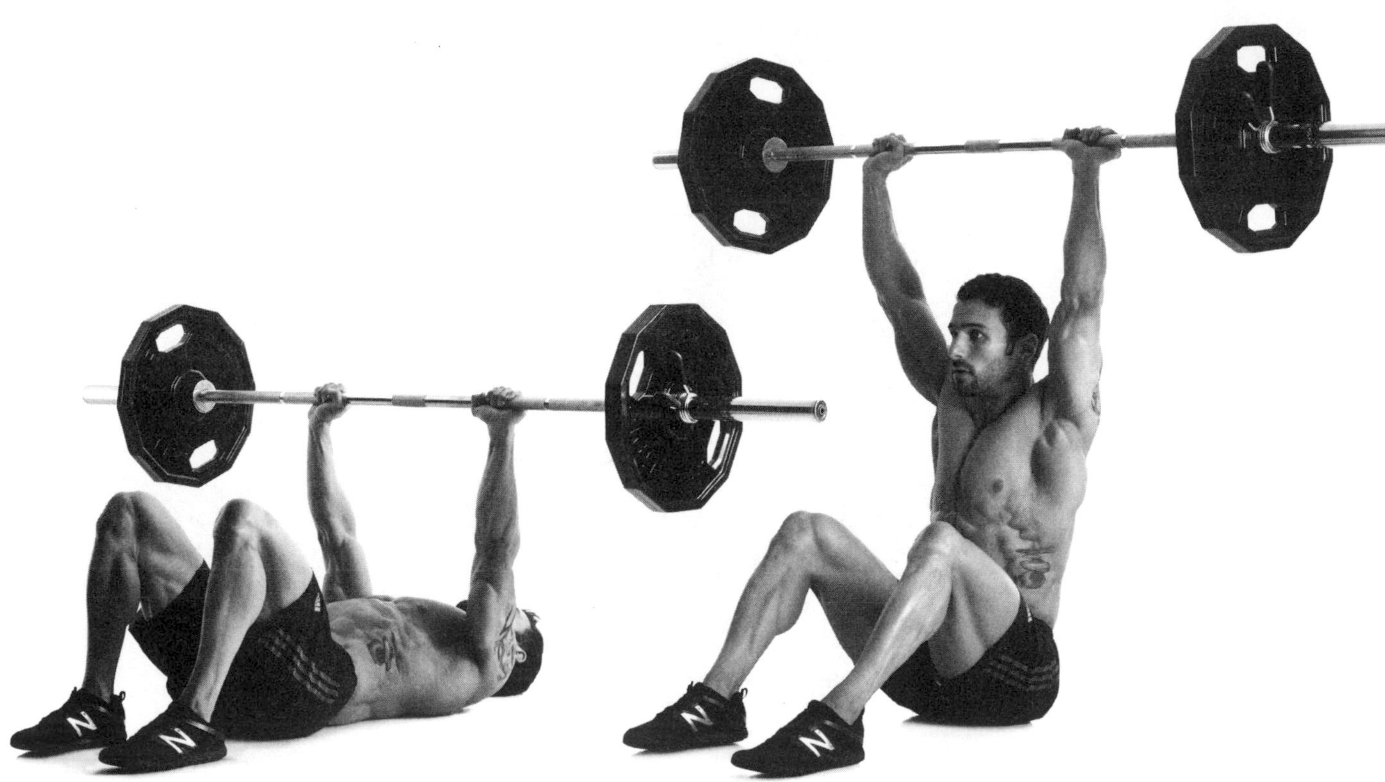

PRESS SITUP

PURPOSE

Target your abdominals.

START

Grab a barbell with an overhand grip and lie faceup on the floor with your knees bent and feet flat. Place the barbell over your chest with arms straight.

MOVEMENT

Using your abdominals, curl your torso to a sitting position by pushing the barbell up toward the ceiling. The motion should be smooth and controlled with the barbell finishing over your head.

FINISH

Slowly lower your torso back to the floor and the barbell back to over your chest.

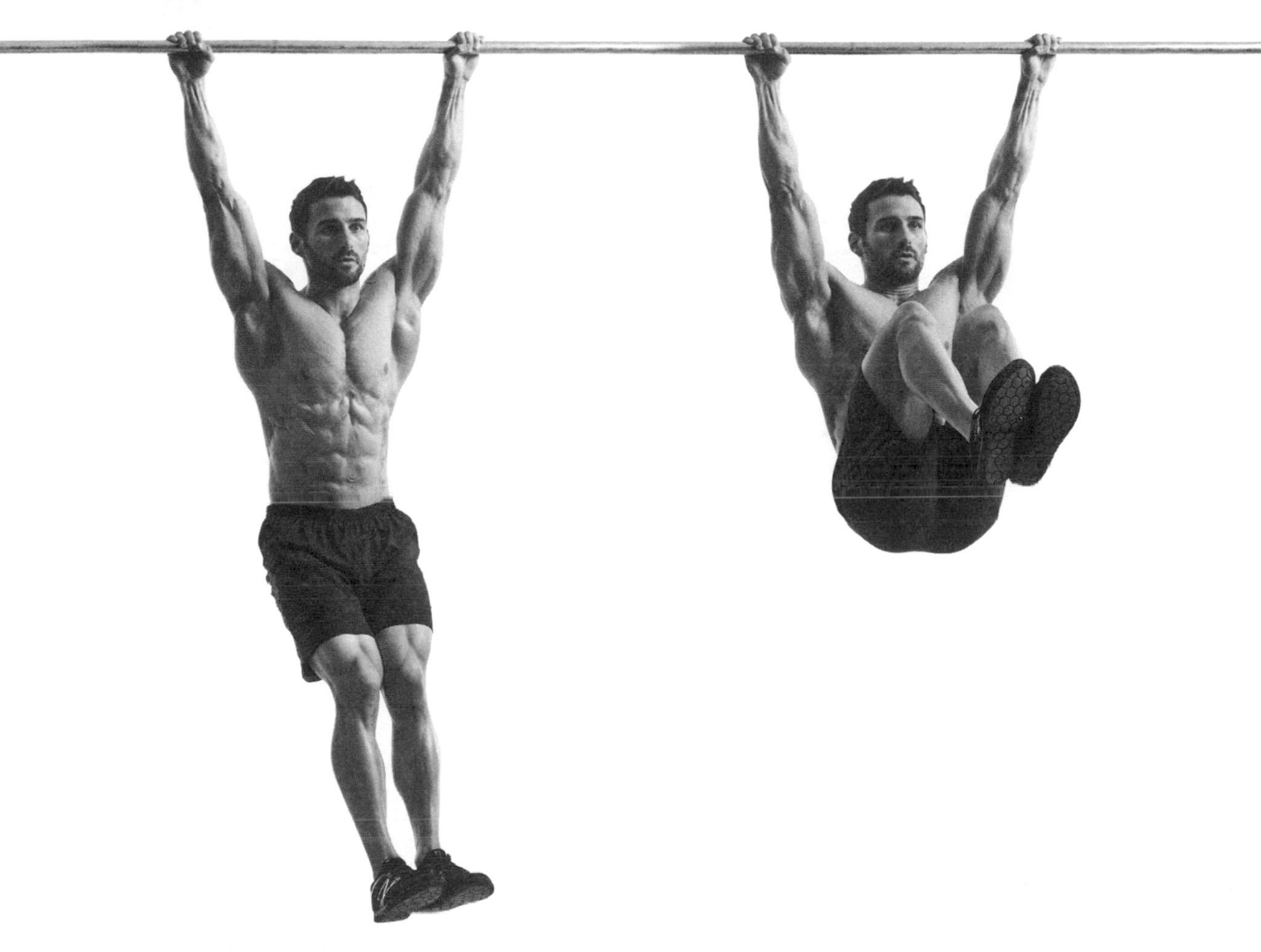

HANGING KNEE RAISE

PURPOSE

Target the abdominals.

START

Grab a chinup bar with an overhand grip that is shoulder width apart. Keep your knees slightly bent and your feet together.

MOVEMENT

While bending your knees, simultaneously raise your hips and curl your lower back underneath you as you lift your knees toward your chest.

FINISH

Pause, then slowly lower your legs back to the starting position.

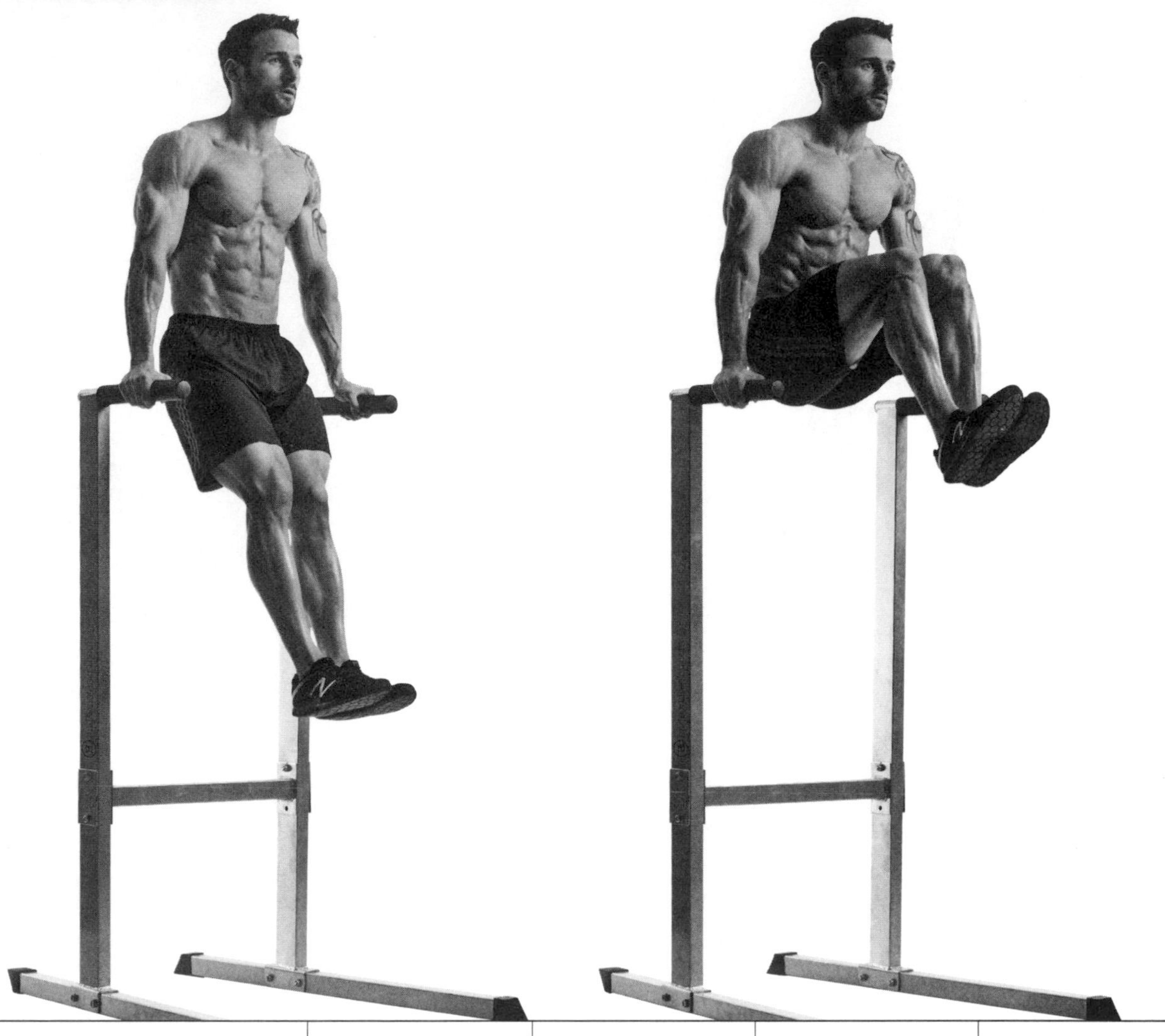

PARALLEL BAR KNEE RAISE

PURPOSE

Target your abdominals.

START

Hold yourself up on a parallel dip bar with arms straight. Keep your knees slightly bent and your feet together.

MOVEMENT

Simultaneously raise your hips and curl your lower back underneath as you bend your knees toward your chest.

FINISH

Pause, then slowly lower your legs back to the starting position.

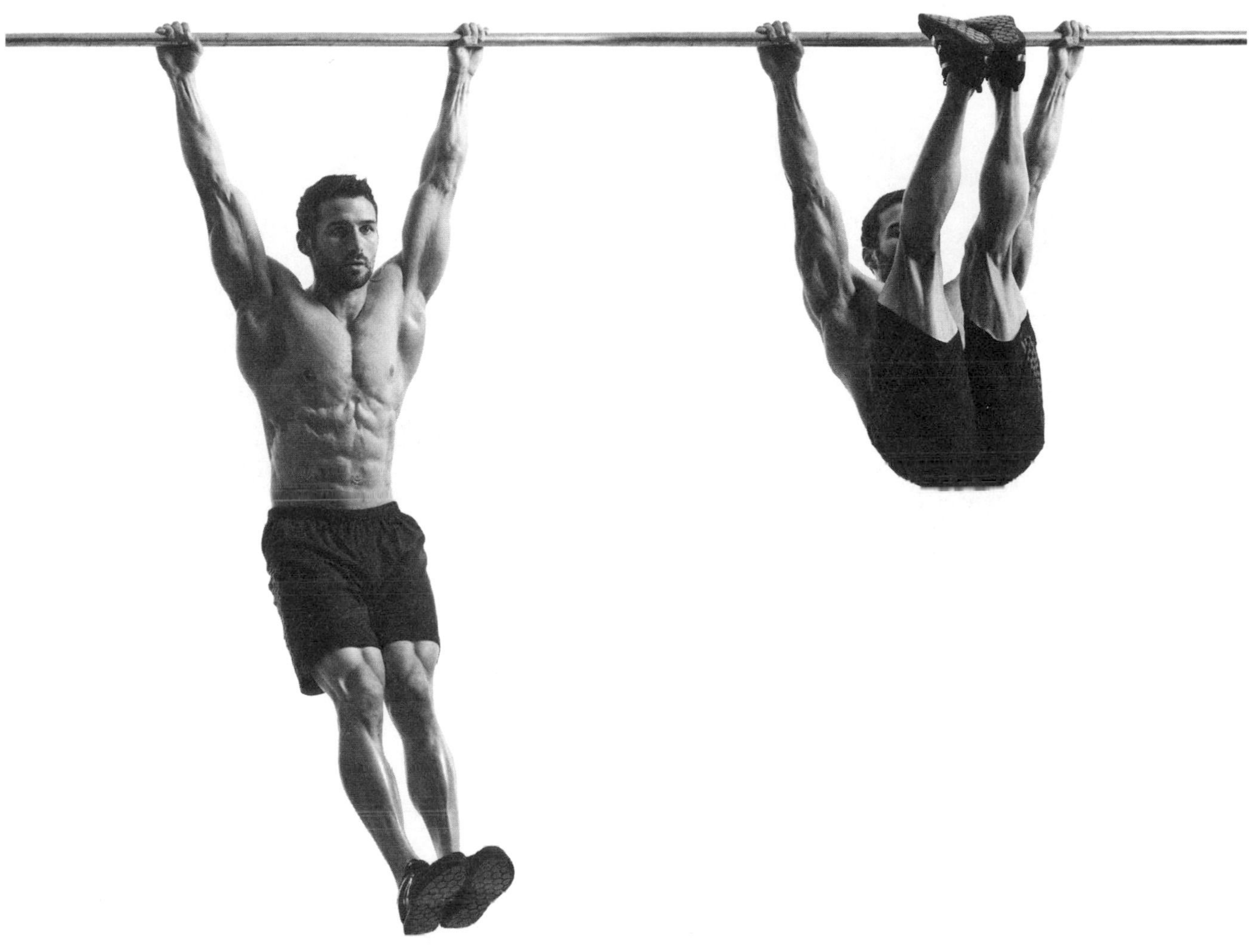

HANGING LEG RAISE

PURPOSE

Target abdominals.

START

Grab a chinup bar with an overhand grip that is shoulder width apart. Keep your knees slightly bent and your feet together.

MOVEMENT

Lift your legs toward the bar while raising your hips and curling your lower back underneath you.

FINISH

Pause, then slowly lower your legs back to the starting position.

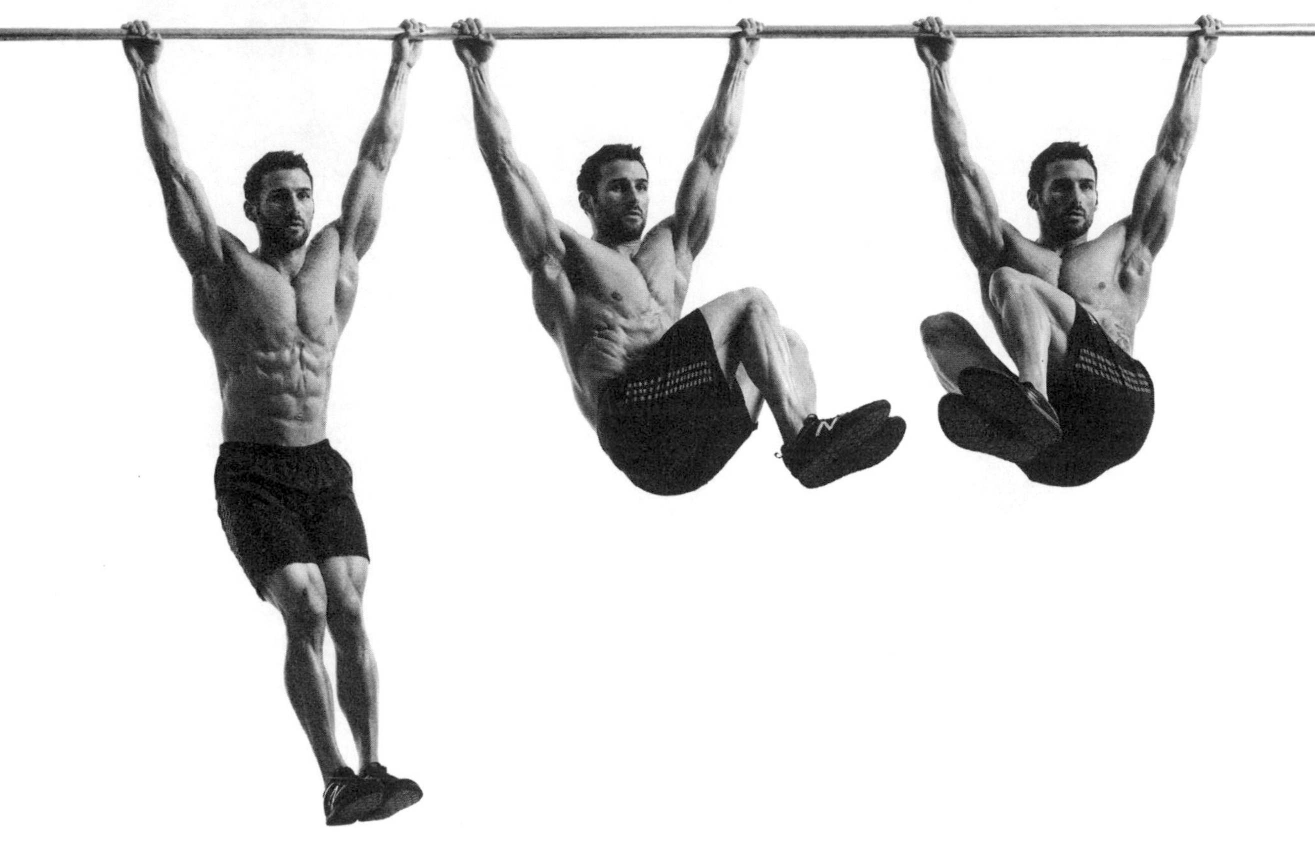

HANGING X-BODY KNEE RAISE (OBLIQUE RAISE)

PURPOSE
Target the obliques and abdominals.

START
Grab a chinup bar with an overhand grip and allow your body to hang at arm's length.

MOVEMENT
Lift your knees until your hips and knees are bent at a 90-degree angle. Raise one hip toward the armpit on the same side of the body.

FINISH
Pause, then return to the starting position before alternating sides.

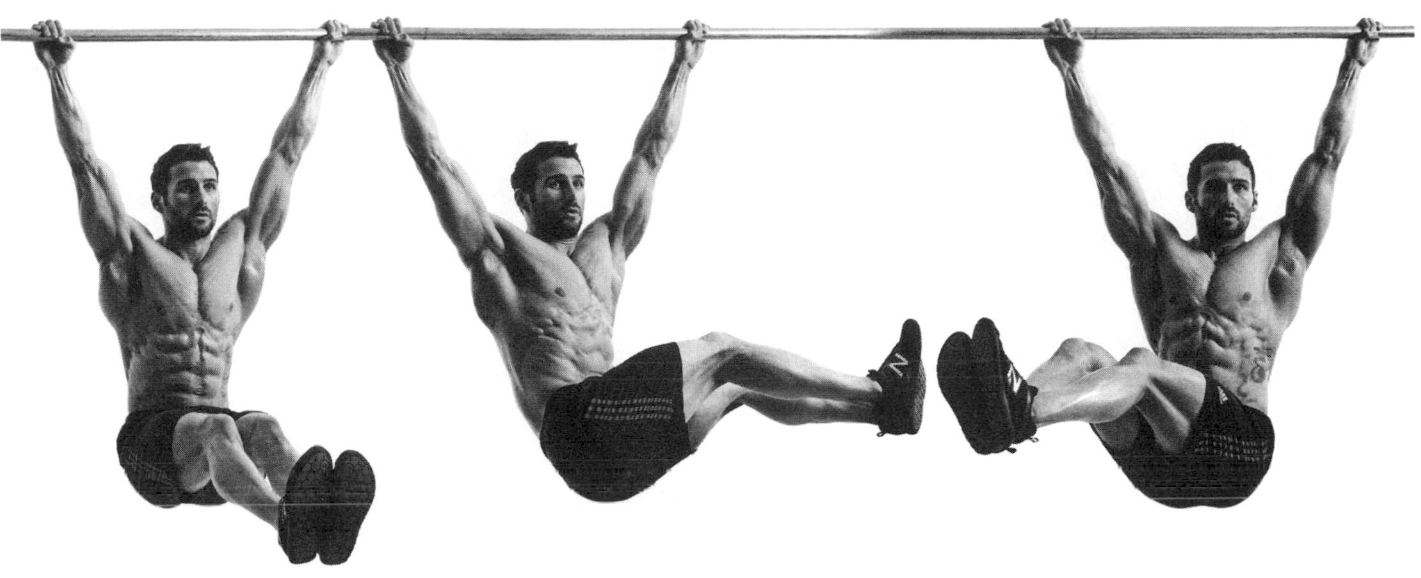

HANGING-LEG WINDSHIELD WIPER

PURPOSE
Target the obliques and abdominals.

START
Hang from a chinup bar with an overhand grip. Keep your feet together and your knees slightly bent.

MOVEMENT
Keeping a slight bend to your knees, lift your legs higher than your hips and across your torso toward the left. Then immediately swing your knees to the right. Repeat back and forth.

FINISH
Pause, then lower to the starting position in a dead hang.

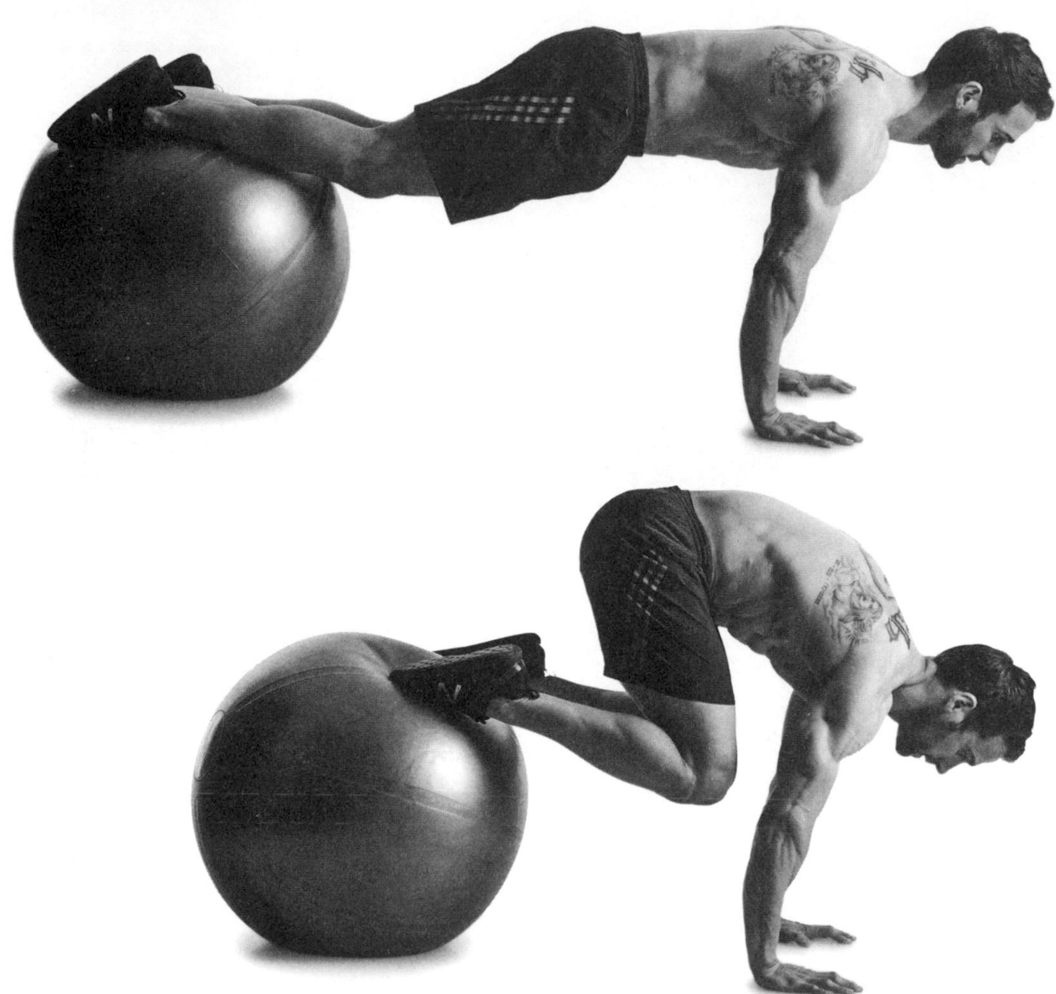

STABILITY BALL KNEE TUCK

PURPOSE
Target the abdominals.

START
Rest your shins on a stability ball and place your body in a pushup position with your arms straight under your shoulders. Keep your body in a straight line. Brace your core and don't round your back.

MOVEMENT
Roll the stability ball toward your chest by bending your knees and pulling it forward with your feet.

FINISH
Pause, then return to the starting position.

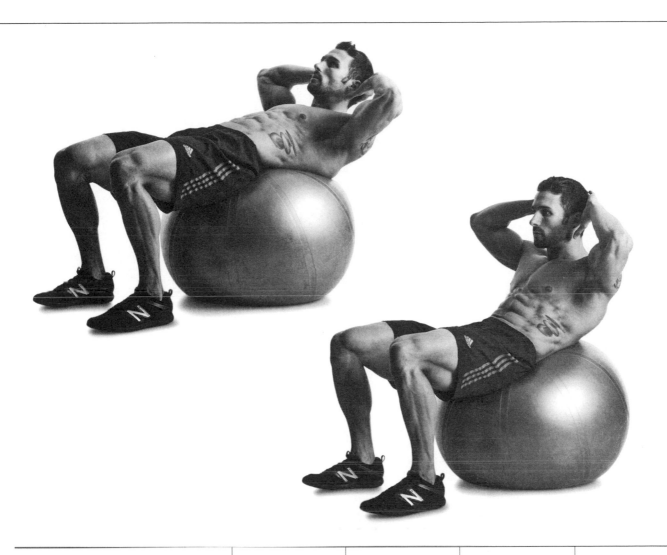

STABILITY BALL CRUNCH

PURPOSE
Target abdominals.

START
Lie with your hips, lower back, and shoulders in contact with the ball. Place your hands behind your head.

MOVEMENT
Raise your head and shoulders off the ball, bringing your rib cage toward your pelvis.

FINISH
Pause, then slowly lower your body to the starting position.

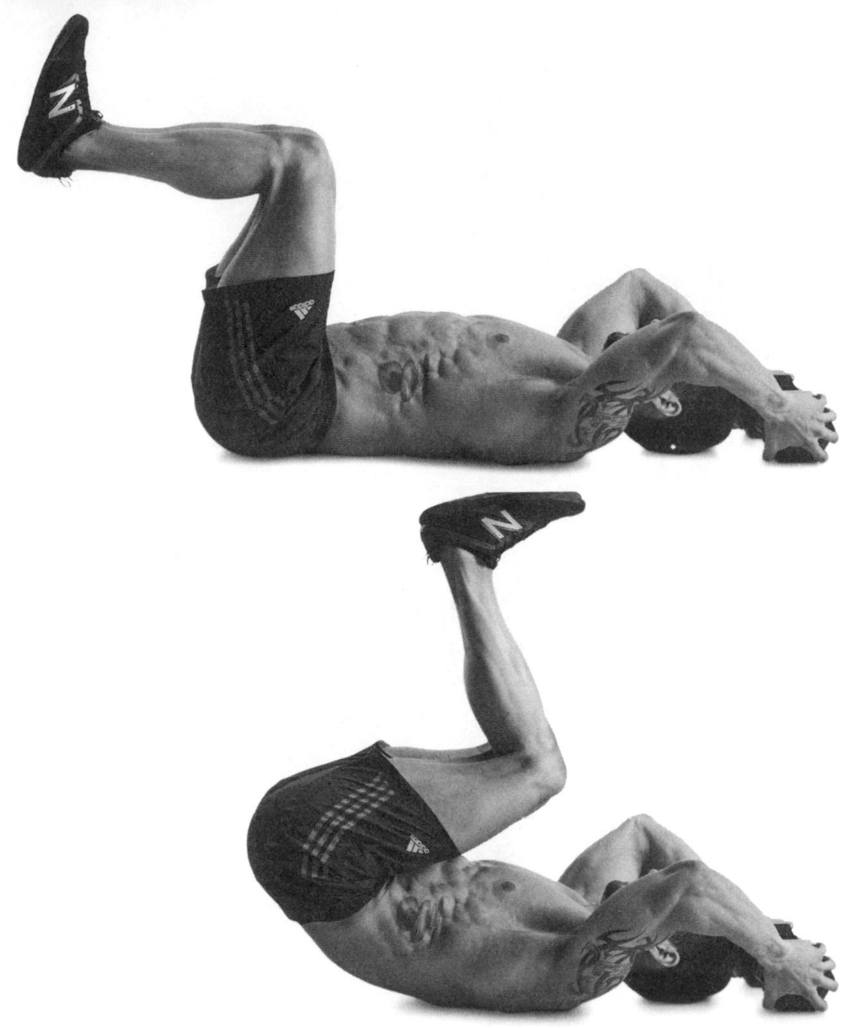

SUPINE REVERSE CRUNCH

PURPOSE

Target the abdominals through hip flexion.

START

Lie faceup on the floor with your hands grasping the ends of a dumbbell over your head. Bend your knees and hips to a 90-degree angle. Keep your feet together and at knee height.

MOVEMENT

Do not lift the dumbbell. Keeping your shoulder blades on the floor, raise your hips and lower back off the floor and crunch your hips inward.

FINISH

Pause, then slowly lower your legs until your heels are just off the floor.

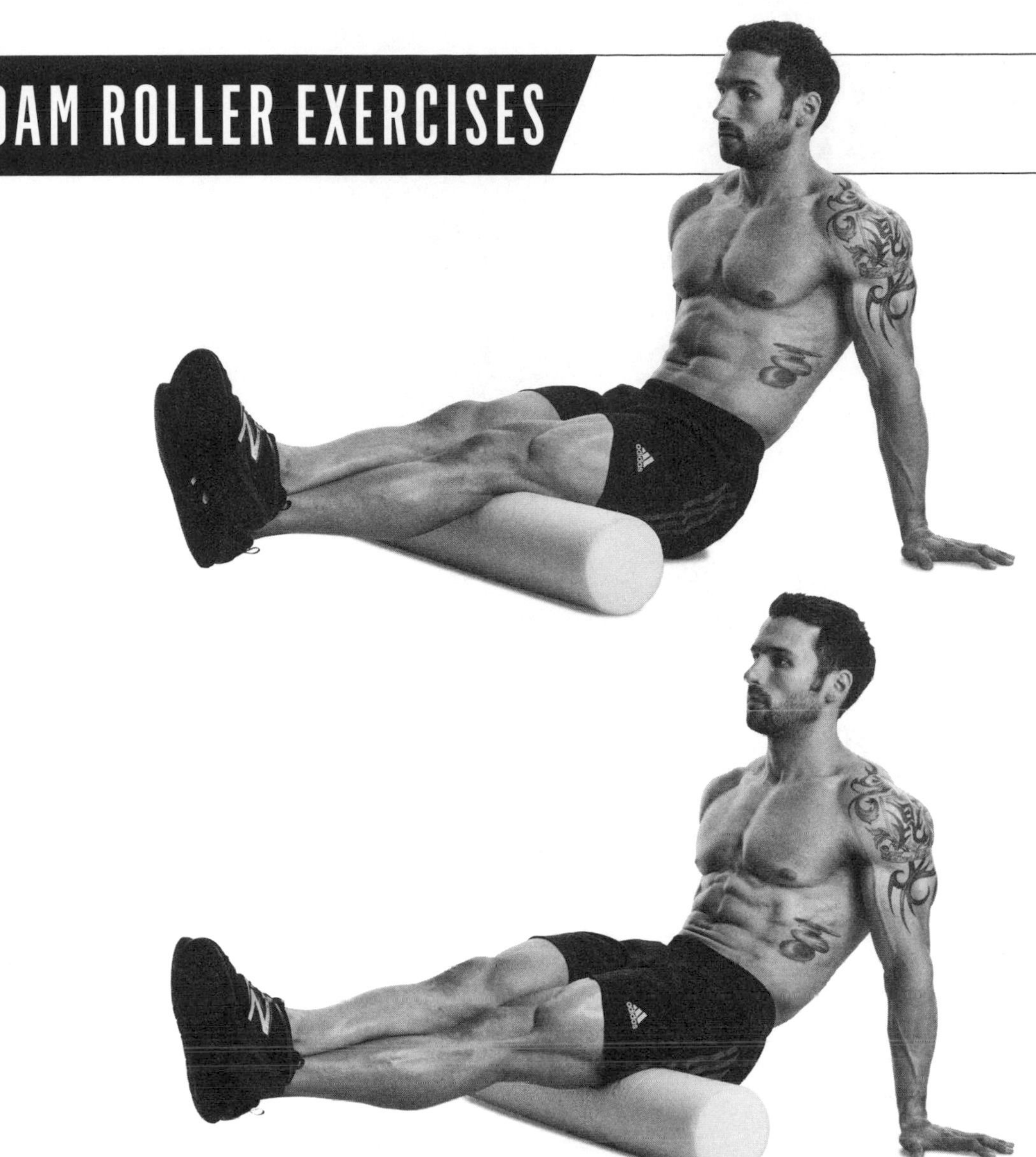

HAMSTRING ROLL

PURPOSE
Loosen connective tissue of the hamstring.

START
Place a foam roller under your left knee with your opposing right leg straight. Cross your right leg over your left ankle. Put your hands flat on the ground behind you.

MOVEMENT
Roll your body forward until the foam roller reaches your glutes. Roll back and forth.

FINISH
Repeat on other side.

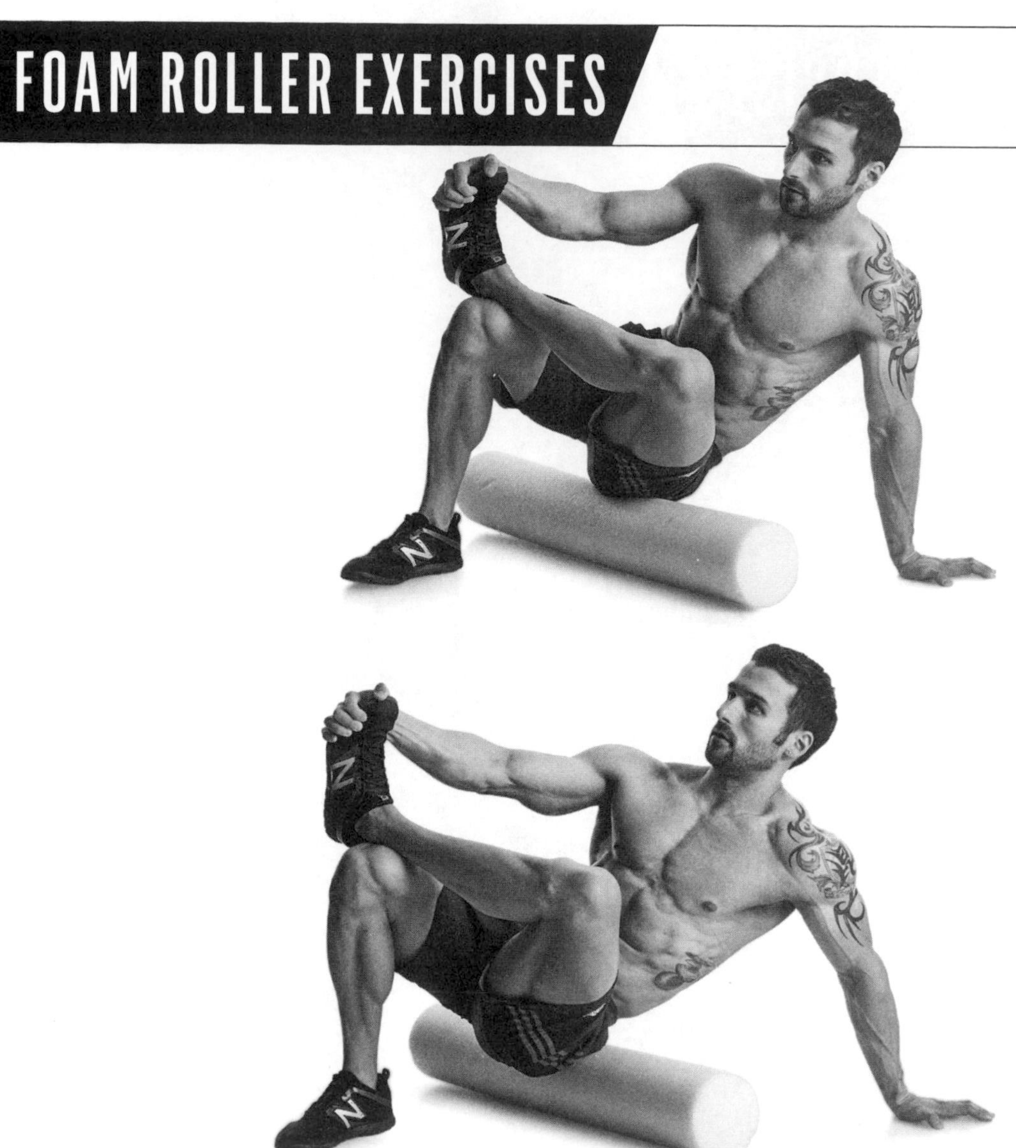

GLUTE (PIRIFORMIS) ROLL

PURPOSE

Loosen connective tissue of the glutes (piriformis).

START

Sit on a foam roller, with it positioned on the back of your left thigh, just below your glutes. Cross your left leg up over the front of your right quad. Keep your left hand flat on the floor for support.

MOVEMENT

Roll your body forward until the foam roller reaches your lower back. Roll back and forth.

FINISH

Repeat on other side.

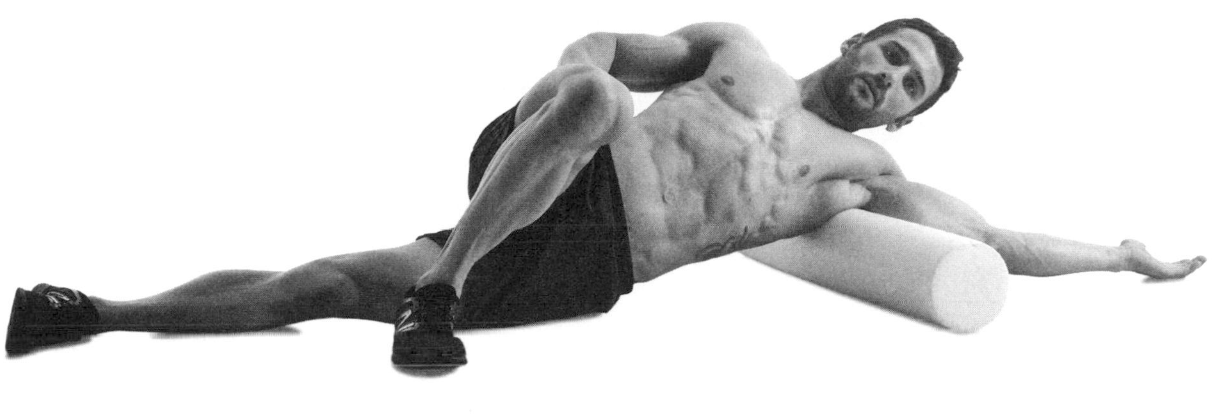

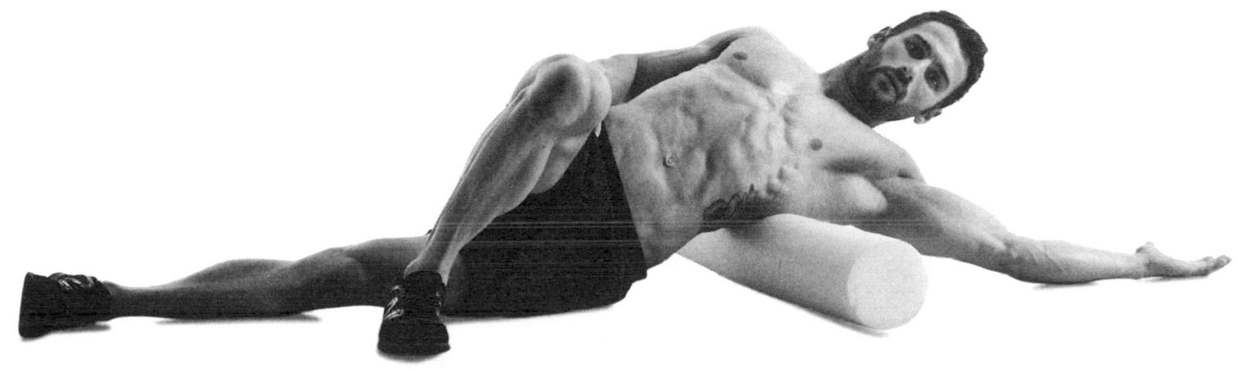

LAT ROLL

PURPOSE

Loosen connective tissue of the lats.

START

Lie on a foam roller on your left side and place your left upper lat on the foam roller. Put your left hand on the floor. Cross your right leg over your left and place your right foot flat on the floor in front of your body.

MOVEMENT

Push your body forward on the foam roller until it reaches your lower lat. Roll back and forth.

FINISH

Repeat on other side.

FOAM ROLLER EXERCISES

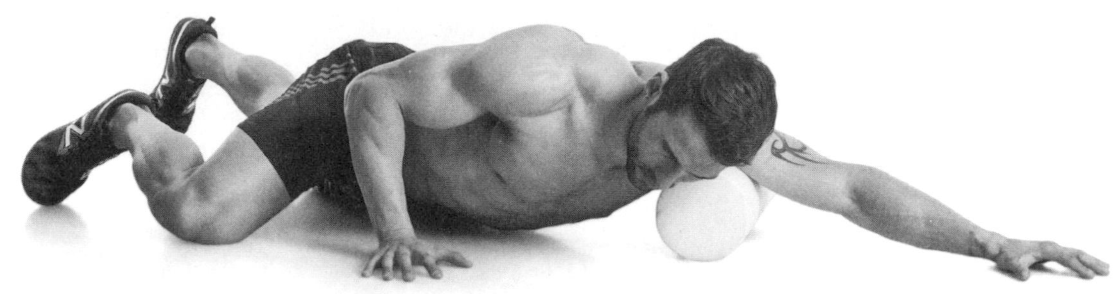

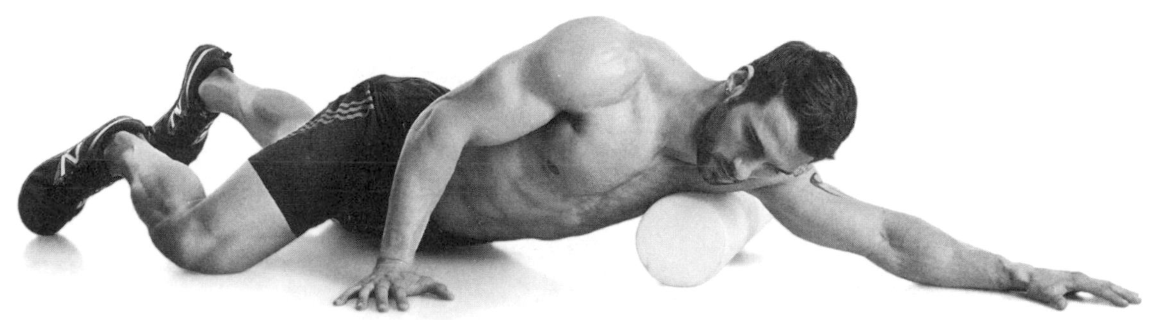

PEC ROLL

PURPOSE

Loosen connective tissue of the pectorals.

START

Lie facedown on a foam roller and place left upper pec (between your armpit and outside chest) on the foam roller. Put your hands on the floor for support. Keep your legs on the ground.

MOVEMENT

Roll your body forward until the foam roller reaches your inner chest. Roll back and forth.

FINISH

Repeat on other side.

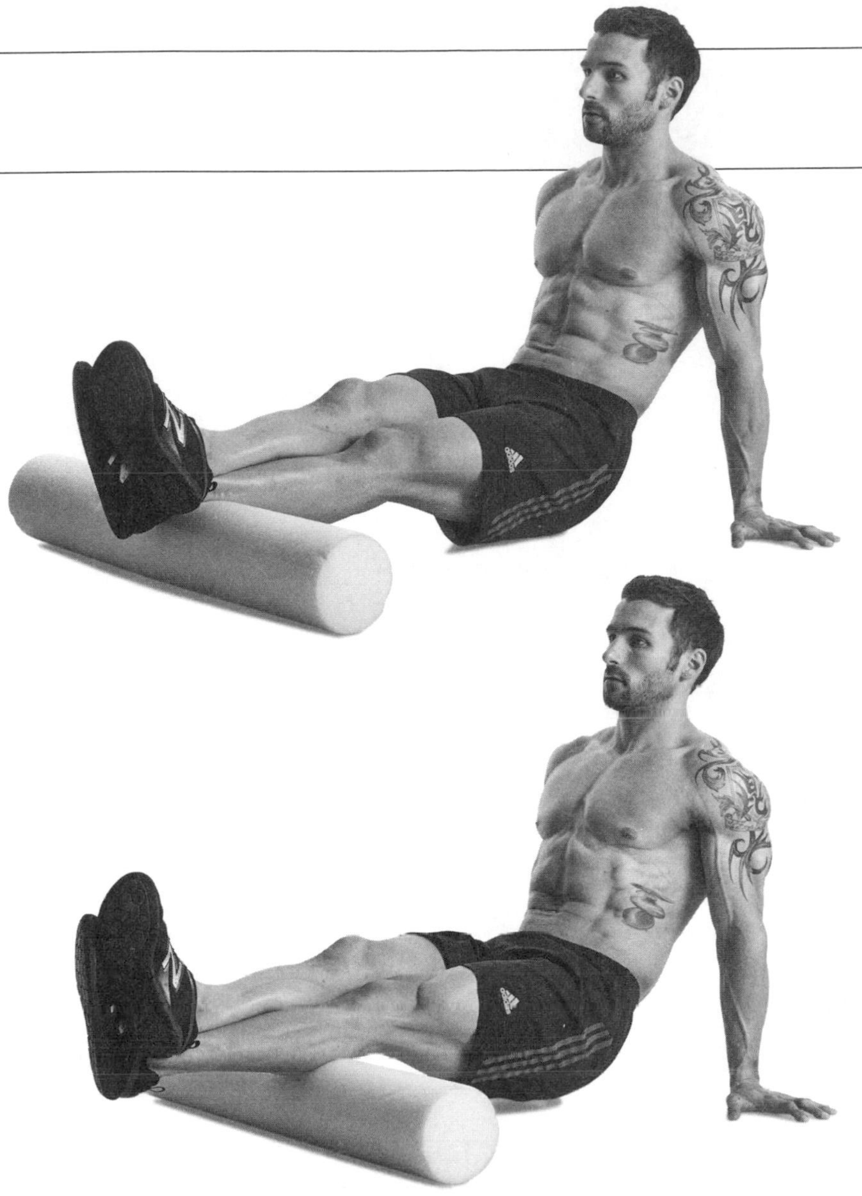

CALF ROLL

PURPOSE

Loosen connective tissue of the calves.

START

Place a foam roller under your left ankle with your left leg straight. Cross your right leg over your left ankle. Place your hands on the ground behind you.

MOVEMENT

Roll your body forward until the foam roller reaches the back of your left knee. Roll back and forth.

FINISH

Repeat on other calf.

FOAM ROLLER EXERCISES

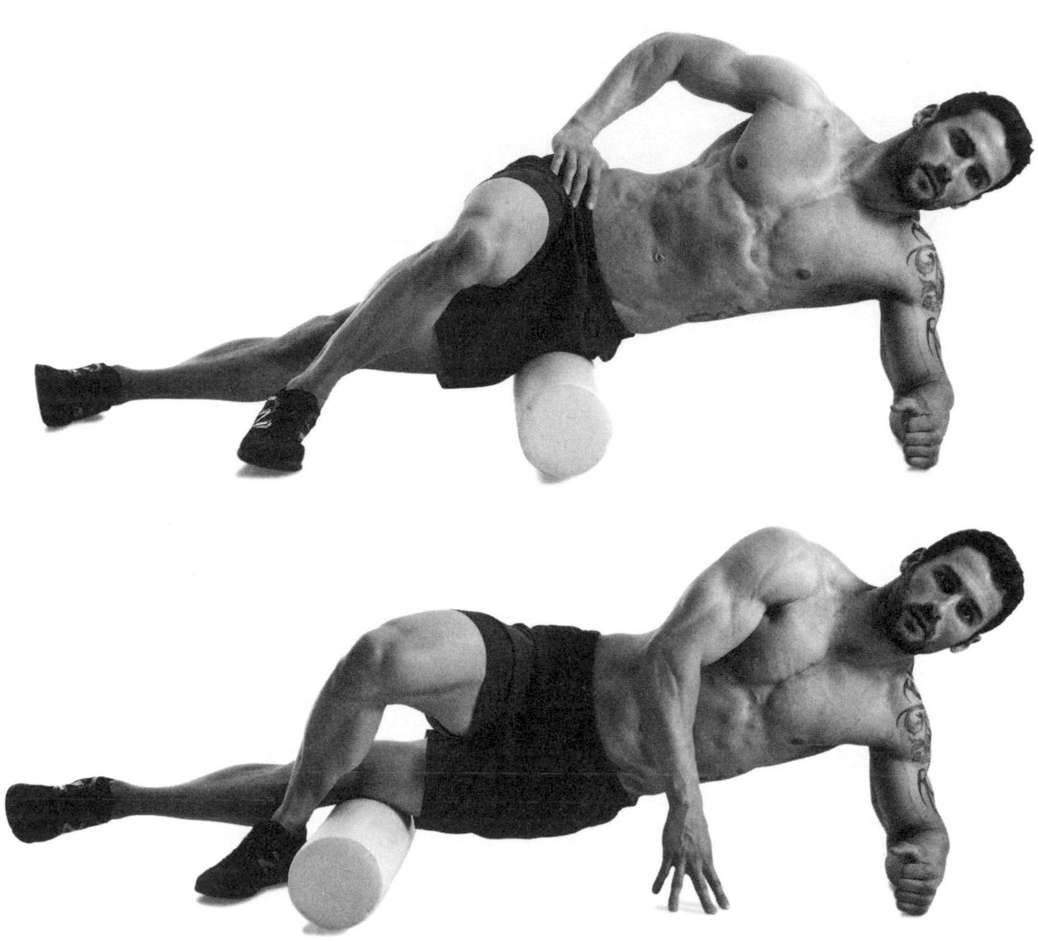

ILIOTIBIAL BAND ROLL

PURPOSE

Loosen connective tissue of the iliotibial band.

START

Lie on a foam roller on your left side and place your left hip on a foam roller. Put your left forearm on the floor for support. Cross your right leg over your left and place your right foot flat on the floor in front of your body.

MOVEMENT

Roll your body forward until the foam roller reaches your knee. Roll back and forth.

FINISH

Repeat on other side.

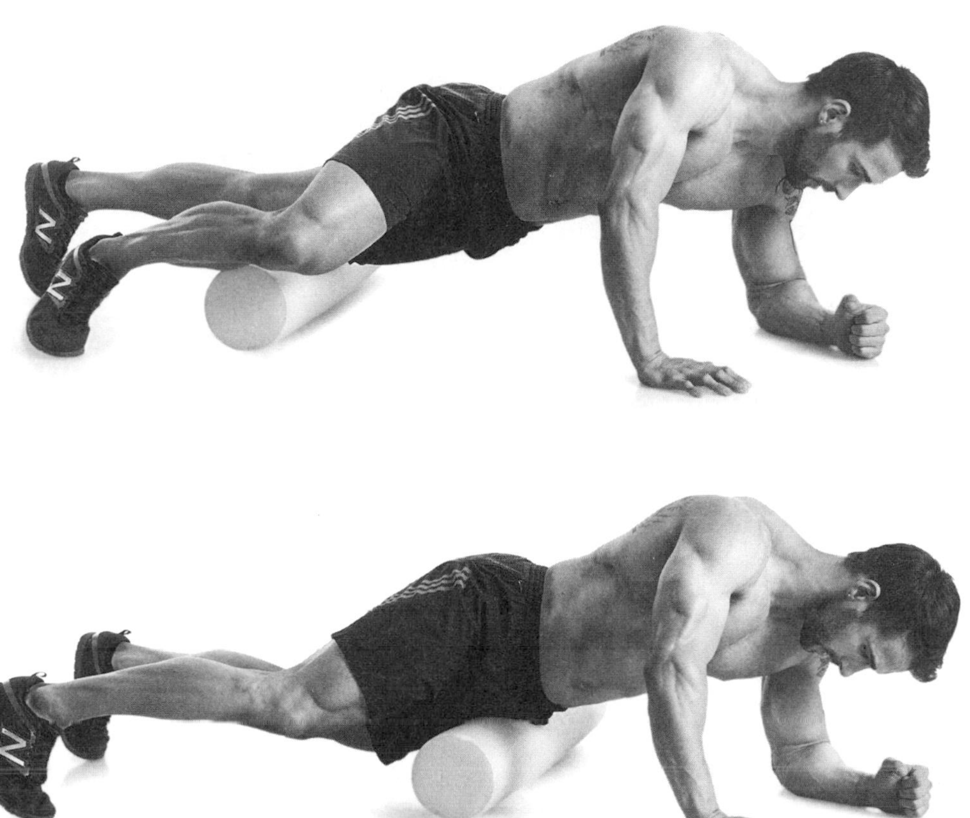

QUADRICEPS ROLL

PURPOSE

Loosen connective tissue of the hips and quadriceps.

START

Lie facedown on the floor with a foam roller positioned above your left knee. Place your left forearm and your right hand on the floor for support.

MOVEMENT

Push your body backward until the foam roller reaches the top of your left quad. Roll back and forth.

FINISH

Repeat on other side.

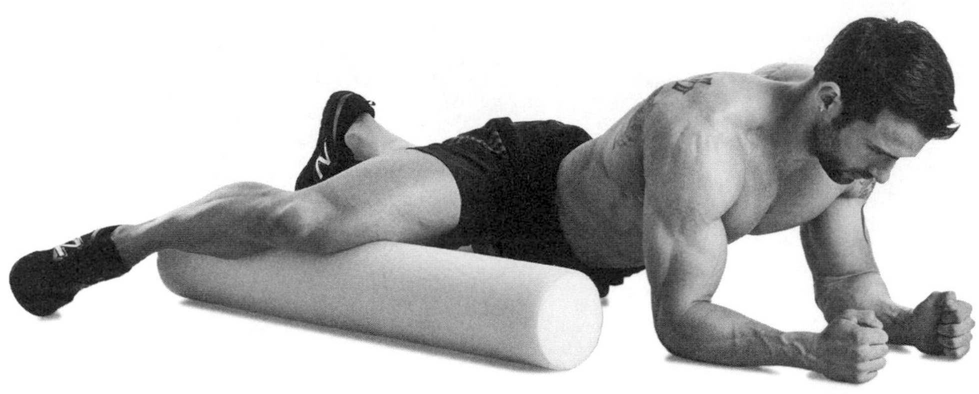

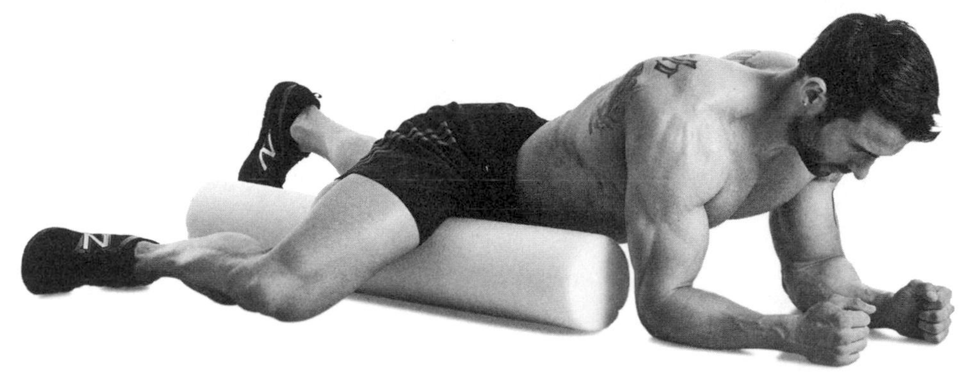

ADDUCTOR (GROIN) ROLL

PURPOSE

Loosen connective tissue of the groin (adductor).

START

Lie facedown on the floor and place the foam roller parallel to your body. Place your forearms on the floor for support. Position your right thigh almost perpendicular to your body, with the inside of your quad on the foam roller, just above the level of your knee. Keep your forearms flat on the floor for support.

MOVEMENT

Roll your body forward until the foam roller reaches your pelvic area. Roll back and forth.

FINISH

Repeat on other side.

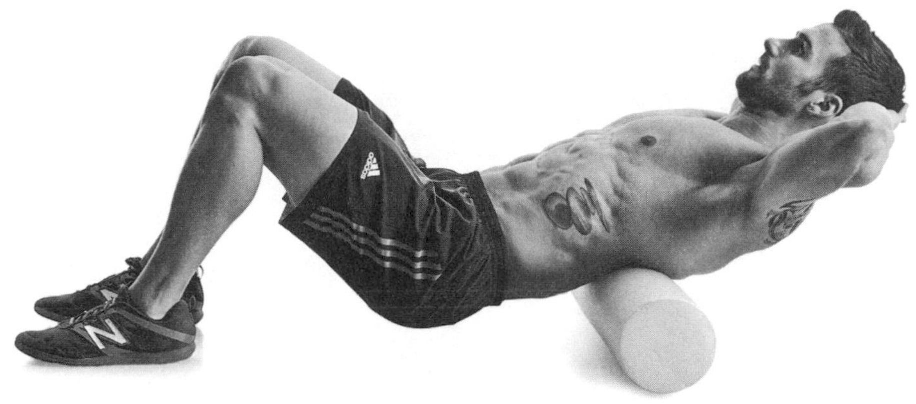

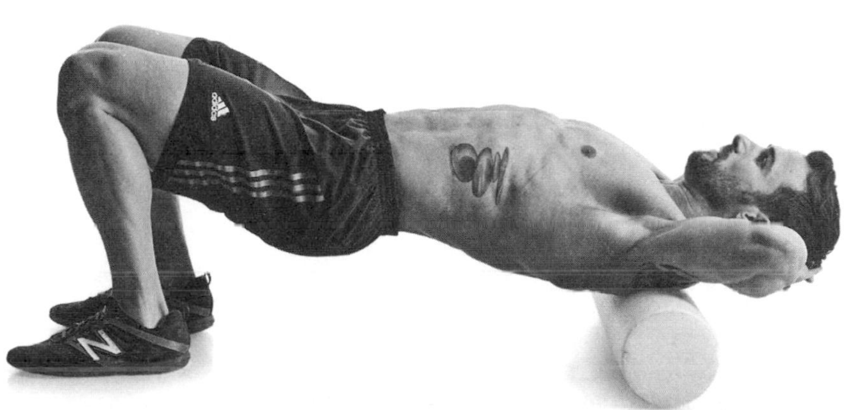

T-SPINE ROLL

PURPOSE

Loosen connective tissue of the thoracic spine.

START

Lie faceup with a foam roller under your mid back (thoracic area) just under your shoulder blades. Cross your hands behind your head and pull your elbows toward one another. Lift your hips off the floor.

MOVEMENT

Roll your body forward until the foam roller reaches your upper back.

FINISH

Roll back and forth a few times.

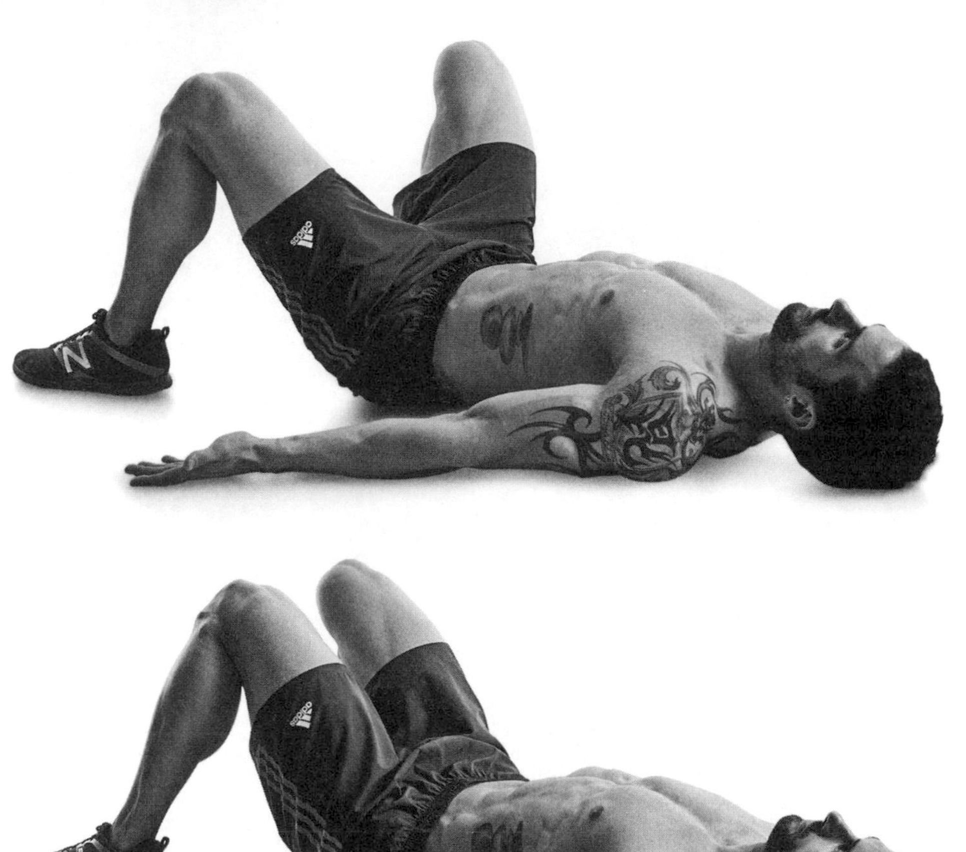

SUPINE HIP INTERNAL ROTATION

PURPOSE

Loosen the muscles of the inner thighs and hips.

START

Lie faceup on the floor with your knees bent at 90 degrees. Your feet should remain flat on the floor and positioned about twice the width of your shoulders.

MOVEMENT

Do not allow your feet to move as you bring your knees inward as far as you can, then hold for 1 to 2 seconds.

FINISH

Return to the starting position.

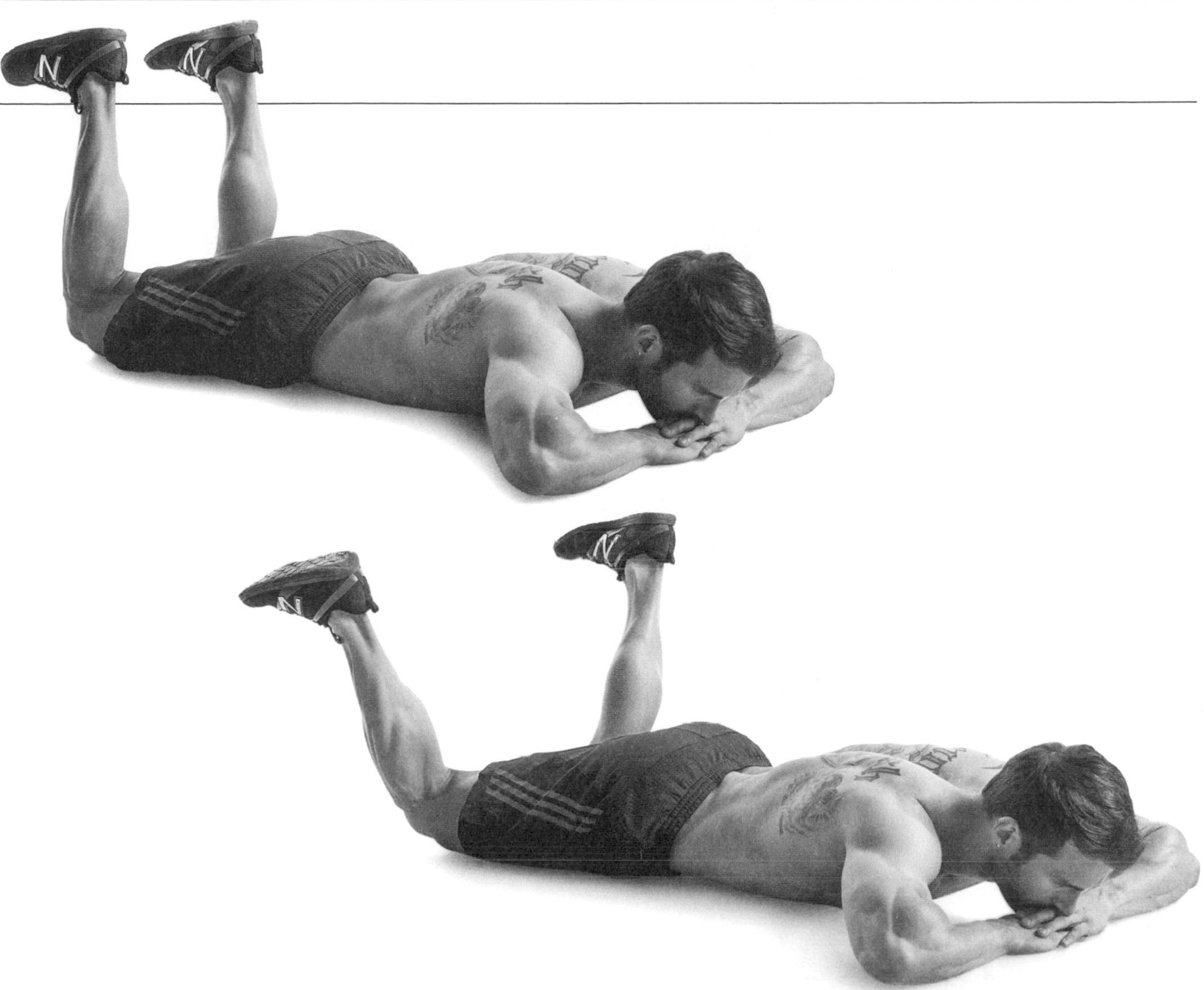

PRONE HIP EXTERNAL ROTATION

PURPOSE
Loosen the muscles of the outer thighs and hips.

START
Lie facedown on the floor with your knees bent at 90 degrees.

MOVEMENT
Do not allow your hips to move off the floor as you lower your feet straight out to the sides as far as you can, then hold for 1 to 2 seconds.

FINISH
Return to the starting position.

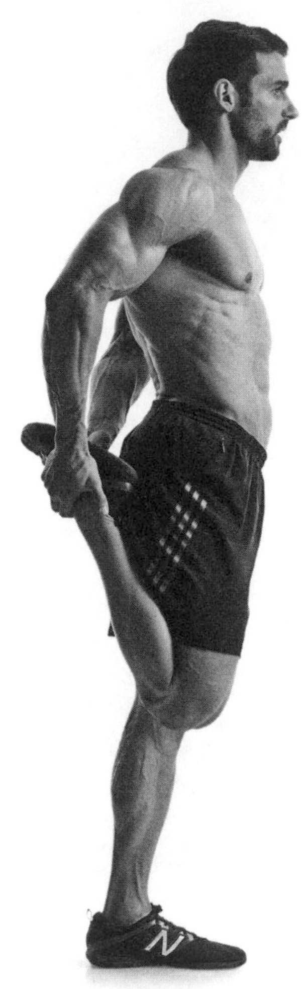

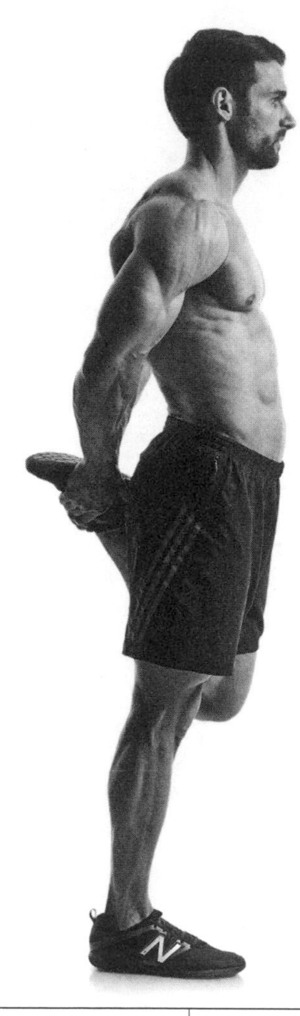

WALKING HEEL TO BUTT

PURPOSE

Loosen the muscles of your quads.

START

Stand tall with your arms at your sides and your feet hip width apart.

MOVEMENT

Step forward with your left leg, then lift your right ankle toward your butt, grasping it with your right hand. Pull your ankle as close to your butt as you can.

FINISH

Release your ankle, take three steps, and then repeat on the other side.

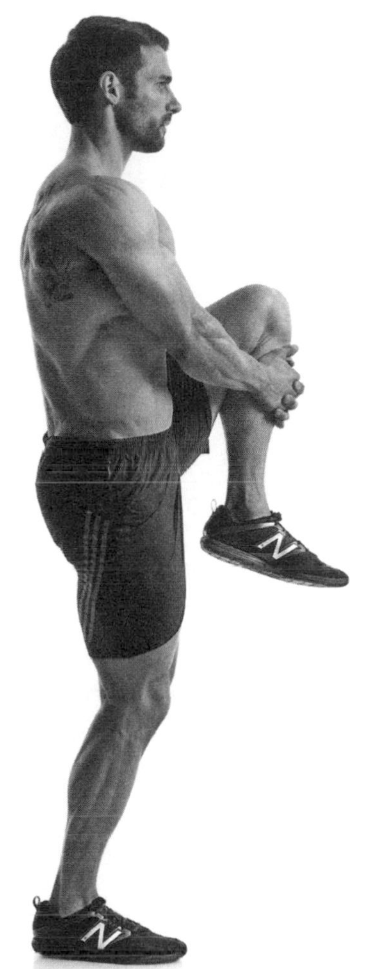

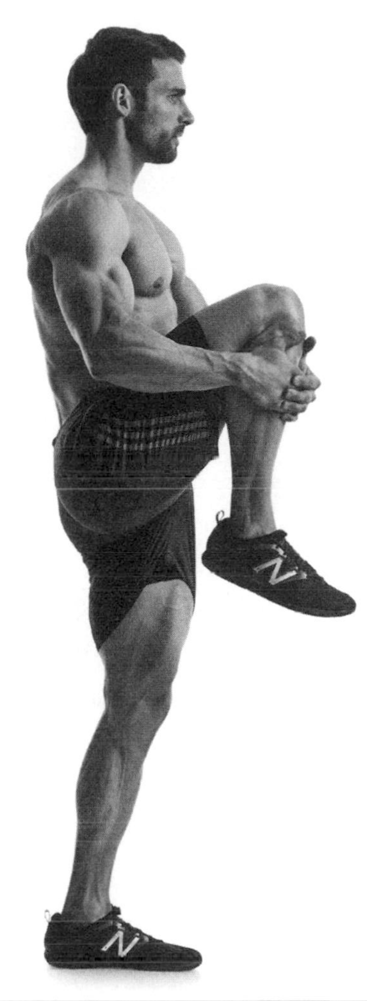

WALKING KNEE HUG

PURPOSE

Loosen the muscles of your glutes and hamstrings.

START

Stand tall with your arms at your sides and your feet hip width apart.

MOVEMENT

Step forward with your right leg and lean slightly forward at your hips. Lift your left knee toward your chest, grasping it with both hands just below your kneecap. Then pull it as close to your chest as you can while continuing to stand tall.

FINISH

Release your leg, take three steps forward, and then repeat on the other side.

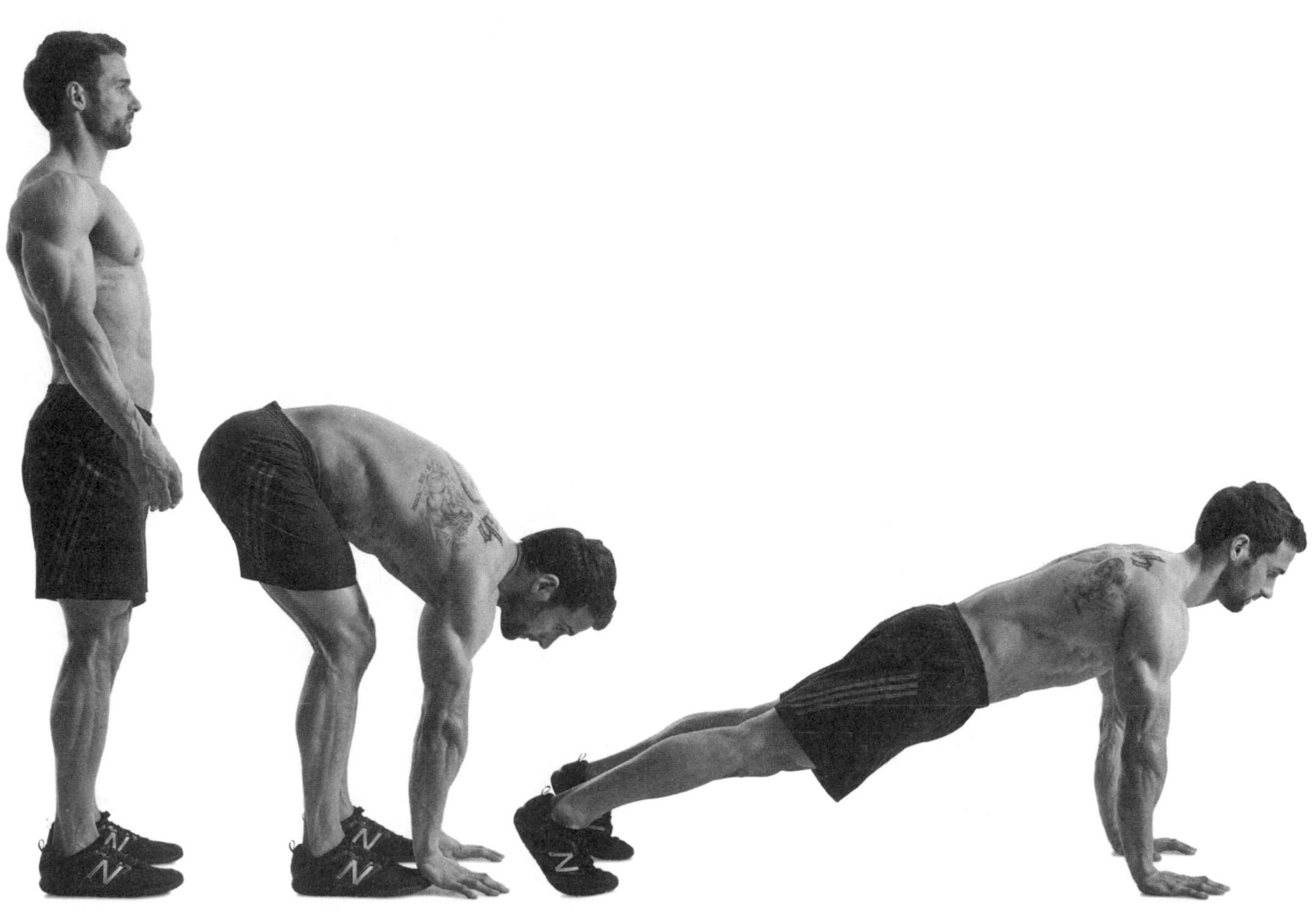

INCHWORM

PURPOSE
Loosen the muscles of your quads, hips, and obliques.

START
Stand tall with your arms at your sides and your feet hip width apart.

MOVEMENT
Bend over and touch the floor with your hands. Maintain straight legs and walk your hands forward. Then take tiny steps to walk your feet forward to your hands. Brace your core and walk your hands out as far as you can, then walk your feet forward.

FINISH
Repeat this motion for the desired number of repetitions.

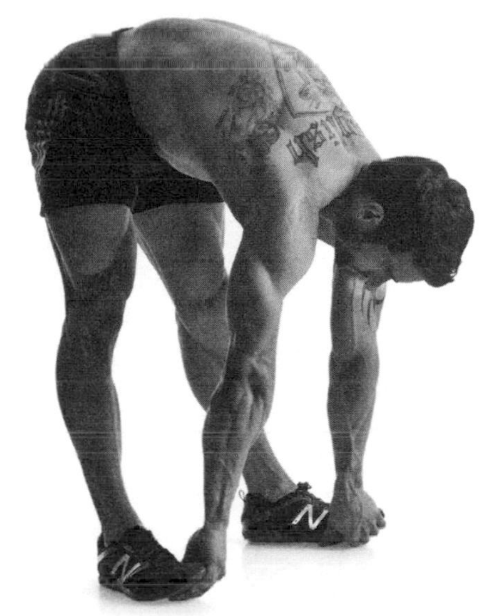

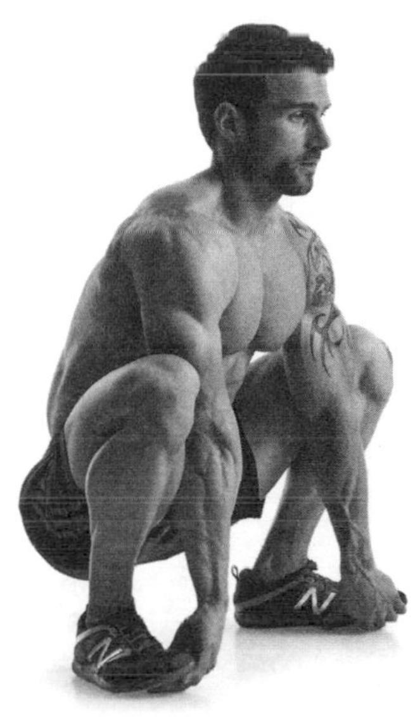

SUMO SQUAT TO STAND

PURPOSE

Loosen the muscles of your quads, hamstrings, glutes, adductors, and lower back.

START

Stand tall with your arms at your sides and your feet hip width apart.

MOVEMENT

Keeping your legs straight, bend over and grab your toes. Without letting go of your toes, lower your body into a squat as you raise your chest and shoulders.

FINISH

Stand up.

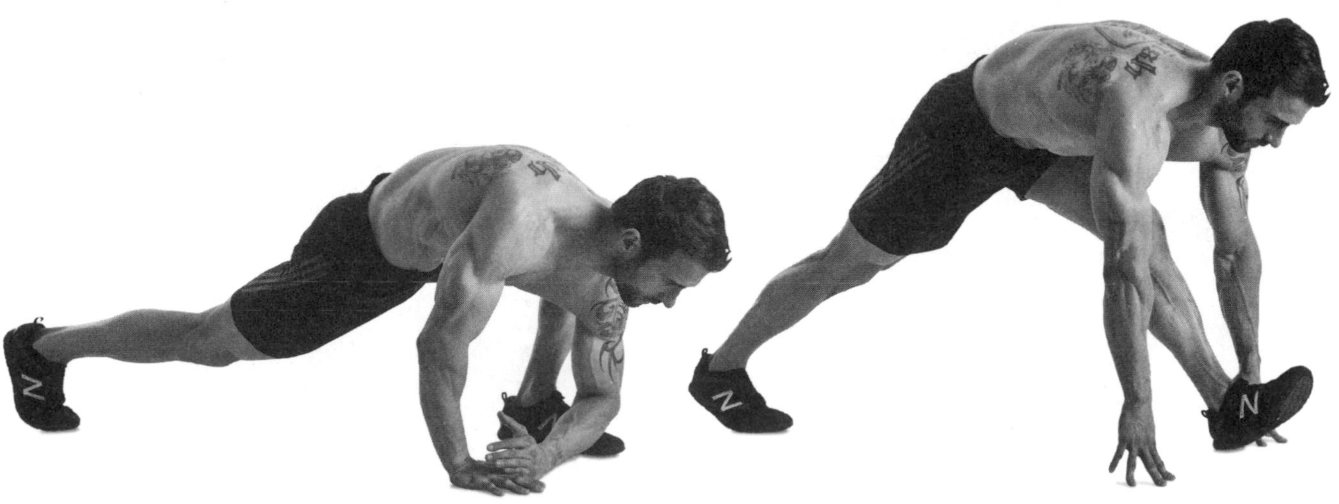

FOREARM TO INSTEP LUNGE

PURPOSE
Loosen the muscles of your quads, hamstrings, glutes, and adductor.

START
Stand tall with your arms at your sides and your feet hip width apart.

MOVEMENT
Brace your core and lunge forward with your left leg. When you lunge, lean forward at your hips and place your right hand on the floor so that it's even with your left foot. Place your left elbow next to the instep of your left foot (get as close as you can) and hold for 2 seconds. Then straighten your left leg and lift your toes to stretch your hamstrings. Support yourself with your fingers.

FINISH
Step forward with your right leg and repeat.

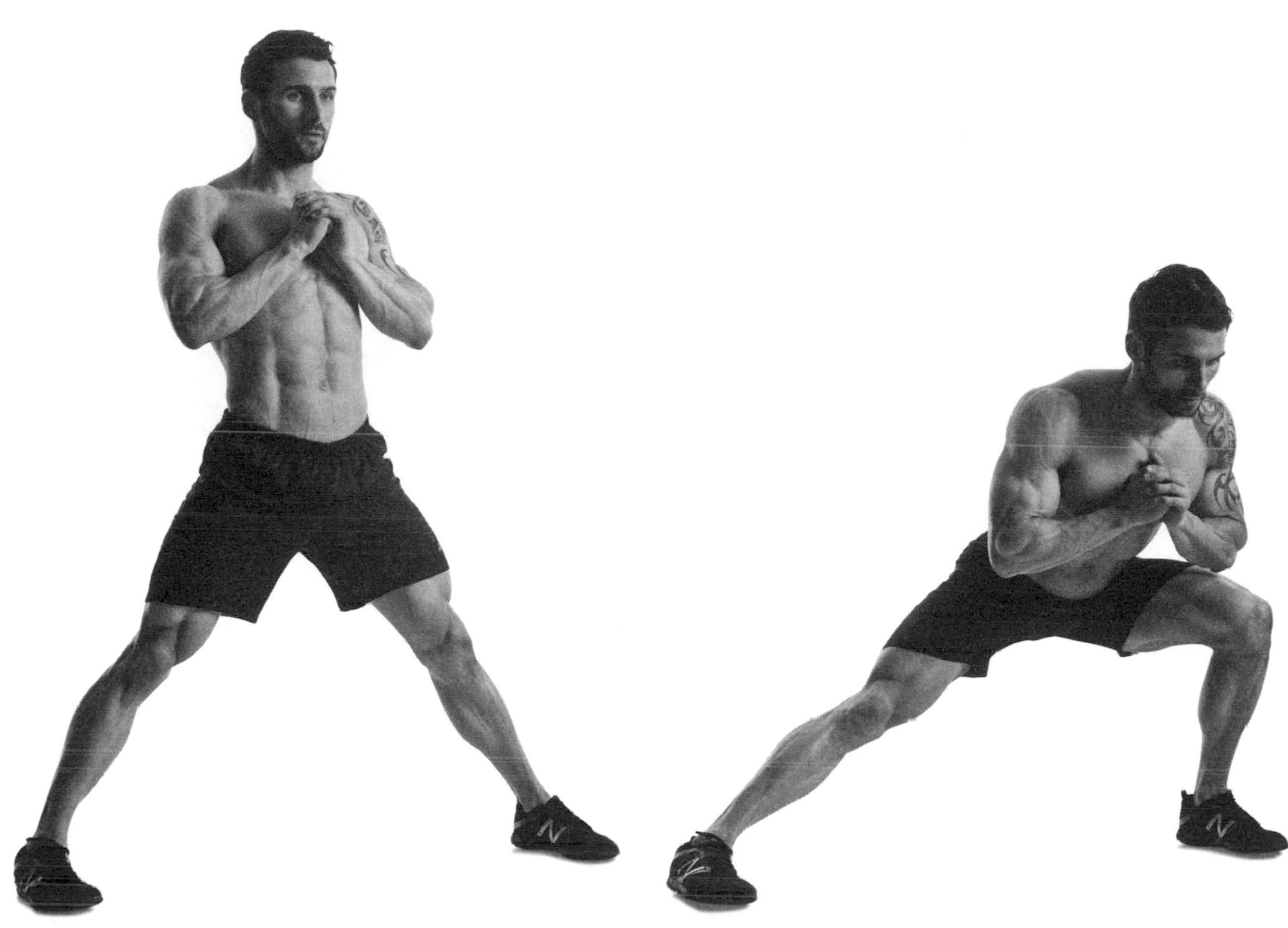

LATERAL LUNGE

PURPOSE

Increase the mobility of your hips and loosen the muscles of your glutes and adductors.

START

Stand tall with your feet twice shoulder width apart and facing straight ahead. Clasp your hands in front of your chest.

MOVEMENT

Shift your weight over the left leg as you push your hips backward and lower your body by dropping your hips and bending your left knee. Your lower left leg should remain perpendicular to the floor. Your right foot should remain flat on the floor.

FINISH

Raise yourself back up and complete the desired number of reps before switching sides.

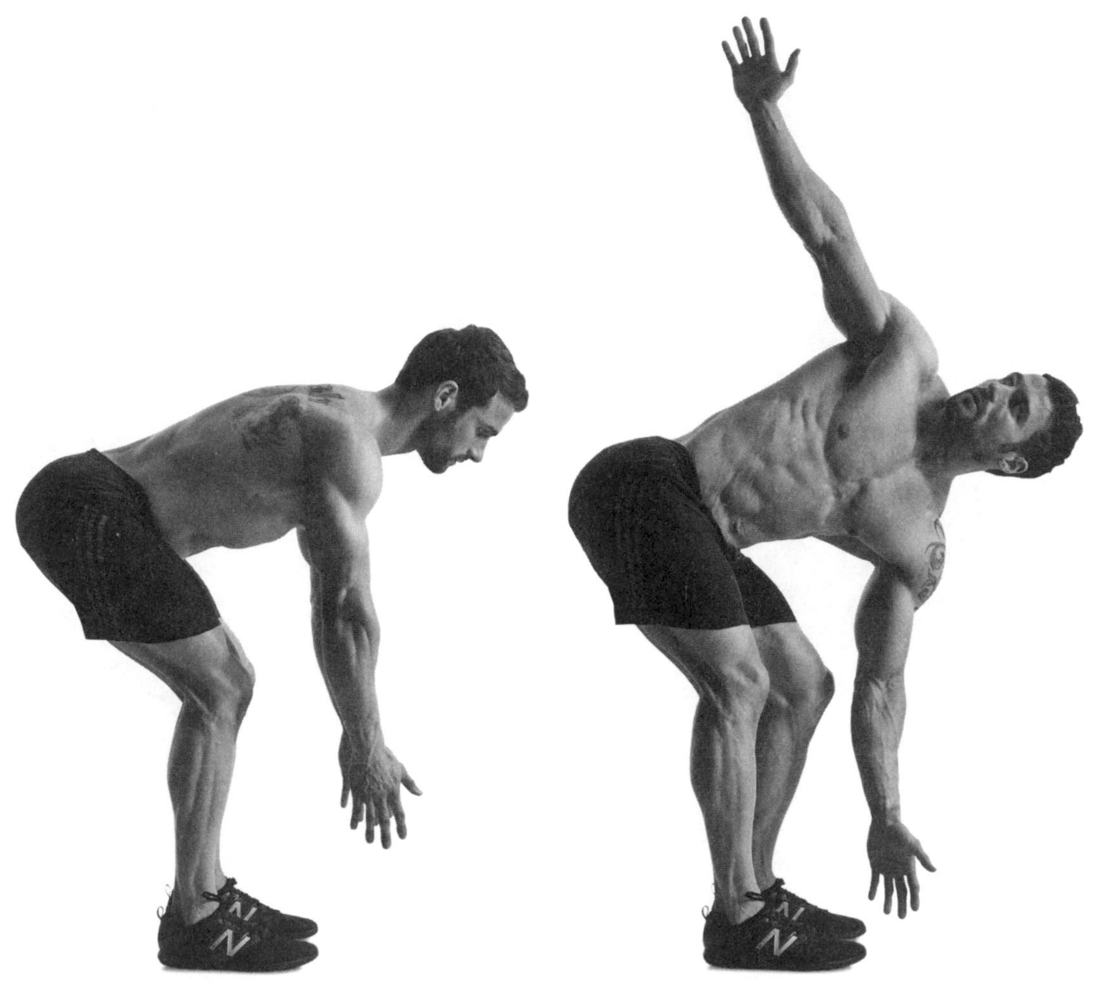

BENT-OVER T-SPINE MOBILITY

PURPOSE
Increase the mobility of your thoracic spine and upper back.

START
Keeping your lower back in a natural arch, bend at the hips and knees and lower your torso until it's almost parallel to the floor. Let your arms hang straight down from your shoulders, palms facing each other.

MOVEMENT
Brace your core and rotate your torso to the right as you reach as high as you can with your right arm.

FINISH
Pause, then reverse the movement to your left.

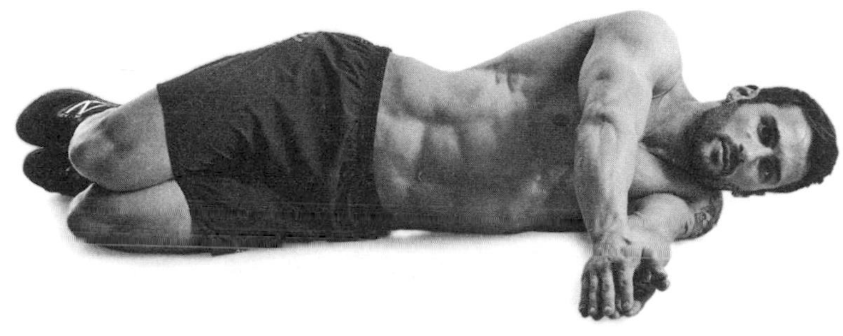

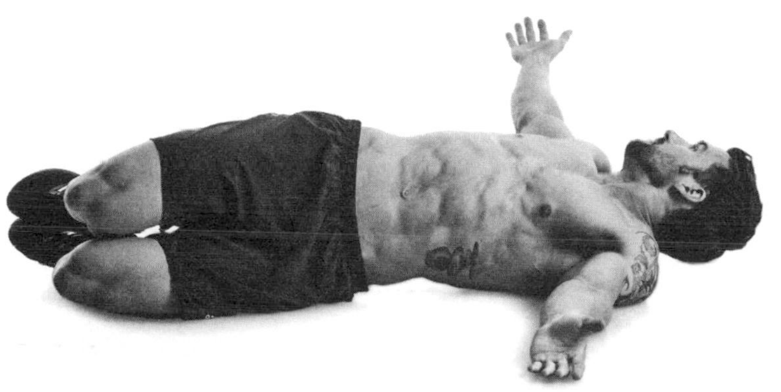

SIDE-LYING THORACIC ROTATION

PURPOSE

Increase the mobility of your thoracic spine and middle and upper back.

START

Lie on your side on the floor, with your hips and knees bent at 90 degrees. Straighten both arms in front of you at your shoulder height, palms touching each other.

MOVEMENT

Keeping your left arm and both legs in position, rotate your right arm up and over your body and rotate your torso to the right, until your right hand and upper back are flat on the floor. Hold for 2 seconds.

FINISH

Return your arm, and complete the desired of reps, and then turn over and do the same thing on the other side.

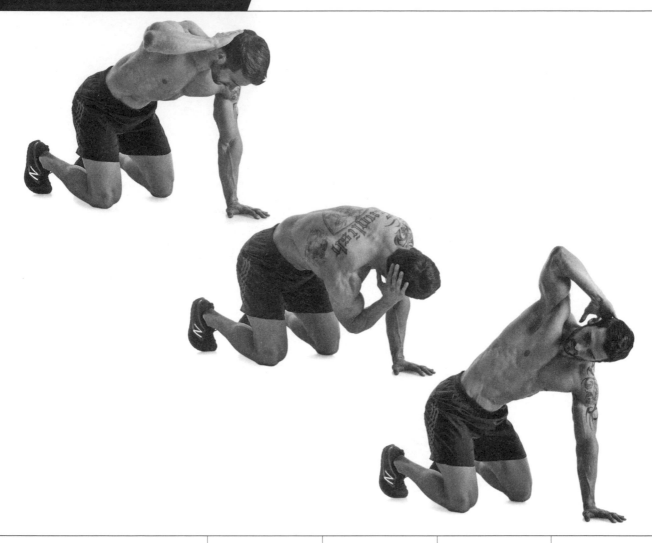

QUADRUPED THORACIC ROTATION

PURPOSE
Increase the mobility of your thoracic spine and upper back.

START
Get on the floor on all fours. Place your right hand behind your head. Brace your core.

MOVEMENT
Rotate your upper back downward so your elbow is pointed down and to your left. Raise your right elbow toward the ceiling by rotating your head and upper back up and to the right as far as possible.

FINISH
Complete the desired number of reps, then do the same thing on your left.

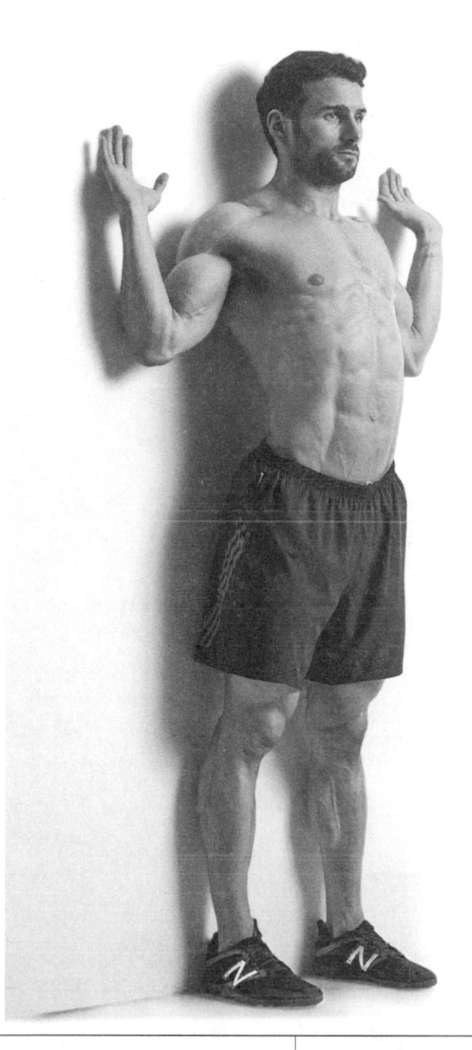

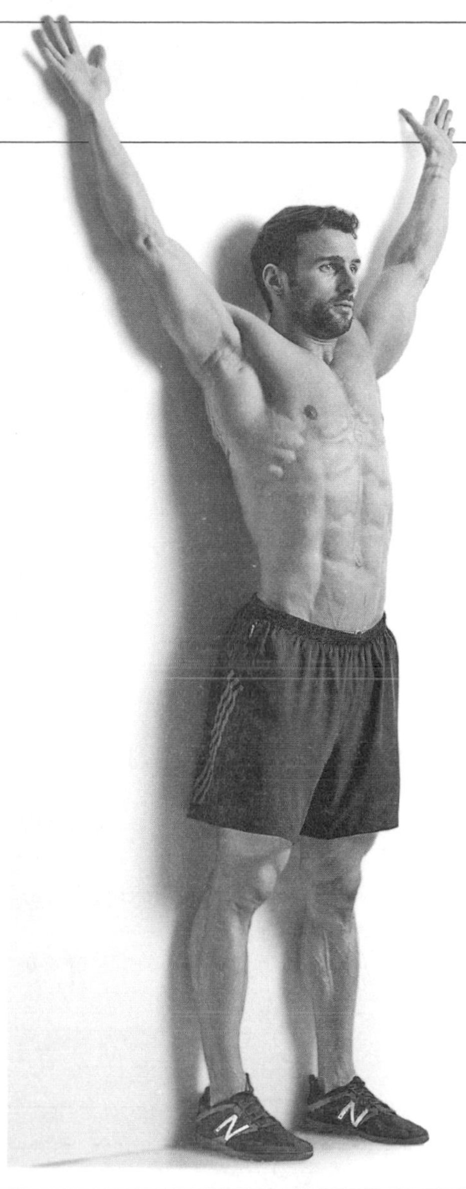

SCAPULAR WALL SLIDE

PURPOSE
Increase the function of your shoulders.

START
Lean your head, upper back, and upper butt against a wall. Place your hands and arms against the wall.

MOVEMENT
Keeping your elbows, wrists, and hands pressed against the wall, slide your elbows down toward your sides as far as you can as shown in the first photograph.

FINISH
Squeeze your shoulder blades together. Slide your arms back up the wall as high as you can while maintaining contact with the wall.

PART 3

CHAPTER 11

The Importance of Cardiovascular Workouts

For extreme lean and good health, metabolic training is a must.

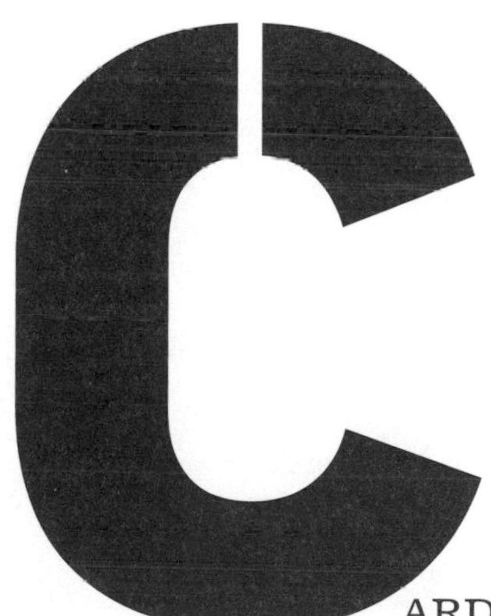

CARDIO WORKOUTS, TO A LOT of bodybuilders, are like kissing your aunt Babushka from the old country—something you'd really like to avoid, but something you're required to do. By and large, bodybuilders hate cardio. Old-school bodybuilders never did much of it because they didn't like it or feel it was beneficial. Some even believed it hurt their muscle-building efforts. Even today it's safe to say if bodybuilders can achieve their desired look through training and diet, they'd nix cardio. But skipping cardio work during the contest preparation will make achieving your desired body-fat level nearly impossible unless you happen to be a freakishly lean ectomorph with an extremely fast metabolism.

The great debate in the bodybuilding world surrounding cardio is whether you should perform cardio at low intensity or high intensity. Even more heavily debated is when the two styles should be performed in conjunction with certain dieting strategies and strength-training workouts.

Let's first consider some facts. Strength training is your number one way to spare muscle glycogen and burn body fat. Strength training in all its different forms has been proven through research to increase your body's calorie burning potential, through a phenomenon known as excess post-exercise oxygen consumption (EPOC). Another term for EPOC is *after-burn,* which describes the calories expended beyond the resting metabolic rate after a bout of intense exercise. The metabolic disturbance caused by all the chemical reactions happening as your body returns to its pre-exercise state—reactions such as lactate removal, increased blood circulation, higher body temperature, and increased oxygen consumption—elevates metabolism and boosts calorie burn while sparing muscle mass. Depending on intensity of effort and your own metabolism, it generally takes between 15 minutes and 48 hours for the body to fully return to a resting metabolism. That's great news for anyone who wants to drop body fat, especially the bodybuilder. But it still doesn't mean that a bodybuilder in contest-prep mode can eliminate cardio training. Diet and weight lifting alone won't do it all. For a bodybuilder to reach optimum body-fat levels of 6 to 3 percent, cardiovascular training must be performed.

But which type of cardio is best? Many bodybuilders assume that low-intensity cardio is the way to go because it's aerobic and as such burns more body fat. High-intensity cardio is characterized as anaerobic because it taps fast-burning glucose stores for fuel. Studies comparing the two have shown that high-intensity cardio burns fewer overall calories but results in more fat lost and muscle spared.

As a person who has utilized both protocols during contest preparation, I'm not here to start a debate. What I can tell you through personal experience and coaching is that high-intensity cardiovascular work is superior and needs to be utilized by the dieting bodybuilder in order to speed up the body-fat-burning process.

A key component to high-intensity cardio is the way the body responds to this training style. Just as strength training does, high-intensity cardio increases your body's insulin sensitivity and causes the release of more growth hormone, IGF-1, and testosterone but without the central nervous system fatigue associated with resistance training. So, your first choice should be high-intensity cardio work. But there are benefits to be reaped from aerobic training, too, if you can fit that into your workout schedule as well.

The best times to perform high-intensity cardiovascular work are on non-strength-training days. Treat the session just as you would a strength-training session, that is, follow the same pre- and post-workout nutrition plan.

The Bodybuilder's Beginning Cardio Prescription

Here again, your body type plays a critical role in your cardio plan of choice.

Ectomorph

Frequency: 3 sessions per week
Length of session: 20 to 30 minutes
Do 1 to 2 sessions as high-intensity cardio

Mesomorph

Frequency: 4 to 5 sessions per week
Length of session: 20 to 30 minutes
Do 2 to 3 sessions as high-intensity cardio

Endomorph

Frequency: 5 to 7 sessions per week
Length of session: 20 to 45 minutes
Do 2 to 3 sessions as high-intensity cardio

Ranking the Different Forms of Cardio

From highest to lowest calorie after-burn or EPOC:

#1: Metabolic Resistance Training (MRT)
What it is: MRT is an intense lifting style that combines aerobic and anaerobic training in an efficient workout that torches calories and will test your cardiovascular endurance. It can be done as circuits, supersets (using compound movements), but it is primarily characterized by very short rest periods.
What it does: An effectively designed strength-training program will create an increase in excess post-exercise oxygen consumption (EPOC) or metabolic disturbance following the workout. MRT promotes the body to maintain lean muscle mass while elevating the post-exercise metabolism.
When to use: If you only have 3 to 4 hours a week to train, perform as part of your strength-training program. Use with alternating sets, tri-sets, or quad-sets.
Specifics: Intensity is key—work can best be performed by following a form of periodization.

#2: High-Intensity Anaerobic Interval Training (HIIT)
What it is: Also known as HIIT, it involves alternating between short bursts of high-intensity effort and recovery segments at lower intensity. For example: In a HIIT running workout, after warming up, you might sprint at an intensity level of 8 out of 10 for 30 seconds followed by 30 seconds of recovery-level jogging (maybe a 4 or 5) and continue to alternate this way for the duration of your run.
What it does: HIIT much like MRT increases EPOC following a training session. HIIT will burn calories during and after the session. Studies show it promotes similar hormonal responses in the body as strength training.
When to use: Do this cardio workout on non-strength-training days if you have 4 to 6 hours to devote to your contest training per week.
Specifics: Be sure to follow up work periods with at equal or longer rest periods, that is, 15 seconds of work, 30 seconds of rest; 30 seconds of work, 30 seconds of rest; 30 seconds of work, 60 seconds of recovery.

#3: High-Intensity Aerobic Training
What it is: Steady state aerobic training, this is sustained at a fairly intense level for a moderate period of time. In other words, it is training at a non-fluctuating or constant speed at high-effort level.
What it does: High-intensity aerobic training will burn more calories than a low-intensity aerobic training session of equal time but won't promote muscle mass or elevate your metabolism following the session.
When to use: If you can devote 6 hours per week in addition to strength training, perform this on non-strength-training days or after a lower-intensity strength session.
Specifics: Work periods will mostly be performed with intervals greater than 45 seconds and up to 5 minutes. For example—bike intervals of 2 minutes of intense work followed by 2 minutes of recovery.

#4: Low-Intensity Aerobic Training
What it is: Steady-state aerobic training, this is sustained at a low-intensity level for a longer period of time.
What it does: Low-intensity aerobic training will burn calories—possibly a good number of calories, depending on how long you perform a session—but it won't help promote muscle mass or elevate your metabolism.
When to use: Only if you are one of those freaks who can devote about 8 hours of cardio training in addition to your strength training, perform this as part of your workout on strength-training and non-strength-training days.
Specifics: This is true aerobic training: running, walking, or riding a bike at a steady pace for 30 minutes to an hour. This puts you in what's called "the fat burning zone" because your intensity is only 60 to 65 percent of your maximum effort.

PART 4

The Competition Phase

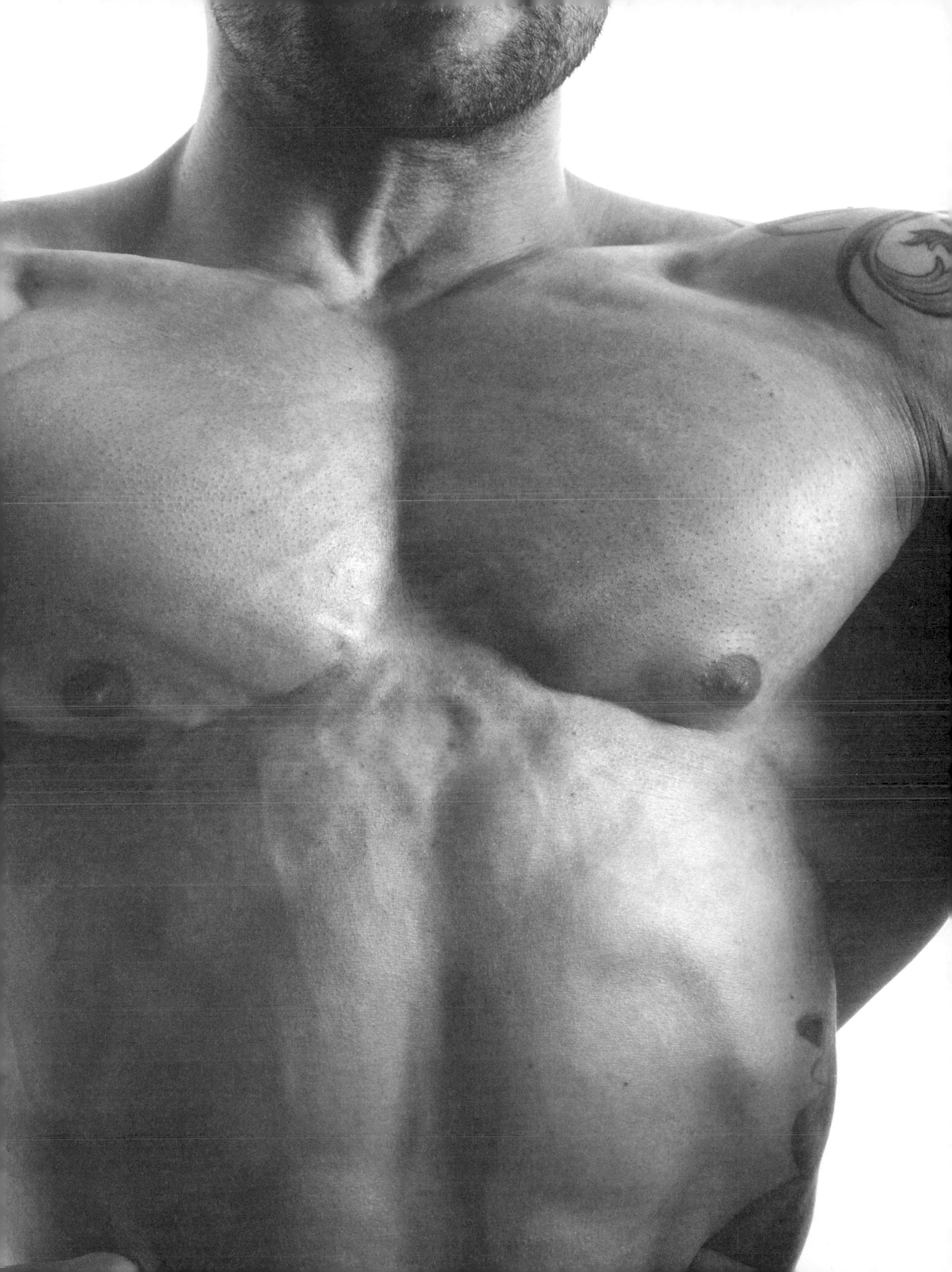

PART 4

CHAPTER 12

The Final Push

How to tweak your training and diet during the last weeks

CONGRATULATIONS. YOU made it this far. You've been diligent. You've worked hard. You're stronger and leaner. You've become an expert nutritionist without the registered dietician degree. Now, don't freak out.

That's what a lot of first-timers do when they get this far along in a bodybuilding program as they prep for their first contest. Instead, pat yourself on the back. Recognize your accomplishment and give yourself some credit. And be realistic. Look, the most dramatic increases in strength and muscle growth occur at the start of a training program. A lot of those initial gains have come from the rewiring of your central nervous system. Now you are beyond that, so don't expect dramatic changes in these final weeks before competition. Now is the time to assess and tweak. There's still much work to do and lots of detail-oriented preparation. And I even have some suggestions for recreating that initial nervous system shock that'll recruit more muscle fibers so you'll be able to maximize your muscle size and definition just before the event. But first, let's review some of the key tenets of bodybuilding as you assess where you've taken your body so far.

The Importance of Condition

How do you look in front of the mirror? Don't worry if you aren't exactly where you want to be. For many bodybuilders their first competition may not bring out their top condition. Usually this is due to not giving themselves enough time to allow their body to reach the top-end condition weeks before competition. I've been guilty of it in my early competition years, as have many other natural bodybuilders. Remember, you are learning. This is a process, a stage to go through in a long journey. Anything worthwhile requires time, practice, making mistakes, and learning from mistakes. Can you play guitar? Were you able to improvise a solo before learning the chords to "This Land Is Your Land"?

Give yourself time to learn and grow. This may be your first contest, but it won't be your last. Learn from it. Part of that learning process is recognizing the truth in what I said back in the beginning of this book: The longer a bodybuilder spends dieting, the greater his chances at achieving the leanest physique possible, full dense muscle, tighter skin, and a consistent and more predictable body. All this is critical to bring you to this stage in contest prep and allow you to make key adjustments leading up to "peak week," the 7 days before the contest.

"Your Peak Week will mean nothing, if you're not lean enough."

—Dr. Joe Klemczewski

Bodybuilders are judged on symmetry, muscularity, and conditioning. A bodybuilder who has come in lean enough can often seem more symmetrical and more muscular when his condition is top-notch. The only way to get lean enough, in my experience, is to track my progress through the practice of food logging.

For many newbie bodybuilders the thought of tracking their every macronutrient can seem daunting. So let's say you choose not to track your food during your contest preparation. I can tell you with full confidence that you're setting yourself up for disappointment.

"Tracking your daily food consumption, isn't just about numbers," says Dr. Klemczewski. "It's about physiology."

Making the commitment to keep a consistent track record of your daily protein, carbohydrates, fat, and calories will set a strong foundation for your progress and ultimately your success throughout each week of contest preparation.

Did you track your daily food? If not, there's not a lot you can do about it now, but learn from this experience. It is that crucial to bodybuilding.

Expect to Make Mistakes

No contest preparation is without error, but leaving room for inevitable error should be a key goal during your journey. Leaving room for error is what can help separate a top-3 finish from a top-5 finish. The subjectivity of the sport of bodybuilding is so crucial that giving yourself the opportunity to slip up early on in your preparation will only allow you the time and work needed to make adjustments or tighten things up.

Life will get in the way, if you are doing it right. Bodybuilding is only a portion of your life, it's not your life. To expect that life won't get in the way is to not allow yourself to be realistic. Give yourself this much-needed room for error.

Think about this: You are going to diet for 16 to 24 weeks for a competition that will only call for 20 to 30 minutes of your time. For you to think that you may not have periods that include an off meal or two, an unbalanced day, or even a series of days, is just plain unrealistic. There will be times of error, which should be expected and embraced as part of your journey. The best solution to an inevitable problem that every bodybuilder may encounter is time. It always seems to come back to allowing yourself enough time to diet. That way you allow yourself the room to get back in line when life does what it does best—gets in the way.

Remember to Have Fun

I'm not sure where or when I first heard this, but I've heard this sentiment echoed by many of my colleagues: "Fit bodybuilding into your life, don't make bodybuilding your life."

As a young aspiring bodybuilder, I made bodybuilding my life, and it negatively affected many parts of my life. Early on in my bodybuilding career I would never eat food unless I prepared it. I avoided social gatherings, family functions were always about what I could or couldn't eat, and I never took the time to work in a specifically calculated "anchor meal," or larger meal, to satisfy my desire for more carbohydrates as the dieting process grew longer.

This lack of balance in my life never allowed me to truly see the bigger picture of what bodybuilding was providing me. Bodybuilding should never "define you," but it should allow you to grow as a person. You need to find the balance required to make bodybuilding a "part" of your life, not your be-all and end-all. Being able to create this balance is a key goal and vision of the successful bodybuilders who choose to maintain this level of competition in their life, year after year. Remember, you are a husband, a father, a friend, a business owner, or an employee before you are a bodybuilder. Learn this small fact and watch all your bodybuilding goals come true.

Bodybuilding Myths Debunked

TO MAKE THE RIGHT CHOICES as contest day nears, it will help to keep your goals and the methods you choose to achieve them in perspective. Here are some common myths about bodybuilding that will help you in your final push toward the stage.

MYTH #1

You Need PEDs to Win

PEDs, of course, are performance-enhancing drugs like steroids, growth hormone, and testosterone. Steroids have become widely used by many bodybuilders. Those organizations that have chosen to bypass drug-testing protocols have made the use of steroids and other PEDs commonplace.

In the natural bodybuilding world the use of any steroids or PEDs is frowned upon and will only get you disqualified. Don't be tempted to try them. A common belief is that all bodybuilders need to take PEDs to reach peak-condition levels. This is a false statement. Natural bodybuilders need only to rely on diet, strength training, cardio, and legal supplementation. There are many of us who have achieved amazing physiques and the awards and accolades that go with them through natural means. The knowledge that you have achieved your goals without cheating makes the wins all the more sweet.

Taking steroids alone does not make or break a top-level bodybuilder. He still has to put in the hard work and dedication to rise to the top against other drug users. So, it's really not that much of a sure win after all. Steroids alone will not get any bodybuilder to the promised land.

The bodybuilder that chooses to use anabolic steroids may choose to use such methods as extreme carb depletion followed by carb loading, depleting or cutting water intake, loading sodium and/or potassium, diuretic consumption, and even laxative use. Sounds like fun, huh? All this torture for the simple purpose of looking right on stage. As a natural bodybuilder, you won't need to use any of these methods to achieve a crisp look.

MYTH #2

Carb Depletion–Carb Loading Is a Must

You've heard about the carbohydrate manipulation that most bodybuilders attempt, right? You've been told that you need to deplete your body of carbohydrates earlier on in peak week so that you can overcompensate carbohydrate uptake to your muscle tissue by carb loading later on in the week. This concept is usually associated with the eventual elimination of water and the belief that this will allow you to appear massively full and hard.

The entire process goes something like this: You deplete your body of carbohydrates early in peak week, leading up to your big competition day, then you slam home a ridiculous amount of carbohydrates the night before and day of your bodybuilding competition to pump your muscles full of glycogen so your physique looks massive on game day. The most common carb depletion–carb loading series always seems to be 3 days of carb depletion followed by 3 days of carb loading with the subsequent elimination of water starting on Thursday and Friday, before competition day on Saturday when a few sips may be your only water intake. So you eliminate water and keep the carbs pouring in.

I tried this early on in my bodybuilding career. I'm sorry to break your heart: This guessing game doesn't work. By extreme depletion or elimination of carbohydrates all together and then ultimately working to overcompensate your carbs and deplete water, you are playing a guessing game. Do you really know how your physique is going to react to the abundance of glycogen-swelling carbohydrates?

Understand this: Your body is smarter than you! You will never "trick" your body into overcompensating for something you should have never eliminated in the first place. By eliminating carbs and then reintroducing them or creating a sense of "super-compensation," your body will experience what's known as a "spillover" effect. That's where your muscles become soft and puffy with water, not hard and defined. It's exactly what you don't want to happen. You want your muscles to remain full, hard, and dense before your stage time. Don't risk spillover.

MYTH #3

Water Depletion Works

For years bodybuilders have seemed to overlook the simple fact that water and carbohydrates must work together to keep you full and hard on show day. They mustn't be separated or eliminated, leaving one or the other to provide some type of magical power that doesn't exist unless the two work together throughout the peaking process.

Your body's muscle tissue consists of around 60 to 70 percent water, and it's your daily water intake that makes the muscle full and hard. While prepping for your first competition and living the life of a dieting bodybuilder, remember all the times you look in the mirror while completely hydrated and seeing how hard your muscles are. By eliminating the intake of water during your peak week, your body will never reach its ultimate fullness or hardness on stage. You can't achieve that goal without enough water, no matter how much glycogen you continue to pour into your muscles. You are essentially telling the muscle to decrease its overall volume because there is no way for the skin to be fully stretched—thus leaving you with a smaller and softer look. With your muscle volume smaller, you lack separation, and if anything, your skin appears thicker. This is not what any bodybuilder wants on the day of a show. The end result is, again, that spillover effect that will leave your physique flat and soft due to the high levels of glucose outside the muscle cell. Any remaining water in your body will find its way here under your skin.

MYTH #4

Cut the Salt

Somewhere along the way the amateur "broscientists" felt the need to tell the bodybuilding world that sodium needed to be eliminated from the contest prep diet during the week leading up to competition.

It's simply not true. You need to account for, plan, and control minerals in your body during peak week. How do you do this? By keeping them very consistent. Studies show that blood sodium remains unchanged even when you consume high-sodium foods or wipe it out of your diet. It's homeostasis—and your body will do what it needs to maintain order and balance because your brain is monitoring millions of chemical reactions per second.

If you plan to follow one extreme or the other, either massive sodium depletion or a massive sodium load, you'll only create instability in your body. The muscle tissue in your body needs sodium to keep water inside the muscle. If you remove this, you take water out and leave your muscles small, soft, and ultimately flat.

Sodium will become a maintained component of peak week, and only small amounts of sodium or high-sodium foods may be implemented in place of a larger supply of carbohydrates to add a fast increase in muscle fullness and hardness.

MYTH #5

Pound the Potassium

I used to swallow 99-milligram potassium tablets at every meal on contest day. Why? Because everyone else was doing it, so it had to work. Right? Well, it doesn't work.

Loading your body with extra potassium to "trick" your body into wringing out the extra amounts of water isn't actually what will happen.

Instead, taking potassium tablets throughout the day will contribute to water retention in your body by creating an instability in how your cells use sodium and potassium to maintain a healthy hydration level. In the worst cases the combination of carb depletion, sodium loading, cutting of water, carb loading, and potassium loading can lead to an overdose of potassium and an elimination of sodium in your muscles. With your heart being a muscle, the worst-case scenario can lead to cardiac arrest. And that would really throw a monkey wrench into your posing routine!

MYTH #6

Train Like a Maniac

Old bodybuilding conventional wisdom says you should fill your last prep weeks with gut-wrenching total-body training sessions to deplete all glycogen from your muscles.

If you want to step on stage with rock-hard muscles, then don't do anything extreme. Instead, cut back the intensity. During your final week of contest prep, you won't lose your muscle by easing up on your training. But if you allow your body to become extremely depleted of carbs following a training session, your body is guaranteed to become carb and insulin sensitive. Any attempt to super-compensate carbs will lead to a spillover. Training in a carb-depleted state will do nothing more than severely flatten you out and leave your muscles soft during peak week. This will be hard to recover from in only a few days.

MYTH #7

Train Very Lightly

Another training fault of many bodybuilders during peak week is to train very easily and allow their bodies to completely rest the last half of peak week.

Remember, your workouts use glycogen and following the workout you replenish that glycogen. This repeated pattern causes water to follow glycogen into the muscle tissue, leaving you fuller and much tighter, and it allows you to control the level of fullness and hardness leading up to contest day. So, don't stop exercising; do moderate workouts, but avoid extreme training during peak week.

PART 4

CHAPTER 13

The Dark Art: Tanning for the Contest

How to make a muscle with color

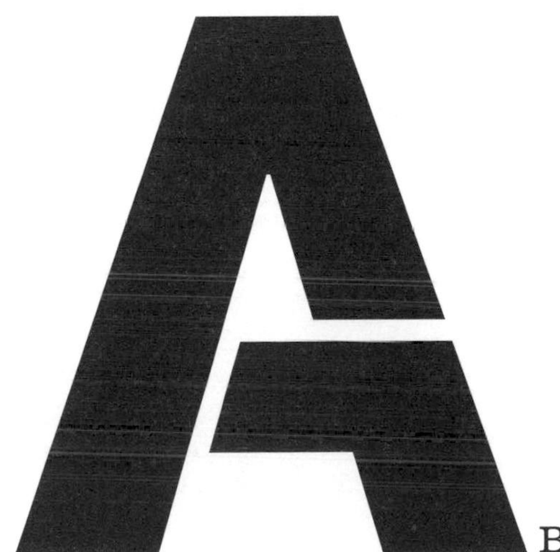

ABS ARE ABS, BUT ON contest day they need to be wearing makeup or you might as well be wearing a T-shirt over them. Being tan is part of the job on competition day. The intense bright lights on the bodybuilding stage will wash out your natural skin color by up to 30 percent. Even if you have a naturally warm brown complexion, the lights won't do justice to your hard-fought muscle. And if you have pale skin, you'll look pasty and flat.

The darker your skin tone, the easier it will be for the judges to evaluate your muscular development and conditioning. A golden or bronze color accentuates the lines of your muscles, allowing the stage lighting to show off your definition to the judges.

Look, I understand this entire approach to competing in a bodybuilding competition may be an overwhelmingly new endeavor, but trust me, your presentation is key, especially on stage and especially to the judges. When competing, I've seen everything from the guy who looked like he just rolled in a mud pit to the guy who was so pasty white, he looked like a bed sheet ghost at Halloween. When it comes to tanning, here's one thing you can bank on: You'll never be too dark.

Here's how to get a look that shows off your 24-week dedication to building muscle:

Stay out of the salon. Don't waste your money trying to get a base tan at your local tanning salon. By the same token, don't spend hours baking your body in the sun either. These methods will never get your skin dark enough. Only stains will.

Remove the hair. Shaving off body hair will allow you to show off more of your muscle definition and allow for a better, more natural tan. You have a few options

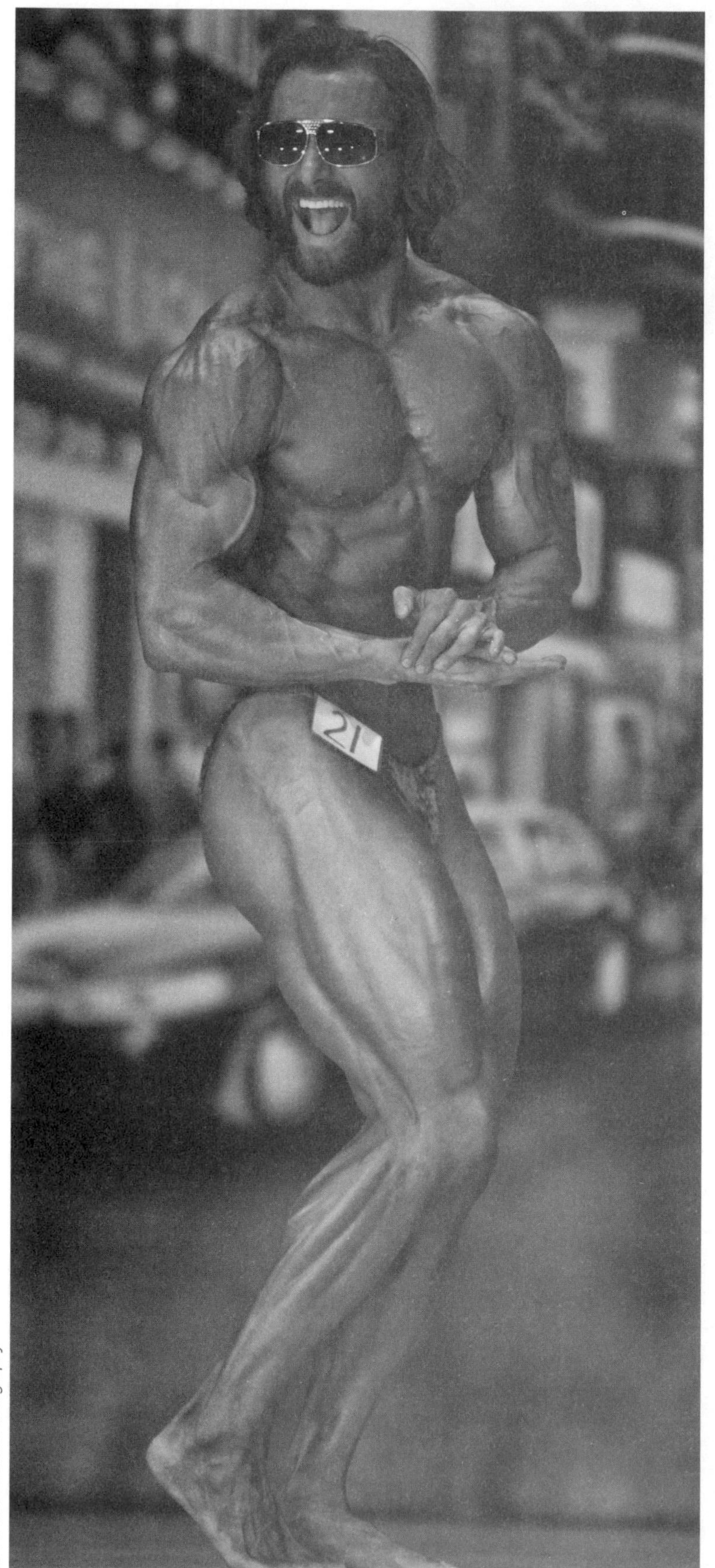

© Jordan Samuel Photography

here: you can use a spray-on hair remover like Nair for Men or a razor and shaving cream. I've always been a fan of a razor and shaving cream and will start prepping my skin weeks or even months before the competition. This method takes practice, so don't wait until a few days before your competition. Start getting ready far in advance.

Apply a stain. One of the most popular tanning products is Pro Tan Overnight Competition Color, which can be brushed or sprayed onto the skin for an instant tan that will become darker in 3 to 5 hours. The application may adhere better if you first buff your skin with an exfoliant. Pro Tan gets darker with each application. Typically, you'll start the process 4 to 7 days before the competition to get your skin dark enough. You may shower during this time frame, but expect that to lighten your overall color. You will need to reapply. Allow to dry for 30 minutes before putting on clothes.

Use a bronzer. Even if you use a stain, you may not be dark enough. The best way to go about getting your skin color to your liking is with a bronzer. Dream Tan is my personal favorite competition color for bodybuilders. The bronzing agent comes in two different shades: a "golden bronze" (Dream Tan #1) and a "red bronze" (Dream Tan #2).

Applying Dream Tan is fast and easy when done right. But it takes some practice. If done incorrectly, it can cause a mess and stain clothes. You should practice applying your color several weeks before the competition. It's a good idea to practice your poses while tanned, too.

Dream Tan will make you much darker than any self-application tan and also adds a better natural shine onstage because it has a natural posing oil mixed into the application.

When applying Dream Tan, you'll need someone to help you rub it on and then pat it down on the skin. You'll want to evenly disperse the tan over your body. The best approach is to tackle your body in segments—chest and abs, arms, left leg, right leg, backside, and upper back. Once the color has been rubbed on, patting of the skin will smooth out any blotches. Apply only a small amount to your face, feet, and hands.

Most Dream Tan applications will only need two coats. I apply three: a coat the night before, one in the morning before heading to the venue, and a third coat before prejudging in the morning. You will need to do touch-ups or can even apply a new coat, over the current coat, before the night show. It will only enhance the color and shine.

Try the new spray-on bronzer. The latest and newest option readily made available at many bodybuilding competitions is stage color Spray Tan. The nice thing about Spray Tan is you don't have to worry about applying your own stage color, as it will be done by a licensed professional right at the competition.

Spray Tan has become increasingly popular with figure and bikini athletes, but I've also seen bodybuilders use it with success. The application usually takes 30 minutes to an hour, depending on the competitor's natural skin tone. You will need to set an appointment with Spray Tan before the show. Typically, you are sprayed on the Friday evening before the show and once again in the morning of the competition. Be sure the competition you are registered for offers Spray Tan, because it is not always made available at all shows.

Companies like Elite Bronzing, which offers Spray Tan, have become staples at many natural bodybuilding competitions across the East Coast and the New England area. For more information, visit elitebronzing.com.

There are a few steps you need to follow to prepare your skin for a professional Spray Tan.

Spray tan preparation:

- Exfoliate gently for a period of 3 days before the competition spray (especially around elbows and knees)
- Use a water-based scrub designed for spray tanning
- On the day of your spray tan, exfoliate gently before
- Do not apply lotion before
- Do not apply deodorant before
- Avoid activity after spray tanning (sweating will create streaks)
- Shave at least 8 hours before your spray tan, and ensure that all waxing is completed at least 72 hours before, if you're accustomed to waxing.
- Otherwise, wax 7 to 10 days before your spray tan appointment.
- After your color is applied, you cannot shave or shower. You must wait until after your competition.

Consider using a posing oil. These products will give you a sheen over your tan. Posing oils can run you from $15 to $30. Personally, I've never used them. I've found that a simple $3 can of spray cooking oil works perfectly. Posing oils can be overused by many competitors. If you choose Dream Tan, you don't need to use a posing oil because, as I mentioned, the solution already contains an oil base that will add to your stage sheen.

Posing Suit Selection

Besides a good tan, you'll also need a posing suit to cover up the parts you didn't tan. A posing suit is an important piece of equipment. It needs to fit tightly, of course. The main issues here are style and color. You want to select the right color for your hair and skin tone. But don't overthink this.

When selecting a suit color, you can never go wrong with a solid, dark color. For one, the dark suit will mask any possible tanning errors that may end up on your suit. I've seen guys with great physiques but with tanning solution all over their light-colored trunks. I've always avoided light colors because they tend to distract the judges' eyes from the more important parts of your body.

Avoid colors like light blue and yellow because they look terrible under the power of the stage lights and will not provide your physique with anything more than a distraction for the judging panel.

If you are new to bodybuilding, go with a dark color; don't try to be too flashy.

POSING SUIT COLOR/SKIN TONE GUIDE

	LIGHTLY TANNED	DARKLY TANNED	BROWN	BLACK
RED HAIR	medium blue to dark green	gold, yellow	n/a	n/a
BLOND HAIR	red, royal, blue, black	burgundy, red, medium blue, orange	n/a	n/a
BROWN HAIR	black, navy, blue	burgundy, brown, purple, teal	black, yellow, chocolate brown	n/a
BLACK HAIR	black, navy, blue, brown, white	yellow, red, gold, orange, baby blue	lime green, kelly green, purple, fuchsia	bright red, red-orange

Selecting a Style

There are numerous styles or "cuts" to the bodybuilder's posing trunks. It's a good idea to pick a cut that fits best and shows off your physique most dramatically.

FRENCH CUT
- Fits high on the hips
- 3/4"-wide sides
- Dips low in front
- Three quarters coverage on back

FLEX CUT
- Same as French cut
- With 1/4" to 3/8" sides

BRAZILIAN CUT
- Fits high on hips
- Thin sides
- Slightly less than three quarters coverage on back
- Accents more of side glutes

AMERICAN CUT
- Fullest coverage of all with 2" sides
- High front and back
- Popular among newbie bodybuilders

EUROPEAN CUT
- Fits lower on the hips, covers most on the back
- Sides are 1 1/4" wide
- Has a high front

PREMIER CUT
- Fits high on hips
- 1/4" sides
- Front dips down a little (narrower than French cut)
- Back shows more of glutes than Brazilian cut

WHERE TO ORDER

Try Jagware Posing Suits. It's a California-based company that does very nice work: jagware-posingsuits.com.

Most posing suits run from $25 to $40, depending on the design, cut, and style.

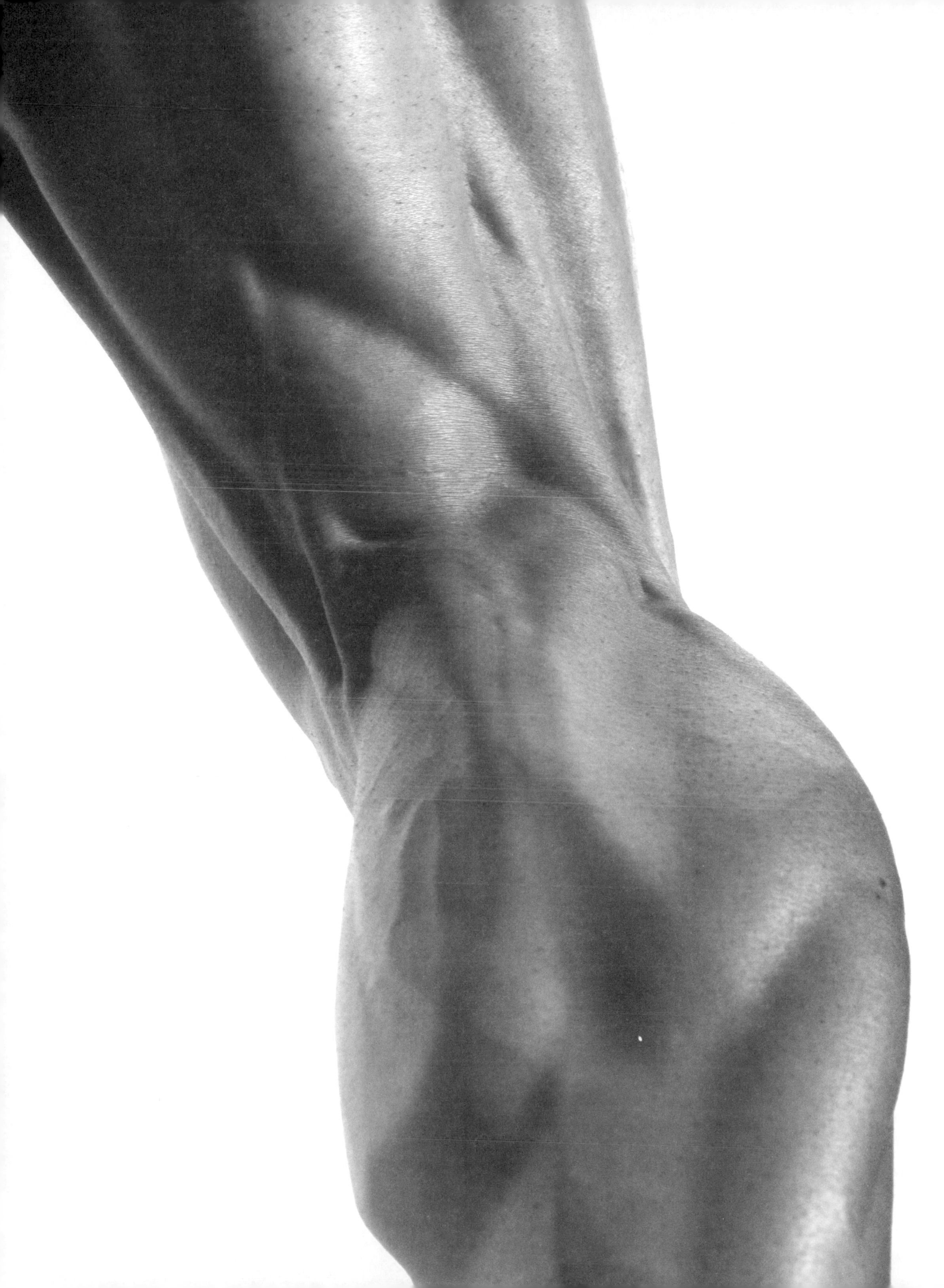

PART 4

CHAPTER 14

Flex Appeal: The Choreography of Contest Posing

Muscle matters, but it's all about how well you show it

THE POSING PART OF PREPARing for a bodybuilding competition is often the last thing people new to the sport think about. That makes sense because posing in a competition is the culmination of all your effort. You spend months dieting, trimming body fat, and building muscle. That's your focus and your priority. But I can tell you this: If you don't know how to present your physique on stage in the mandatory poses, you can hurt your ability to showcase the body you've worked so hard to sculpt. The best posing will always beat the best physique.

The reason bodybuilding competitions are often called "shows" is for the simple reason that the event is more of a show than a contest. You are showing off your physique, and you do that through posing. So perfecting your posing is critical to your success, and as such it should be a regular part of your training from early on, not just at the end of your 24-week buildup to competition day.

Posing is an art that must be practiced over and over and over so that it feels natural, because in a competition you won't have the benefit of mirrors to use to adjust your pose. The pose you strike needs to be perfect the first time because there's nothing between your body and the judges' eyes. Practice is also important because it allows you to perfect the art of illusion. The bodybuilder who knows how to present his physique properly can often use a pose to showcase his body's strengths while hiding any weaknesses from the judging panel.

On stage, posing is not comfortable. The stage lights are incredibly hot. You will start to sweat the moment you step onstage. You should try to mimic this in your practice by turning up the heat in your room and adding bright lights as you pose. Judges can immediately tell those bodybuilders who have spent time honing their performance and those who did not practice enough. The more you rehearse this difficult and uncomfortable task, the more it will look natural, smooth, and fluid, a performance that showcases the body's form and aesthetic. Through proper practice, you will convince the judges that you are having fun up there because you really will be enjoying yourself.

When should you practice? Throughout your contest prep training. Do it during and after workouts as an active part of conditioning your muscles. Keep these tips in mind as you plan your posing:

Perfecting your posing:
- Practice constantly, for a minimum of 15 minutes per day (more is better)
- Increase your practice time slightly each week
- Pose in front of the mirror only half the time because you won't have mirrors to use onstage
- Eliminate the mirror 4 weeks before show day
- Posing takes endurance; practice holding each pose for 10 to 15 seconds
- Condition your muscles by posing during training
- Start from the bottom up, that is, start with your legs even when striking an upper-body pose
- Hold each pose for a minimum of 15 seconds
- Remember that judges can only judge what you show them
- Practice your routine to accent your physique
- Choose your music to complement your routine; do not pick the music you like and "attempt" to pose into it

During the weeks leading up to your contest, practice as if you were posing in competition. Visualize your contest posing. Don't just practice individual poses, but practice the entire routine and pay keen attention to your transitions into your poses. They are as important as the poses themselves, and practicing them will improve your endurance. If you can't control your poses because you lack endurance, your muscles will begin to shake, a telltale sign that you are not completely ready and the judges will notice.

Tips for posing presentation:
- Transition smoothly
- Make your poses slower and steadier than you think is necessary. A common beginner's mistake is to go too fast.
- Remember to have fun
- Smile
- Avoid grimacing (I'm guilty of this)
- Have confidence

Judging Rounds

A TYPICAL BODYBUILDING COMPETITION is broken up into three different rounds of posing. In each, the judges are looking for something different that will be considered as a whole when they tally their final scores.

The first of these is the symmetry round. Judges will be looking at how well balanced your muscles are from top to bottom and from side to side. The better balance your physique presents, the more symmetrical your muscles look, the better you will score. For example, having wide shoulders and a tiny waist will give the bodybuilder a greater chance of scoring well in a symmetry round due to the balance of muscle throughout his physique. Judges are looking for a balance between structure and muscularity. Even though your overall conditioning is not scored in this round, your body-fat percentage can impact your score. It helps to be as lean as possible so judges can see your muscles.

"Good posing will always be rewarded. All too often as a judge you'll say to yourself, 'If only this competitor did this, they would have scored higher.'"

—Nancy Andrews, four-time WNBF World Champion and natural bodybuilding legend

The second round is the mass round, where judges are looking for overall muscularity and muscle mass. The judges ignore symmetry here. They are judging the overall size of your muscles, looking for a large, wide back and well-developed shoulder, chest, and arm muscles. The "more muscular" the competitor, the better he will score in this round.

In the conditioning round, competitors are basically judged on how lean they are. Although bodybuilding is not a dieting contest, being lean is important because it's an indication of your overall physical conditioning and it will enhance the appearance of your muscles.

The following are the mandatory poses you will be required to perform in almost any natural bodybuilding competition.

Symmetry Round—Quarter Turns

These poses—front standing relaxed and side-standing relaxed—are standard poses you will strike between the main judging poses. Call them interim poses. They are designed to show off the symmetry of the bodybuilder's physique. The symmetry round is all about the balance of a bodybuilder from top to bottom and from side to side. If your physique presents better balance throughout, it will score better.

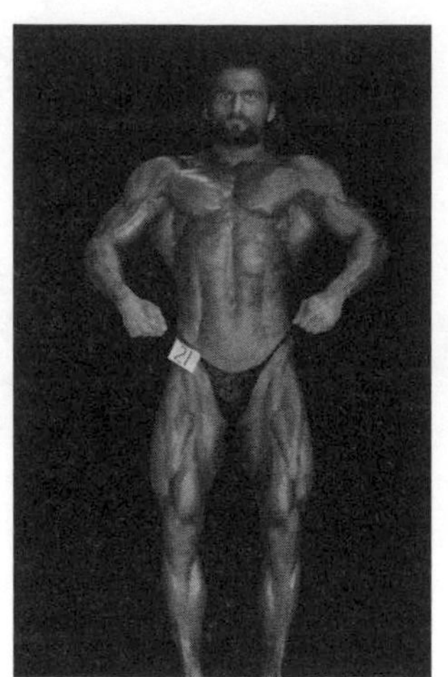

Front Standing Relaxed

This is the pose that you will take for most of your time onstage, but by no means is it really "relaxed." It takes effort and you will be contracting your muscles. This is the pose that bodybuilders will come back to between any front-facing mandatory poses.

Your knees should be slightly bent, to keep your quads flexed. The chest should be made to look larger as you widen your back, giving your physique the look of being wider and larger. Keep your abdominals tight, but not truly flexed or drawn in. Bodybuilders with extremely good abdominals can keep them flexed, but make sure you don't burn out before the real posing begins. By keeping your chest, lats, and shoulders engaged you'll make your upper body appear larger and give the illusion of a smaller waistline.

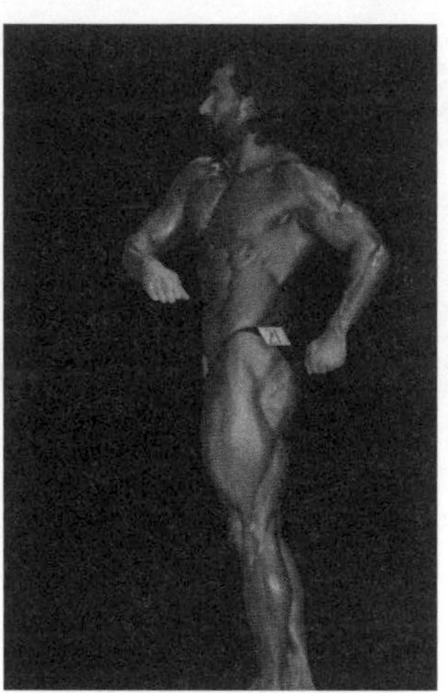

Side Standing Relaxed (left and right)

Turn to face the side of the stage. Slightly flex the arm that's nearest the front of the stage. Hold it just over your posing suit and glutes. Press the other arm on your chest to create the appearance that your chest is larger. You can almost imagine creating a "tea cup" position with your arms, as you twist your torso to keep your obliques flexed and visible to the judges.

Slightly stagger your legs with your back knee pressed up against the hamstring of your front leg to give the illusion that the hamstring of the front leg is larger. The key is to keep the sweep of your quad, glutes, and calves tight, while keeping your feet grounded. Be sure to face the side of the stage, and not the judges, during this pose to keep your side shot looking narrow with a big leg sweep, tight midsection, and large chest and shoulder area.

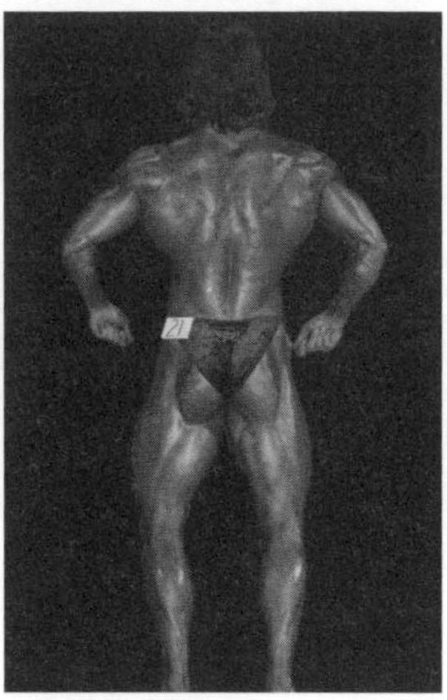

Rear Standing Relaxed

While you face the back of the stage, you will start tensing your muscles from the legs up by keeping your feet a few inches away from each other and slightly externally rotated. The setup is essentially the same as the front relaxed from the ground up until you focus on the essentials.

As you face the curtain (back of the stage), flare your lats to become as wide as possible while keeping your rear deltoids flexed to display back width, thickness, and shoulder definition. Leaning back slightly is okay, as long as you avoid overly squeezing your shoulder blades together, which will hide definition and make your back seem narrow. Squeezing extra tight is not always the best route because it may cause you to bring your shoulder blades together and lose that width and definition. Your glutes, hamstrings, and calves should remain tight. A bodybuilder can separate himself in terms of definition by keeping striated glutes flexed during this pose.

Photos © Jordan Samuel Photography

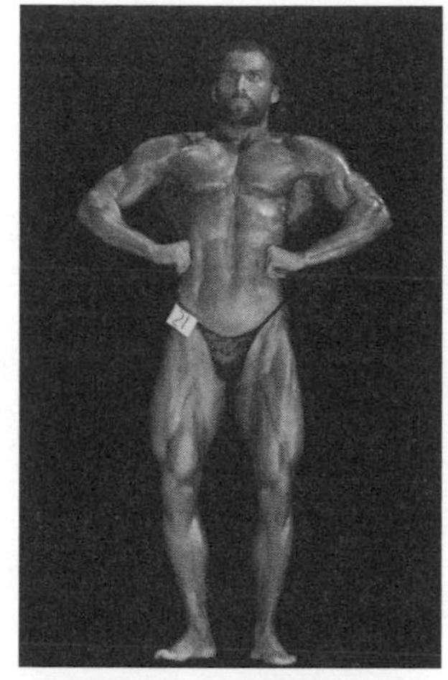

Mandatory Poses

Front Lat Spread

Facing the judges and crowd, place your hands on your torso above your hips, flex your quads with a slight knee bend, and spread your elbows forward to bring out the width of your lats. Keep your chest up and avoid leaning back too much; this will give you a larger look. Don't flex your abs during this pose.

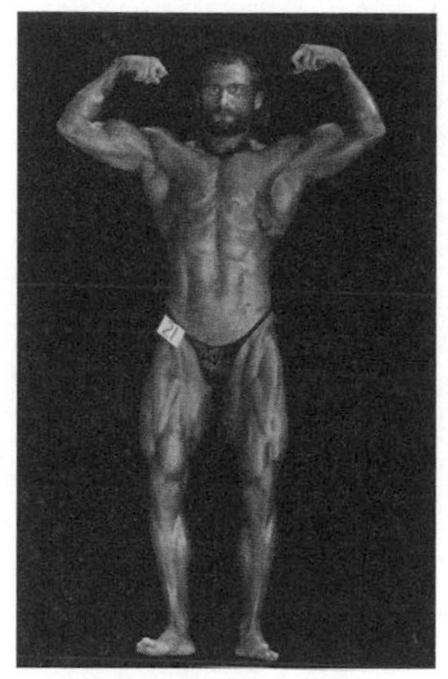

Front Double Biceps

Start from the ground by keeping your feet slightly separated and turned out slightly, and your knees bent to show off your quads. Raise your arms so your forearms are just slightly higher than shoulder level. As you raise your arms, pull your forearms back slightly while simultaneously pulling your upper arms forward to bring out your lat and chest development. Be sure to keep your chest up and your lats engaged, and flex your biceps.

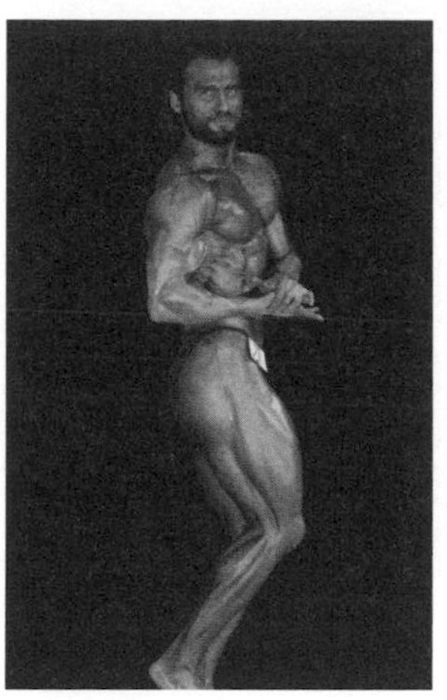

Side Chest

Bring the leg closest to the judges up against your other leg to allow your front leg to appear larger. Push up on the ball of your front foot to spike the calf of the front leg. Fill your lungs with air to lift your chest up and out. Grab the hand or wrist on the arm closest to the judges with the opposite hand. The arm farthest from the judges should be pushed up against the pectoral that is farthest from the judges while flexing that pec and simultaneously flexing the biceps on the front arm. Be sure to keep your chest up and display your inner costal obliques and abdominals. If you are tall, you'll want to squat down a bit once you fall into the pose. This will allow you to look thicker. If you are a shorter bodybuilder, stand up as tall as possible to look a bit larger compared with your taller competition.

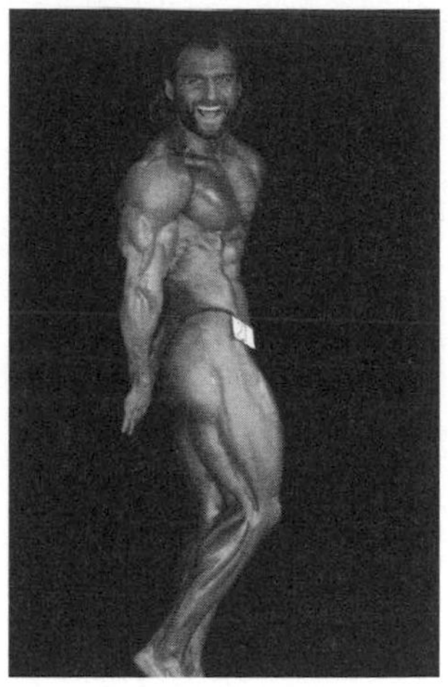

Side Triceps

Stand facing the side of the stage and bring the leg closest to the judges up against the other leg to allow your front leg to appear larger. Push up on the ball of your front foot to spike the calf of the front leg. Now, the arm that's closest to the judges will be the arm you'll display. Keep it straight down. Reach behind your back with your other arm and grab the wrist or inside hand of the front arm and flex your triceps downward. Press that arm against your torso to make it seem even larger. This is a great pose to accent your abdominals and obliques, so be sure to emphasize these during this pose by keeping them tight and pulled in.

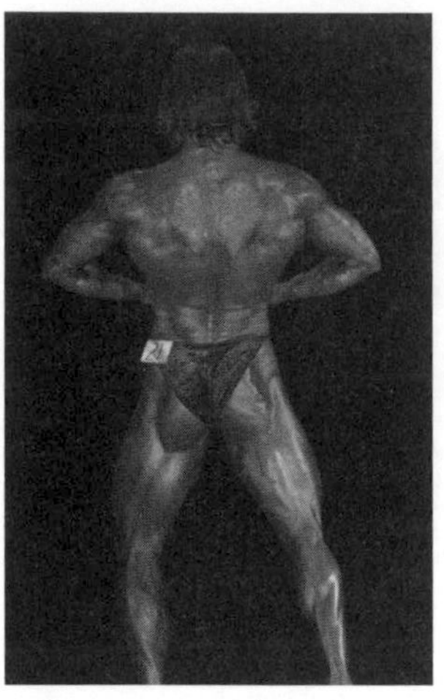

Rear Lat Spread

With your back facing the judges, spike the calf of one leg while simultaneously flexing your hamstring. Be sure to lean back slightly to bring out your lower back muscles. Place your hands on your lower lats, hands in fists, and spread your lats as wide as possible while driving your elbows toward each other in front of your body.

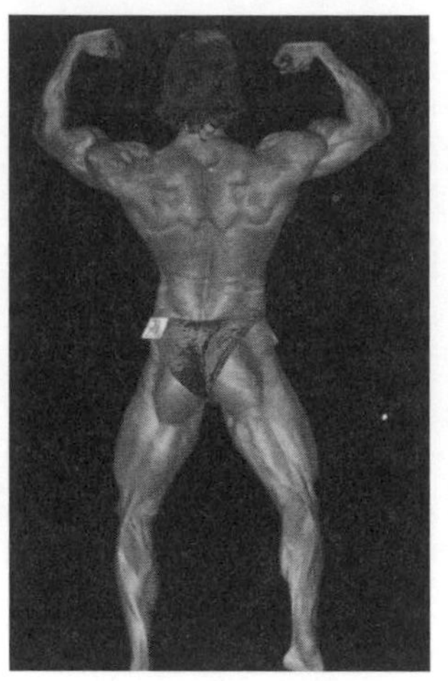

Rear Double Biceps

With your back toward the judges, spike the calf of one leg while simultaneously flexing that leg's hamstring. Be sure to lean back slightly to bring out your lower back while raising your arms to flex your biceps. Avoid squeezing your shoulder blades together. Raising your elbows higher than your chest will enhance the look.

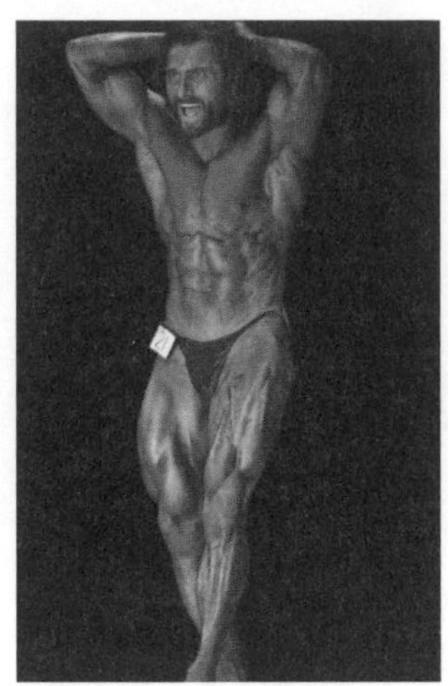

Hands-on-Head Abdominals

This pose is meant to accent your abdominals and quad muscles. The easiest way to get into it is to place one leg slightly forward or staggered in a T in front of your other leg while placing your hands behind your head and flexing your abdominals.

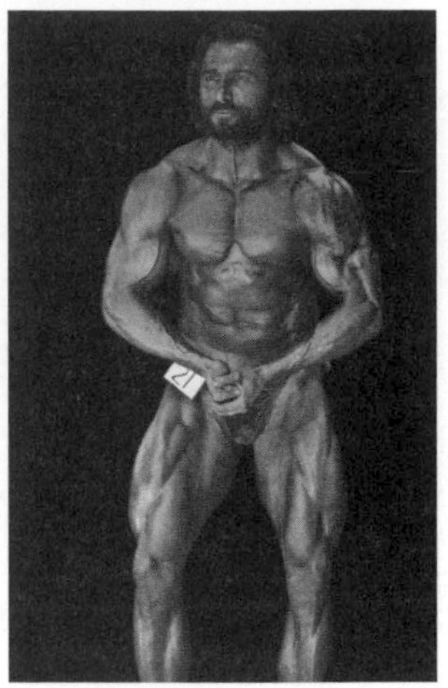

Most Muscular

There are a few variations of this pose. You can have your hands together (as shown above), your hands behind your hips, and your hands on your hips (as shown at right). The ultimate goal of this pose is to demonstrate the most muscle mass on your upper body. The most popular way to perform "most muscular" is to set your feet shoulder width apart, with a slight knee bend, and bring your hands toward each other in front of your lower torso. This brings out your chest, arms, shoulders, and traps, showcasing just how much muscle mass your body holds.

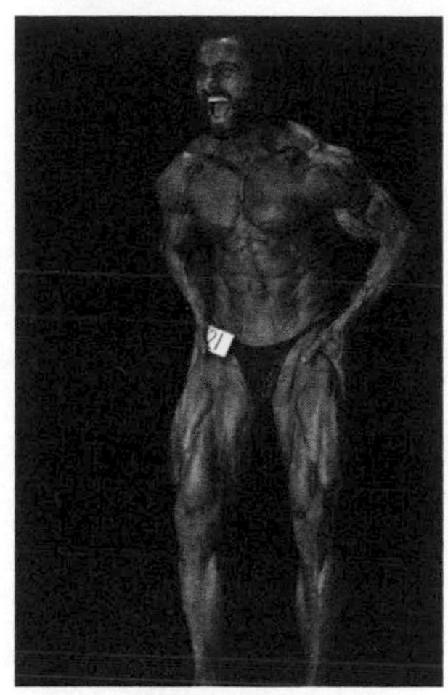

Hands-on-Hips Most Muscular

Here's a look at the hands-on-hips variation, which I find to be the more aesthetic "most muscular" pose. Keeping your knees slightly bent and quads flexed, place your hands on your hips. As you bring your hands onto your hips, push your elbows forward, flexing your chest and shoulders while bringing out your traps and abs.

Optional Poses

These poses are usually requested by the judges when a class of competition is very tough to decide and the judges need additional poses in order to help them decide between two bodybuilders whose scores are nearly identical. The optional poses help judges select for specific placings.

Side Serratus Pose

This is much like the side triceps pose but with the arm closest to the judges overhead, exposing the obliques and abs. The farthest arm presses up against the rear chest muscle from underneath.

Calf Raise Pose

Face the rear of the stage and then slowly rise up on the balls of your feet, exposing your calf muscles.

Hamstring Curl Pose

Face the rear of the stage and add a slight angle to your body. Lift one leg and flex, displaying your hamstring muscle as you would in performing a partial leg curl.

Your Posing Routine

- Select 10 to 20 poses that are your best poses and that are most effective for showing off your physique
- Pick music that choreographs nicely with your selection of poses
- Music should be 60 to 90 seconds (depending on the requirements of the organization holding the competition)
- Perform a routine that has meaning
- Songs with clear beats and guitar riffs make posing transitions easier
- Create a good flow from one pose to the next
- Practice your routine to accent your physique
- Practice even more
- When there's nothing good on TV, practice some more!

If you are not technically savvy or just not good at mixing your own music, hire a professional to do so. I've paid too much money for music and then have had it not play or skip when I've tried to do it myself. Trust me when I tell you there is no worse feeling than being onstage by yourself and having something go wrong with the audio. I've used my friend Jason Piper, owner of Mastermindz Productions (http://mastermindzproductions.com/body_building_music.html) since 2005. It's well worth the expense to hire a pro.

PART 4

CHAPTER 15

Peak Week

Fine-tuning before you step on stage

BODYBUILDERS PUT A LOT of importance on the week leading up to competition—peak week—and for good reason. Most of the work is done; now is the time to fine-tune your body and your routine and prepare yourself mentally for the stresses and challenges of your performance.

The good news is that if you have been disciplined about your dieting and training and have given yourself adequate time to get ready, this week's preparations will feel natural and easy. Your emphasis during peak week—the week that your body peaks—should be on nutrition. Continue to track your protein, carbs, and fats all the way through competition day. By now you most likely have the drill down pat, but just in case you thought you could stop paying attention to your diet, understand that it's important to be even more precise this week.

The best advice I can give you is to plan. Build your entire week's nutrition and training template before the week begins so you maintain a good structure. Having that confident base will allow you to adapt your carbohydrate consumption as you monitor your body. Let's look at the key considerations for optimum peak-week preparation.

Carbs and Water

Remember that it is the combination of carbohydrates and water that will ultimately decide how full and tight your physique will appear on stage. Your protein and fat intake can remain stable and unchanged during peak week. We will shift your focus to the roles of carbohydrates and water for their power in the peaking process. Contrary to bodybuilding dogma, the fewer moving parts during peak week, the better. Focusing your attention on only your carb intake and your continued hydration will allow you to achieve your desired full, dry, and tight look.

As I said before, do not reduce your water intake during peak week. Doing so even the slightest will make your muscles appear smaller while losing density. That's not a desired look for any bodybuilder. Water remains a staple in your peak-week prep and won't deviate outside of the regular daily intake you followed throughout your dieting process.

Consider an analogy from

Dr. Joe, which goes something like this: Think of a balloon that is full, and then one that lacks air. The fuller the balloon, the tighter and rounder it looks. If it's lacking air, it will appear soft, loose, and thick.

Your muscle separation can be controlled drastically by how hydrated the muscle is. The muscle gets flat and smaller if it's dehydrated and thus lacks volume to stretch your skin. The skin will sag against what is now a smaller muscle, lack separation, and look dull.

Be sure to continue to drink 8 to 12 (8-ounce) glasses of water a day. Manipulating your carb intake will also affect your body's hydration.

During the first few days of peak week, increase your carbohydrate intake by 25 to 50 grams to place a good amount of glycogen storage in your muscle tissue. By doing this early in the week, you won't risk any chance of spillover. As you continue your training throughout the week, the workouts will use up the glycogen, and you'll need to replenish it. Therefore, we will continue to bring carbs to the muscle each day of peak week. It makes no logical sense during the most critical time of your contest preparation to eliminate carbs. Remember, carbs are anabolic and eliminating them only to reintroduce them in a supercompensation format just before the contest can actually increase insulin sensitivity, making it much easier for you to spill over.

"Over-carbing" is another common mistake among bodybuilders during peak week. It can make your body convert excess glucose to new body fat, something you certainly don't want. Depletion is not the answer, but there are ways for you to deliver glycogen into the muscle without causing spill over. It's called carb cycling.

How to Cycle Your Carbs

As you begin entering your peak week, your current level of carbohydrates will be different from the next bodybuilder. Even though there may not be an "exact formula" for the start of a peak week, for each person we can take a certain consistent approach.

During the weekend before the weekend of your contest, taper back your carb intake slightly (this can be by as much as 100 to as little as 25 grams depending on carb sensitivity) to allow your body to recover and prep your muscles for an influx of carbs on Monday, your highest carb day of the week. On Monday, you should consume 25 to 100 grams more than a regular dieting day of carbohydrates to force glycogen to be stored in your muscle tissue. This is predicated on your ability to consume carbohydrates.

By the middle of your peak week, around Wednesday and Thursday, your body will have reached a peak hardness look. For an ectomorph both Thursday and Friday may be used to increase carbs and increase muscle fullness. What's worked well for me is to have Thursday be a day in which I consume more carbs, allowing me to taper back on Friday and regain a bit more tightness.

On the day of the show, you'll use specifically timed meal combinations of protein, carbs, fat, water, and when needed, small additions of sodium to keep your muscles full, hard, and tight.

Monitor your physique, carb sensitivity, and make the necessary tweaks. After all, by now you are lean enough and understand the level of carbs your body can or can't handle.

How to Monitor Sodium, Potassium, and Water

Contrary to popular bodybuilding folklore, you don't have to manipulate your water, sodium, and potassium intake any differently from what you've been doing all through your training and dieting process.

If you've been drinking a gallon to a gallon and a half of water a day for weeks, keep right on doing so. Remember, the water and carbs will work together to give you the dry, full, and tight appearance that we bodybuilders desire on game day.

Sodium is a component of peak week that is misinterpreted and mismanaged by many competitors. Your body will store water either inside or outside the muscle. What we want is water inside the muscle, allowing it to appear full. Balancing out the extracellular water, or water outside the muscle, and the intracellular water, or water inside the muscle, is the game that most bodybuilders lose when toying with sodium, potassium, and water levels during peak week. Keeping water coming is crucial to the balance—to losing extracellular water and to the filtering of intracellular water.

When considering sodium and potassium, we need to know to keep them consistent throughout peak week. As your body consistently monitors millions of chemical reactions per second in an effort to maintain homeostasis, it's important during peak week to keep these minerals stable.

The average adult needs 2,000 to 2,500 milligrams of sodium per day. As a bodybuilder, you'll use more while training, sweating, drinking water, and performing cardio.

For example, if your body is regularly consuming 3,000 milligrams of sodium per day during contest prep, there is no reason to eliminate this consumption during peak week and attempt to super-compensate by adding more sodium later in the week. Your blood sodium will remain constant whether you eliminate it from your diet or consume sodium-rich foods.

Sodium is a requirement for your body to keep water in the muscle tissue—hardly something you will want to eliminate. If you eliminate sodium, your muscle tissue will push water out, but at the expense of leaving muscles flat, tiny, and soft. By cutting sodium and loading potassium, you'll also shift the ratio of potassium to sodium way too high and increase the levels of aldosterone in your body.

Aldosterone is a hormone in the body that causes the reabsorption and retention of water and sodium. This increase in aldosterone will lead to water moving under the skin and giving your body a soft appearance, not the goal during peak week. Once you've depleted your sodium levels, it will also become nearly impossible to deliver carbs to the correct place. The lack of sodium will limit your body's ability to absorb glucose by having it remain in the small intestine while bringing water to that area, causing a bloated look in the midsection.

The best route on peak week is to keep your sodium and water intake the same as you have throughout the dieting phase. If you are drinking 2 gallons of water a day, keep it there. If you are consuming 2.5 to 3 grams of sodium a day, then that is where you'll want to remain for peak week. The same can be said for potassium—consistency with sodium and potassium will keep your muscles full and tight. Throughout your contest prep diet, monitor the amount of sodium you consume during the day. For many bodybuilders this number will remain 2,000 to 2,500 milligrams during peak week. Doing so will keep the cellular balance of water equal, a healthy hydration level along with full, tight muscles.

Training During Peak Week

Training during peak week is important because you don't want to lose any muscle and you want to keep working through the glycogen stored in your tissues. Stick to the same workouts you've been doing before peak week, keeping each session intact, but reduce your volume and intensity to 80 percent of what you have been doing and do not do any forced reps. (A forced rep is a rep which you can't complete by yourself—a training partner must assist you.) With forced reps, you risk injury and overtaxing a muscle. You shouldn't do that during the week before a competition.

Remember your workouts will use glycogen, and the last thing you want to do during peak week is rest or train too light. By working out hard enough, you will ensure that your body uses glycogen. And if your body is using glycogen, then it also gives you the opportunity to replace it. This simple step allows your body to create a dynamic use of fluid. Continuing to train at a good intensity and consistency will cause the water you consume to follow your glycogen into your muscle cells. The end result is fuller, tighter muscles throughout peak week.

You should have two main training goals on the week of your contest:

1. Stimulate your muscles to allow them to keep enough glycogen in the tissue and water where it is supposed to be.
2. Keep your muscle cells full and tight.

Training continues every day of peak week through Friday. If you feel you need to use some extra glycogen on the day of the contest, do a morning training session.

Cardio During Peak Week

Cardiovascular exercise during peak week is not designed to burn the last amounts of body fat. Instead, it should be used to regulate your glycogen stores in your muscles, allowing you to keep the carbohydrates and water coming in all week. For that reason, these workouts shouldn't be high-intensity sessions or marathon runs. If you regularly do HIIT workouts, just keep these short enough to allow your body to fully recover for competition day.

Practice Your Posing

By now you should have a strong foundation for posing. If you don't, then shame on you! But this happens all the time. Bodybuilders are notorious for getting so hung up on their diet, training, cardio, and everything else that comes with bodybuilding that they neglect to practice their posing enough during the earlier weeks of training and they try to cram during peak week. Others practice throughout training only to stop rehearsing during peak week, which makes no sense. You should make posing practice (without a mirror) part of your peak week routine, just as you do with your meals, training, and cardio.

I've found it best to practice for 10 to 15 minutes first thing in the morning before, say, a cardio session, and again for 10 to 15 minutes in the evening after a training session. These short consistent blocks of posing practice will not deplete your body of too much glycogen in the days leading up to the competition, nor will they wear you out as some of your previous posing practice sessions may have. The ultimate goal of each of these sessions should be to keep your posing game tight and fresh up until show time.

How you choose to plan and structure your peak week is really up to you. It should be based on your individual needs and how well you have trained during the previous 24 weeks. How successful you are this week will depend upon how well you know your body. And each time you compete you will learn more about what works best for you. Hint: Use a notebook and take good notes. Record everything you do and how your body feels. It will be an amazing resource of detailed information for the next time you enter contest preparation. That's what I do and I find it to be very valuable. Here's a look at the details of my peak-week preparation for the 2010 World Natural Bodybuilding Championships.

Saturday

- Protein: 300 g
- Carbs: 300 g
- Fat: 45–50 g
- Water: 1.5–2 gal. (I can increase)
- Sodium: 2.5–3 g
- Cardio: 30 min.
- Training: rest
- Posing: 15 min.

Sunday

- Protein: 300 g
- Carbs: 300 g
- Fat: 45–50 g
- Water: 1.5–2 gal. (can increase)
- Sodium: 2.5–3 g
- Cardio: 30 min.
- Training: rest
- Posing: 15 min.

Monday

- Protein: 300 g
- Carbs: 350 g
- Fat: 45–50 g
- Water: 1.5–2 gal. (can increase)
- Sodium: 2.5–3 g
- Cardio: warmup for workout only
- Training: legs
- Posing: 15 min.

Tuesday

- Protein: 300 g
- Carbs: 325 g
- Fat: 45–50 g
- Water: 1.5–2 gal. (can increase)
- Sodium: 2.5–3 g
- Cardio: 20 min.
- Training: calves
- Posing: 15 min.

Wednesday

- Protein: 300 g
- Carbs: 300 g
- Fat: 45–50 g
- Water: 1.5–2 gal. (can increase)
- Sodium: 2.5–3 g
- Cardio: warmup for workout only
- Training: chest, shoulders, triceps
- Posing: 15 min.

Thursday

- Protein: 300 g
- Carbs: 400 g
- Fat: 45–50 g
- Water: 1.5–2 gal. (can increase)
- Sodium: 2.5–3 g
- Cardio: 20 min.
- Training: abs
- Posing: 15 min.

Friday

- Protein: 300 g
- Carbs: 300 g
- Fat: 45–50 g
- Water: 1.5–2 gal. (can increase)
- Sodium: 2.5–3 g
- Cardio: warmup for workout only
- Training: back, biceps
- Posing: 15 min.

Saturday—Contest Day

In the next chapter, I'll offer advice and insight into what to do to prepare mentally, physically, and nutritionally on the day of the bodybuilding competition.

PART 4

CHAPTER 16

It's Show Time

Bring your game face (and body) to your first physique competition

CONTEST DAY HAS ARRIVED. Welcome to one of the longest days of your life, a day that can go on for 10 to even 18 hours. It will also be one of the most exhilarating days of your life, brief highs when you're on stage followed by long hours of boredom as you wait and wait for the next round of posing. Knowing what to expect on the day of the bodybuilding competition will help ease some of the natural anxiety you'll be feeling, but it certainly won't eliminate it. Let me take you through the day, from the time you get up, until after the awards ceremony, and offer some tips based on my experience.

The Night Before the Contest

Prepare your meals and pack the duffle you'll take to the contest. Planning the next day's meals is critically important. In general, you'll want to keep contest-day meals smaller and frequent, partitioned out during the day. Aim for 20 to 30 grams of protein, 30 to 50 grams of carbs, and 5 to 10 grams of fat, with each meal. This, of course, should be altered according to your individual needs and diet leading up to the show. You should have been using trial and error to determine your body's response to certain types of foods during your pre-contest training, so you should now know exactly what you'll need on contest day and be able to dial it in precisely. Still, bring extra food like Gatorade, a slice or two of pizza, a few muffins, candy bar, extra chicken, steak, and rice, as you may need them.

There may be the need for a combination food of protein, carbs, fat, and sodium to help you fill out. In my experience, the slice of pizza has done the trick. Come prepared with extra food and you won't have to rely on what may or may not be available for purchase at the contest.

Contest Morning: Wake up at 5 a.m.

How did you sleep? Probably not that well. That's typical. I always have a tough time sleeping before a show because my mind is racing. I always set an alarm clock even though I don't need one, just in case. You always want to give yourself enough time to get to the venue without rushing.

Upon waking, take a deep breath and remember how far you've come. You've worked extremely hard for a period of months to showcase all your hard work to your family, friends, and coworkers. Remember this key component: It's time to enjoy every moment of the day. This is a sport that can chew people up and spit them out faster than it takes for someone to perform a posing routine. The reason you made this commitment is larger than any contest trophy. Remember the bigger reasons for embarking on this remarkable journey of self-improvement.

Training That Morning

Don't deviate from your routine. Consume your typical light pre-breakfast snack like a simple rice cake with a small amount of natural peanut butter and 32 ounces of water. After that snack and before eating breakfast, perform a light pump-up if you believe you may be holding a little extra water, then a short training session—about 80 percent of your normal effort. I rarely do this, as a simple upper body pump-up using my exercise bands works just fine for me. But every bodybuilder is different. You may need to do more.

After your light pump-up, take a short 10- to 15-minute walk to loosen up your legs and create a small amount of glycogen depletion before consuming Meal 1. After this brief morning exercise routine, it's all about timing your meals until you pump up before your stage time.

Meal 1—6 a.m., right after your 15-minute walk

Each of your contest-day meals should contain protein, carbohydrates, and some fat. Your protein will come from chicken, sirloin, whey protein, and trace amounts from peanut butter. Carbs will be supplied by starchy sources (rice, fruit, vegetables), and trace amounts of fat will come from the meat and nut butters. Make Meal 1 a smoothie blended from the following:

- 1 scoop protein
- ½ cup oats
- 1 banana
- 10 ounces water
- ⅛ teaspoon Morton Light Salt

It is important to keep carbohydrates and water filtering into the muscle cells to allow you to remain full and hard. For that reason, you'll need to be very deliberate about drinking water with every meal and in between meals in measured amounts. By timing water consumption and the addition of sodium throughout the day, you'll be able to reach your peak for those moments when you are on stage.

Anxiety and Cortisol (the Stress Hormone) Management

It's common for a bodybuilder, especially one new to the sport, to be anxious on contest day. But everyone gets nervous, even the seasoned pros. You'll constantly feel the need to urinate. Part of that comes from all the water and carb consumption, part from nervous energy. "Your body changes, stress levels change, cortisol levels increase, and now your "perfect" plan, isn't so perfect anymore," says Dr. Klemczewski. Expect all this to happen and you will be better prepared to deal with it and keep cortisol from stifling your peaking plans.

There are numerous ways to combat this anxiety. Try these:

- Remember that you decided to do this, and for the right reasons.
- Keep your attitude positive and upbeat.
- Have fun and make friends.
- Listen to music.
- Relax, put your legs up, and chill out.
- Mingle with friends, coaches, etc.
- Visualization (sit down, close your eyes, take deep breaths, and visualize your stage presentation).
- Sip 12 ounces of water between meals all day long; good hydration will help ease stress.

Arrival

Plan to arrive at the contest venue about a half hour before the time suggested so that you aren't rushed and to allow for traffic or other unforeseen delays. And be prepared to hurry up and then wait. Bodybuilding competitions are notorious for running very slowly only to speed up to meet time requirements and deadlines. Schedules and times are very erratic, so be prepared for unpredictability and a lot of waiting around.

Check in with your paperwork. If you arrive early enough, you can secure a comfy place to plop your cooler of food and duffle of clothing where you can stay and rest the better portion of the day. During the morning hours, you may be moved around. Take it in stride. Remember to control the things you can control and go with the flow when you can't control the situation. Having this attitude will help you keep your stress level down.

Meal 2—About 9 a.m.

Between 2½ hours and 3 hours after Meal 1, eat Meal 2. You'll be at the show venue. Try to schedule time when you can eat leisurely without having to wolf it down. Recommended: Eat 5 ounces of sirloin steak, ½ cup of cooked rice, and 12 ounces of water. (You will have prepared your meals the day before, put them into labeled plastic containers, and then transferred them from the fridge to your contest cooler that morning.)

Meetings

Most competitions will hold a meeting sometime during the morning of the contest for all competitors. This will be where you will weigh in and get your number, which will be worn on your posing suit. (Place the number in a secure location.)

You'll most likely need to hand in your music at this time. If not, you'll be handing it in before jumping on stage, so keep it secure. The next meeting you have will most likely be just before the evening show. So if the evening show is set to start at 5 p.m., expect the competitors' meeting to be held around 4 p.m. Schedules for different shows can vary widely, so be prepared mentally to "go with the flow."

Meal 3—2 hours later

- ½ protein bar (with glycerol, containing 20 to 30 grams of protein, 30 to 40 grams of carbohydrate, and 10 to 15 grams of fat)
- 8 ounces water

Meal 4—Prejudging meal, just before pump up

Timing of this meal depends on your scheduled prejudging time.

- 2 rice cakes
- 1 teaspoon of peanut butter on each
- 16 ounces water (sip while eating, during pump-up, and right until stage time)

(Depending on how my body looks, I may eat more than this.)

Prejudging—Anywhere from 12 p.m. to 5 p.m.

This is the first of two posing parts to the competition. The second is the evening show before an audience. Prejudging is held during the morning or afternoon, and it is the most important part of the competition. It is both a rehearsal for the evening event and the key opportunity for the judges to really evaluate you and the other bodybuilders alone without the distraction of a live audience.

As such, prejudging is typically where the judges choose the winners. Prejudging is divided into several different rounds of posing, such as the symmetry round, compulsory poses, and individual posing routines set to music. Sometimes, the latter are not held until the evening show.

Prejudging can take many hours, all depending upon the number of competitors. There may be 100 or more bodybuilders at a typical competition. But during prejudging, there may seem to be even more competitors because many competitors try to improve their chances of winning by crossing over into other competition classes. For example, you may have open class competitors crossing over into master class and figure competitors crossing over into the fit body class.

Following prejudging, scores are tallied to determine the placings of each class of competitors. In most organizations, the winners are determined following prejudging, and the night show posing routines are simply for entertainment of the crowd. In amateur events, posing routines are not scored.

Meal 5—After prejudging (immediately after leaving the stage)

- 5 ounces chicken breast
- 1 cup sweet potato
- 1 cup salad greens with vegetables
- 16 ounces water
- ⅛ teaspoon Morton Light Salt

Meal 6—3 hours later

- 5 ounces sirloin
- ¾ cup rice
- 8 ounces water

If there are at least 2½ hours before the evening show, I will eat Meal 7 just before my pre-show pump-up.

- ½ protein bar (with glycerol, containing 20 to 30 grams of protein, 30 to 40 grams of carbs, and 10 to 15 grams of fat)
- 1 banana, optional
- 12 ounces water

Meal 7—Just before finals show routine

- 1 rice cake
- 1 tablespoon peanut butter
- 14 ounces water

Finals—7 p.m. to finish (9 p.m. to 11 p.m. depending on show)

Finals are held in the evening in front of the same judges and usually a large audience. The symmetry round, compulsory poses, and individual posing routines done in prejudging are repeated. The show culminates in a "pose down," where the top competitors chosen by the judges do freestyle posing together on stage. Following the pose down, judges announce the placings and award the trophies and medals.

There are usually anywhere between five to nine judges (both male and female) who judge a bodybuilding contest. Each judge has been evaluated and certified. Contests are scored using a ranking system. After each round, the judges rank the competitors from first to last. At the end of the contest the competitor with the lowest score wins. This system means that a competitor doesn't have to win every round, but must have the lowest overall score.

After the Competition

A winner is chosen. The places have been awarded. Maybe you were invited to that party. Maybe you weren't.

That's okay. A lot of other bodybuilders in the competition are in the same boat. Don't get down. Don't get angry. I've met plenty of bodybuilders who feel like they were screwed by the judges and deserved a higher placing at the competition. All these emotions are part of human nature. It may help you to put things into perspective. There will always be a winner and just because you weren't the winner, doesn't mean that you aren't good enough or that the judges were out to get you or that they're incompetent. Bodybuilding is a subjective sport. And there are many, many factors that come into play in the judges' decisions: your conditioning, the sharpness of your poses, the richness of your tan and how it accentuates the separation of your muscles, the smoothness of your transitions, even your smile. All these elements are weighed, and they are considered against the entire field of competitors. You need to recognize that your physique and presentation are not being judged in a vacuum; your performance is judged against all the other bodybuilders' physiques and performances.

I've competed in many bodybuilding competitions, as many as seven in a year. Sometimes I didn't place. Sometimes I was only good enough to take second place. A few of those placements were questionable. One contest was decided by a single point, and I was on the losing end. But with each disappointment or victory, I learned something new. I pushed forward and I fine-tuned. I worked on the things later in the year that were missing earlier that year. I tweaked my diet, increased my cardio, took my training to new levels, tightened up my conditioning, practiced my posing more effectively, and came back stronger. Remember, a bodybuilding competition isn't about winning or losing, it's about the journey and the real reasons behind achieving your goals. So regardless of how you fared in the competition, you're already a winner because you made it to a place that very few people experience. You've achieved an incredible physique through hard work and self-discipline, a body that is very, very, very rare in our culture of overindulgence, inactivity, and poor physical health. It's a body to be proud of.

Avoid the Sponge

The day after your competition, your work isn't over. Most important is to "diet out of a show," that is, continue your dieting discipline to avoid the overcompensating on carbohydrates that your body may be craving after peak week. When your body is as lean as it is after a show, binging on carbs can turn your body into a glycogen sponge. You need to stay disciplined to maintain a healthy lifestyle and allow yourself the ability to transition back to normal hormone levels.

Overeating after a competition is something that every bodybuilder will battle with. "After a show you feel a letdown of, 'now what,' and 'I don't know what to do with myself,'" says Kori Propst, a certified mental health counselor, exercise physiologist, and founder of The Mental Edge, a program that provides mental and behavioral training for bodybuilding contest preparation.

Recognizing that post-competition blues and even depression are common among bodybuilders after a show can prepare you to expect swings in emotions and deal with them. It is normal for your weight to increase a little after the show, which makes it even more important to keep a routine as you transition out of contest-prep mode, advises Propst. You were the one who became that Type A personality and prepped like a lunatic for weeks and weeks on end. So now that the ride is over, don't stop cold turkey. "Use the tools you've mastered during this journey to maintain a healthy lifestyle," says Propst.

Here are some tips she suggests will help you post-contest:

- Define what motivates you.
- Inquire about what you put on the back burner and transition back into "normal life."
- Set goals for friends, family, and work.
- List the people, places, things, and animals (yes, they count, too) that supported you throughout your journey.
- List your previous struggles, and be specific.
- Identify what changed when the show ended. Keep a record of how you changed behaviorally, cognitively, and emotionally.
- Identify the present behaviors that are sustaining you (what is working right now?).

Binge Eating and Mindful Eating: Striking the Balance

Even if you make it over the post-competition hump without binge eating, you can still fall prey weeks and even months later when you have returned to your "normal" life. You have probably experienced this at some point in life: Your mind and body are consumed by the thought of food, you overeat and then immediately feel guilt and remorse. This is common for anyone who has lost significant body fat and weight, but it can be even more dramatic for the bodybuilder after a competition. The solution is to develop a mindful approach to eating, and post competition is the perfect time to learn this because it will make it easier to transition into your next round of dieting.

Mindful eating is nothing more than being more cognitively engaged when you select your food and when you eat it. Some mindful eating tips:

- Eat slowly. Give your brain time to register the fullness in your belly and send signals of satiety. By eating fast, you can consume far more calories than your body requires. The old techniques of chewing your food thoroughly and taking sips of water between bites really do work.
- Savor the taste and texture of your food. This signals satiety and helps you reduce the quantity of food you need to eat.
- Enjoy a "Relaxed Meal" not a "Cheat Meal." The typical cheat meal is often considered a free pass to binge eat something processed and high in empty calories. Instead, treat yourself with a relaxed meal, that is, a meal in which you allow yourself some small satisfying indulgences.
- Become a research scientist of your body. Learn and understand how food affects it and which types of foods you enjoy and how they make your body feel.

Take Time to Celebrate

Before you embark on your next contest preparation program, take time to savor the journey you've just completed and reflect on it. For at least 16 weeks, you have dedicated yourself to dieting and training to achieve a competition-ready body, a body you can be proud of. What motivated you to achieve the pinnacle of physical success? Your goal. Your dream of taking a body you painstakingly crafted to the highest level to compete against others in a natural bodybuilding competition. There is no nobler dream.

Remember that bodybuilding isn't a sprint; it's a marathon, a long process requiring years of commitment. In that sense it's more of a lifestyle than a sport because to be successful you need to live the bodybuilder's life daily by maintaining extra-vigilant nutrition habits and a regimented workout schedule.

I've said it before and I'll say it again. The journey I've described in this book is but one man's story; your story will likely be different. My hope is that I've given you the direction and required inspiration to enjoy bodybuilding for the finer things it offers.

Enter into bodybuilding for what it will offer you physically, mentally, and spiritually. Bodybuilding is not about winning or losing; it's about learning about yourself. Enter the sport with this mind-set, and you'll have no other option than to enjoy yourself and gain a rare sense of self-satisfaction. Bodybuilding has given me more than I could ever imagine, and I hope the same for you.

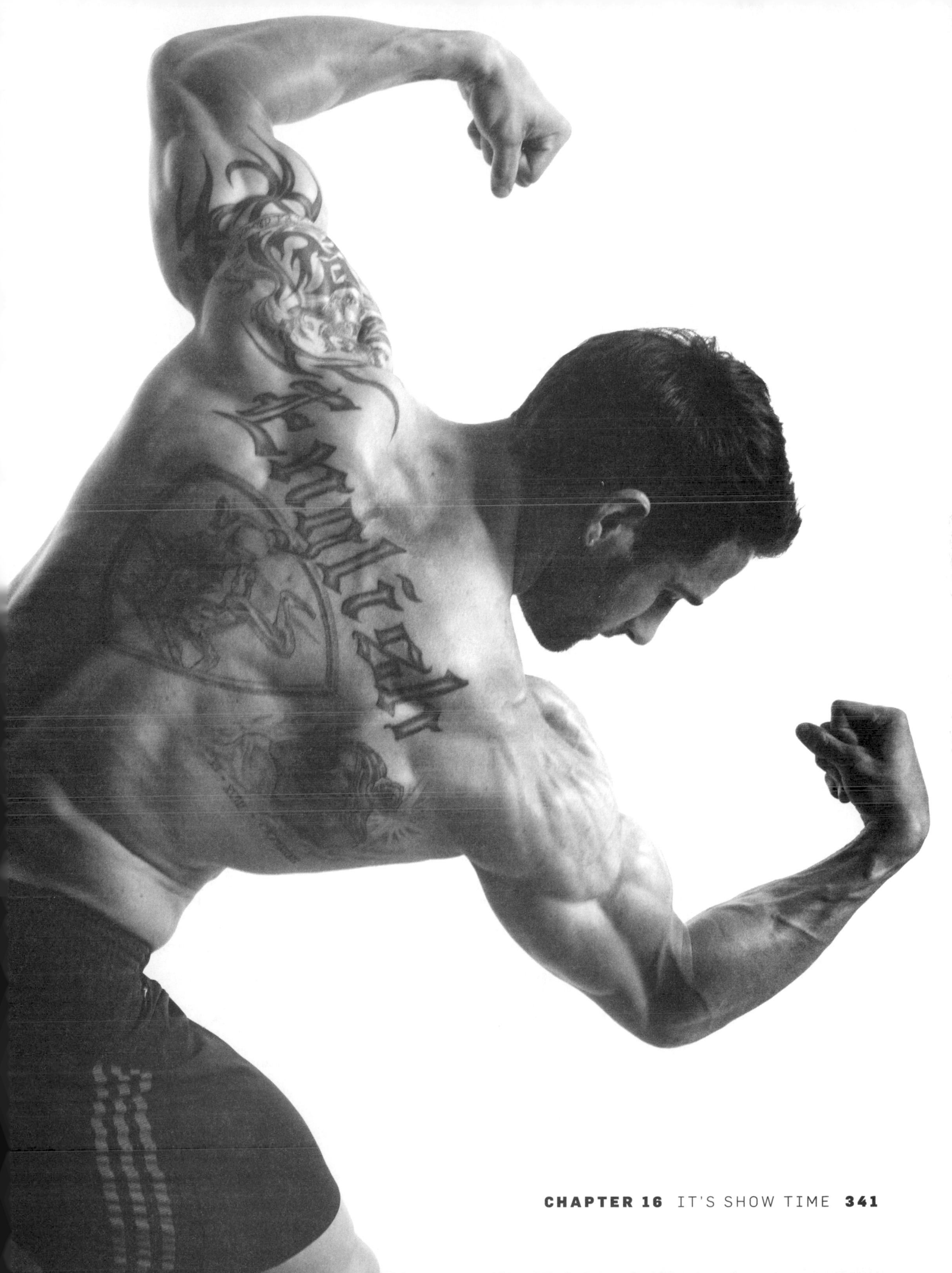

Index

Boldface page references indicate photographs and illustrations. Underscored references indicate boxed text.

C

E

F

G

H

I